Community Paediatrics

Community
Paediatrics

Leon Polnay
MB, BS, MRCP, DObstRCOG, DCH
Senior Lecturer in Child Health, University of Nottingham;
Honorary Consultant Paediatrician, Nottingham District Health
Authority

David Hull
MSc, MB, FRCP, DObstRCOG, DCH
Professor of Child Health, University of Nottingham

ILLUSTRATED BY GEOFFREY LYTH BA

CHURCHILL LIVINGSTONE
EDINBURGH LONDON MELBOURNE AND NEW YORK 1985

CHURCHILL LIVINGSTONE
Medical Division of Longman Group UK Limited

Distributed in the United States of America by Churchill
Livingstone Inc., 1560 Broadway, New York, N.Y. 10036,
and by associated companies, branches and representatives
throughout the world.

First published 1985
Reprinted (twice) 1987
Reprinted 1988
Reprinted 1990

ISBN 0 443 02743 9

British Library Cataloguing in Publication Data
Polnay, Leon
    Community paediatrics.
    1. Paediatrics.
    I. Title   II. Hull, David
    618.92   RJ45

Library of Congress Cataloguing in Publication Data
Polnay, Leon.
    Community paediatrics.

    Includes index.
    1. Community health services for children.
2. Community health services for children — England —
Nottingham (Nottinghamshire) I. Hull, David.
II. Title. [DNLM: 1. Child Health Services—
Great Britain.   2. Pediatrics. WA 320 P777c]
RJ101.P58   1985   362.1′088054   84–19992

Printed in Great Britain by
Butler & Tanner Ltd, Frome and London

Preface

This book is the third in a series written for doctors who care for sick children. The first, *Essential Paediatrics* describes the diseases which affect children. It is intended for undergraduate students and is based on the teaching packages used in the Nottingham Medical School. The second, *Hospital Paediatrics* outlines the management of paediatric problems as they present in hospital. It was prepared to assist residents in their work and in their studies for specialist qualifications. It is based on the practice guidelines used in the various departments in the Nottingham Hospitals. This third book is concerned with the care of the child within his home, school and community. It is based on experience in the community of Nottingham and surrounding districts. The data and examples used are the best we could find relevant to our practice. Much of the information and the approach is taken from the teaching material prepared for the Community Paediatric course which has been run by the Department of Child Health University of Nottingham, for the last eight years. This material has been prepared and modified many times by many people. The Editors are happy to acknowledge the contribution that everyone who has been concerned with the course has made to the book.

The book may, therefore, be of interest to a doctor working within primary care who has a special interest in preventative paediatrics and/or school health, or a hospital clinician who has responsibilities in the community as well as hospital departments, or a specialist concerned with the complex problems of identification, care and education of children with handicaps or chronic ill health and who provides a secondary care service within the community.

We hope that health visitors and school nurses will also find the book of value, particularly if it is read in conjunction with another book in the series, *Nursing Sick Children* (Edited by Adamson and Hull), which deals with the nursing care of individual conditions.

We are conscious that this book is little more than a series of pointers — community paediatrics is as yet ill defined. Even if it were not, it would still be necessary for each practitioner to know about his or her local conditions and resources.

The authors are indebted to the contributors listed on the following page who offered expert advice regarding the accuracy, relevance and balance of sections related to their special interests, in some cases completely rewriting them. Mr Geoffrey Lyth produced the illustrations, which say more than words. We would particularly wish to record our thanks to Miss Kath Reed for interpreting the messages and typing them so efficiently. Finally, to Janet and Carol thank you for 'coping' with us.

Nottingham   L. P.
1985   D. H.

Contributors

Elizabeth R. Perkins
MA, Cert Ed
Senior Research and Development Officer.
Nottingham Health Authority, Health Education Unit

Eleanor More
MB, ChB, DPH, MFCM
Specialist in Community Medicine (Child Health),
Nottingham Health Authority

Connie Pullan
MB, BS, MRCP
Senior Clinical Medical Officer (Paediatrician),
Nottingham Health Authority

Angus Nicoll
MB, ChB, MRCP
Lecturer in Child Health,
Nottingham University

Shirley Lewis
MB, ChB, DPH
Senior Clinical Medical Officer,
Nottingham Health Authority

John S. Fitzsimmons
MB, FRCP (E), DCH
Consultant in charge of the Clinical Genetic Service,
City Hospital, Nottingham

Contents

1

Services

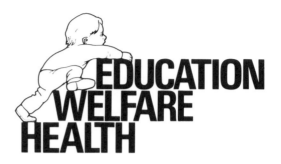

The paediatrician is but one of many professionals whose work is concerned with the care and development of children. Education, social work, nursing, psychology, speech therapy all have major roles. It is important for each to understand the background and training of the other disciplines and the resources of the organisations in which they work. Only with this knowledge is it possible to adopt a shared approach to children's problems and obtain the benefits of a multidisciplinary approach.

STRUCTURE OF CHILD HEALTH SERVICES

Reality is by no means as tidy as the diagram of child health services may suggest. Patterns of service are subject to individual and local variation; the boundary between primary care (open to self referral) and secondary care is not clear cut.

Medical Services

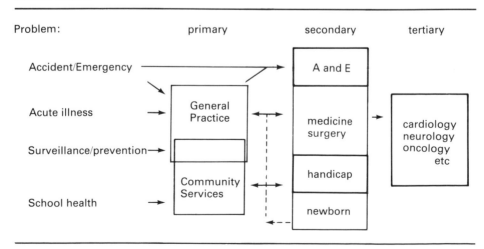

However, the service must respond to three basic needs, the management of acute illness, surveillance, prevention and health education, and the care of children with chronic and handicapping conditions.

Home care or hospital care for sick children?
The hospital as an environment for children has improved in many ways: accommodation is provided for parents to live in, visiting is unrestricted, the nurses are 'children's trained' and play is actively encouraged. However, hospital care is expensive and can still bring with it anxiety for the child. Many children are admitted to hospital who do not require the medical and nursing care that only hospital can provide. The concept of the paediatric home care team is attractive but hardly practised in the United Kingdom. It still offers promise for providing parents and primary care physicians with the necessary support to enable more children to remain at home or to be discharged earlier. Home care provides an opportunity to help parents to manage chronic or handicapping conditions in their own home. However admission to hospital may still be required to relieve parents of stress or enable them to take a holiday. Community based units would be a more appropriate solution.

The primary health care team
Vocational training for general practitioners and the concept of the primary health care team of GPs, health visitor, midwife and district nurse, has led to many practices setting up child health clinics to provide preventative services, as well as surgeries which respond to acute illnesses. The integration of these two aspects of medical care and the concept of care for the whole family, is in keeping with the philosophy of the Court Report 'Fit for the Future'. The principle is most difficult to apply in inner city areas where there is not a tidy catchment area for the practice and where liaison with schools and social work departments might involve too many individuals to make the policy practicable.

Health Service administration

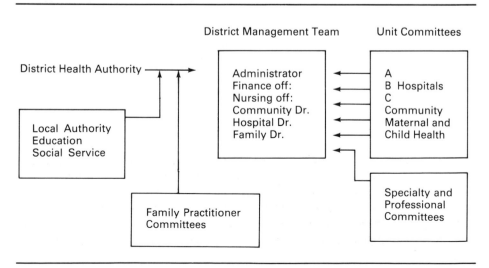

Objectives of community child health services
These are summarised in the Court Report as:
- oversight of health and physical growth of *all* children.
- monitoring the developmental progress of *all* children.
- providing advice and support to parents and when necessary arranging treatment or referral of the child.
- providing a programme of effective infectious disease prophylaxis.
- participation in health education and training in parenthood.

Those involved in the identification of a child with a health problem

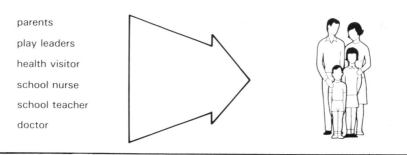

parents

play leaders

health visitor

school nurse

school teacher

doctor

Child health clinics, schools, school clinics and the home
The 'inverse care' law states that those most likely to have problems are least likely to attend child health clinics. Home visiting by health visitors and by doctors is required to reach this important group of non-attenders. However, imaginative development of the clinic can make it a much more attractive service for parents to use, not only accessible but acceptable. To this end we have introduced the following into our child health clinics in the inner city area of Nottingham.
- a playgroup leader to set up activities for children
- a toy library open at the same time as the clinic
- health education classes and English language classes for immigrant mothers.

Clinics may give treatment for common problems and can also be visited by other staff such as a social worker, a physiotherapist or a speech therapist. In separate sessions other hospital specialists such as paediatricians, otolaryngologists, ophthalmologists or dermatologists may attend which enables them to give consultations to the patients nearer their homes which is particularly valuable to those who have difficulty travelling to a district hospital. They are also able to work more closely with colleagues in primary care. A pattern of joint sessions with general practitioners in their own premises is one which is being increasingly favoured by both general practitioners and paediatricians as an alternative to outpatient referral.

The role of the health visitor

The health visitor is a nurse (SRN), with obstetric training who also has had post-registration training and qualifications to enable her to perform the following tasks within either a general practice or within the community child health services in a 'geographical' area

— the prevention of mental, physical and emotional ill health and its consequences
— early detection of ill health and surveillance of high risk groups
— recognition and identification of need and mobilisation of appropriate resources where necessary
— health education
— provision of care; this will include support during periods of stress, and advice and guidance in cases of illness as well as in the care and management of children. The health visitor is not, however, actively engaged in technical nursing procedures.

(Ref. Council for the Training of Health Visitors).

District handicap teams

District handicap teams and assessment centres have been set up to co-ordinate services for handicapped children and their families and to provide continuity between assessment and day to day management.

The basic staff of a district handicap team as recommended in the Court Report is a consultant in community paediatrics, a nursing officer for handicapped children (health visitor), a specialised social worker, a principal psychologist and a teacher. These are usually supported clinically by physiotherapists, occupational therapists, speech therapists and the consultant in mental handicap. The functions of a district handicap team are:

— to provide investigation and assessment of certain individual children with complex disorders and to arrange and co-ordinate their treatment
— to provide their parents, teachers, child care staff and others who may be directly concerned in their care, with the professional advice and support that can guide them in their management of the children
— to encourage and assist professional field-work staff in their management and surveillance of these and other handicapped children locally, by being available for consultation either in the district child development centre or in local premises
— to provide primary and supporting specialist services to special schools in the district
— to be involved with others in epidemiological surveys of need; to monitor the effectiveness of the district service for handicapped children, to present data and suggestions for the development of the services: to maintain the quality of its institutions
— to act as sources of information within the district about handicap in children and the services available
— to organise seminars and courses of training for professional staff working within the district.

STRUCTURE OF SOCIAL SERVICES

The diagram shows the range of general and specialised social services that are provided for children. It also shows the important role of medicine and education in these activities. Statutory duties stated in law or assigned by the courts to individual children come into most of these areas of work. These are more fully discussed in the chapter on the 'Protection of Children'. Social services by their provision develop a framework of aid, advice and supervision where an individual's or family's own resources are limited. Social work training covers 2–4 years with further post-qualifying study being available. Basic courses consist of either a degree course, for example social science, followed by a 1 year qualifying course with practical experience, or relevant experience and a 2–3 year qualifying course. The degree of professional independence and responsibility, for example decisions on the personal liberty of clients, is related to the qualification and experience of the social worker.

The aims of social work are to:
— identify personal and social problems and family breakdown and poverty which cause emotional and social stress
— resolve these problems and reverse their harmful effects, if possible
— or, if this is not possible, ensure that the situation does not deteriorate
— prevent as far as possible those conditions in which problems thrive, such as family stress, bad housing or poverty
— promote favourable conditions which encourage the personal and social enhancement of individuals, families, groups and community.

Structure of Social Services

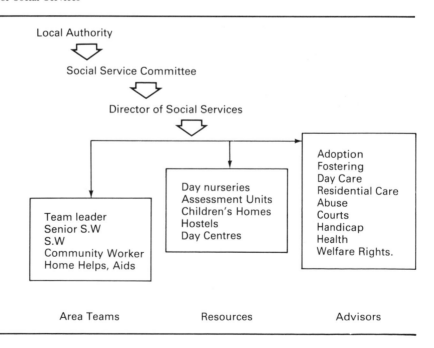

Day care

Great demands are being made for facilities for day care for pre-school children. Some arise from the financial need of many mothers to work, some from a lack of an extended family and some because of perceived inadequacies of the care of the child at home. In other instances handicap in the child or the parents produces special needs for the family. Because of the importance of the pre-school years for later educational progress and social interaction, the substitute care must be of high quality to provide appropriate experience and stimulation and the element of nurture and continuity of care necessary for normal emotional development. Problems arise when the approach in the 'home' and during 'day care' differs and the child is unable to understand.

Childminders have to be legally approved and registered with social service departments. In spite of this requirement much illegal and unsatisfactory child-minding still takes place with the emphasis on income for the minder rather than the needs of the child. Overcrowding, and lack of toys or stimulation may be common in such arrangements, the children leading a dull, uninteresting life. There may be frequent changes of minder and the failure of a close relationship to develop between minder and child. The provision of training courses for child-minders and appropriate support services can ensure a much higher level of care. Most surveys of childminding have been very critical of this system. The child who is quiet and withdrawn is perhaps particularly vulnerable in the childminding setting, the childminder not having the skills, the 'licence' or sometimes the motivation to explore the origins of the child's problems in his natural home.

Day nurseries are generally run by social services departments, but others are run privately or by various voluntary organisations. They all have to obtain registration and approval by the local authority social services department. Day nurseries are staffed by nursery nurses (who have undergone a 2-year training) and have an experienced matron and deputy in charge. In general the nurseries escape many of the criticisms levelled at child minders. However, some operate on a 'custodial system' with a high standard of physical care but lacking the important individualisation of care. Others may be given the grandiose but well earned title of 'therapeutic day care centre'. In this situation, the nursery nurse acts as a proper substitute mother, providing a programme of activities special to that child's needs. Parents are involved in activities in and outside the nursery and hence continuity is established between nursery and home. Many nurseries have units for handicapped children and have additional input from physiotherapists, speech therapists, etc.

Family centres. Day nurseries, even in optimum conditions, cannot meet all the needs of severely disadvantaged children and their parents. The needs are not simply to provide an alternative to home or provide continuity with the home, but to improve the child care skills of parents and their attitude towards the family. The family centre is essentially a day care setting in which parents attend as well as their children and in which a number of programmes are set up to teach parenting skills and to increase the confidence and self-esteem of parents. The Radford Family Centre in Nottingham is staffed by a social worker, health visitor, playgroup leader, community teacher and ancillary workers.

It works with the following stated aims
— to promote practical parenting skills related to play and stimulation, day-to-day physical care, and awareness and management of health problems
— to promote better home management through a home economics programme
— to promote literacy
— to provide insight for parents into the needs of children, both in family life and in education
— to promote satisfaction for parents in parenting, to help parents to enjoy their children
— to reduce dependence on agencies for day-to-day care and acute problems.

Playgroups are run by trained playgroup leaders and the playgroup movement is represented by the Pre-school Playgroups Association. They also need to be approved and registered with the local authority. Attendance may be from one to five mornings a week. They provide an opportunity for children to meet, play and socialise and for parents to meet too. Playgroups may be held in church halls, community centres, private premises or attached to schools, health centres or various social work agencies. Although to some extent restricted compared to a nursery school, the value of playgroups compares very favourably with other resources for pre-school children.

Mother and toddler groups are for younger children. The mother is expected to stay with her child. They often 'graduate' to the playgroup. Mother and toddler groups not only provide play facilities for the child but also important support for the mother who may be lonely, isolated and harrassed.

Combined nursery centres combine the merits of the day nursery which is able to provide extended whole day care for the children of working mothers with the advantage of a nursery school for that part of the day that the child would normally attend. This combination of education and social service provision is a pattern that is being implemented more frequently.

Agencies involved in education

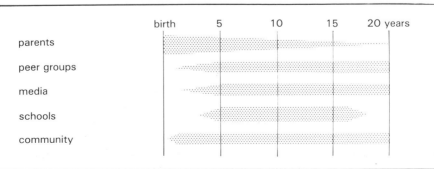

EDUCATION SERVICES

Aims

Education in its wider sense goes far beyond the narrow definition of schooling: it aims to prepare a child by teaching knowledge and skills and influences his behaviour so that he will be happy in the work, recreation and social life of his own community. The information transmitted enables society to retain its character and maintain social stability and permits each generation to build on the knowledge of its predecessors.

Education in schools must be available for all, including those with special needs, and so the systems must be flexible and respond sensitively to the varying talents or aspirations of individual children, yet at the same time provide the balance of skills that the society requires.

Special education

Blind	Maladjusted	Tutorial Classes
Partially sighted	Moderate learning difficulty	Remedial Classes
Deaf	Severe learning difficulty	Language Units
Partially hearing		Diagnostic Units
Physically handicapped		

Structure of educational services

Director and supporting staff is responsible for overall administration, policy, planning and allocation of resources. He is responsible to an education committee which represents locally elected authority.

The curriculum is an outline of the subjects taught. It is uniform between education authorities, and is influenced by national bodies such as the Schools Council and Examination Boards.

The Inspectorate is responsible for monitoring the standards within schools and usually each inspector confines himself to a particular age group or category of education.

Education services

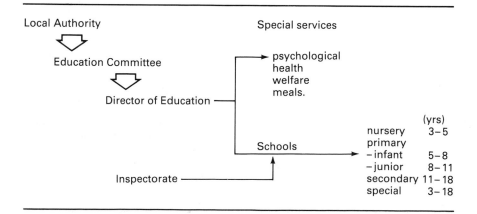

Schools usually accept children according to age, thus nursery 3–5, infant 5–7, junior 7–11, secondary 11–18 or 'first' 3–8 years, 'middle' 8–13 years and 'upper' 13–18 years. Head Teachers are responsible for the day-to-day organisation and administration of the school. In secondary schools department heads are responsible for teaching specialist subjects, whilst heads of year are responsible for a particular cohort of children and have additional pastoral or administrative duties.

Special schools continue to fulfill a need for children with handicaps or learning difficulties. However, the current trend, supported in the UK by the 1981 Education Act, is to integrate, wherever possible, handicapped pupils within ordinary schools and to provide these schools with the necessary support and advice to enable them to do this.

Schools psychological service. This is often combined with the child guidance service. The former is staffed by educational psychologists and provides assessment of children with learning difficulties as soon as they are identified and advice to schools on remedial programmes of management. In a more general

Training for education service

	Normal age at entry	Number of years in training	Comments
Nursery Nurse	16+	2	Qualification (G.B.) N.N.E.B National Nursery Examination Board.
Nursery Teacher Infant Teacher Junior Teacher	18+ 18+ 18+	3 or 4 3 or 4 3 or 4	Qualification: 3 year. Certificate of Education. 4 year B.Ed. (Hons.) Training involves courses on child development, educational psychology and classroom techniques. There is practical experience in school and the opportunity to study in depth particular areas of the curriculum, e.g. music, maths.
Secondary Teacher	18+	3 or 4	Qualification: First degree and postgraduate certificate of education 3 or 4 years B.Ed. (Ord) or B.Ed (Hons).
Remedial Teacher	18+	3 or 4	Qualification: Initial teacher training and diploma in education (learning difficulties)
Special Education Teacher	18+	3 or 4	Qualification: Normal teaching and supplementary course taken after a few years experience.
Educational Psychologist	18+	7	Qualification: Hons. degree in psychology, postgraduate certificate of education, 2 years (minimal) teaching experience, postgraduate professional training in educational psychology.
Education Welfare Officer	25+	4	Qualification: Certificate of qualification in social work (CQSW). Not all EWO's are qualified with the CQSW

context, schools may be helped with activities and programmes for individual groups of children, and parent counselling services may also be offered. The child guidance service is staffed by child psychiatrists and psychiatric social workers. It provides assessment and treatment for children with behaviour problems.

School health service is staffed by doctors, dentists, nurses and technicians. Currently in the UK the medical staff include clinical medical officers, senior clinical medical officers and specialists in community medicine with administrative and planning duties. It is the part of the health service responsible for surveillance of school children. It advises the education department on the relevance of medical conditions to a child's school progress and employment, and arranges for investigation and treatment of children where this is needed. Medical examination of children is carried out both in schools and in specialist clinics, e.g. paediatric, dental, ophthalmic, ENT. The school health service is involved in health education and it works closely with medical, teaching and social work colleagues in the management of children with social, emotional, learning and medical problems.

Education welfare service is responsible for ensuring that the legal requirements for school attendance are met and for assisting families with any domestic problems which might interfere with education, such as the provision of clothing, transport, free school meals or general support.

School meals service which is subsidised out of the education budget, provides a suitable midday meal for school children and special diets if they are required.

WORKING IN TEAMS

Much current thinking on the organisation of services for children rests on the structure of the multidisciplinary team such as the primary health care team or the district handicap team. Such teams have been set up in abundance, often without attention to the underlying problems of integration of professional work.

The essentials for successful team work are as follows:
— an understanding of the training and available skills of each team member, by each other
— a commitment by each team member to work within the team framework and communicate effectively with others

Teams?

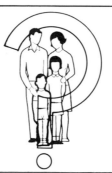

Primary health care team	Area social service team
District handicap team	Mental handicap team
Hospital paediatric team	Child guidance team
Community paediatric team	Family centre team

— a definition of the role of each team member which permits flexibility rather than the construction of rigid professional boundaries
— personal and professional respect for one another
— personalities that work well together
— the ability to reach and stick to joint decisions.

Teams need time to evolve as a group of people who can work effectively together. They certainly do not work from day 1 and some not even from day 100. Time needs to be provided for informal group discussion and the development of team policies, and team identification. Support is needed both within the team and from their own discipline outside the team in terms of individual professional issues or because of stresses innate to the type of work undertaken. Leadership and a democratic process whereby decisions are made are needed. Some may be unable to work within the team framework, others may be able to work in one particular team but not in another. The personalities of individuals are just as important as their professional qualifications.

From the consumer's point of view, they need to be able to identify a key worker within the team with whom to communicate. This 'key worker' needs to be accessible to the family using the service.

Some teams are not multidisciplinary, but bring together persons belonging to the same discipline, for example the area social services team. Some may have a highly hierarchal structure and line management, which can become inflexible and unwieldly. However, it does provide a degree of security and protection to an individual within his own 'professional tradition' which may be important, for example, in police work. It does not leave him exposed to criticism. However, this lack of exposure to criticism from outside can lead to the continuing

Team work?

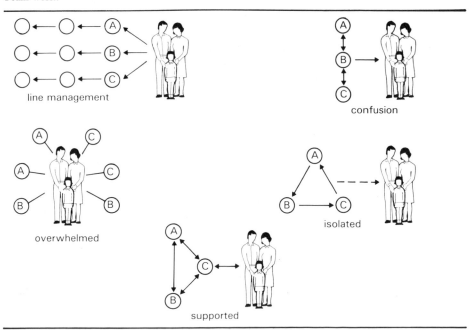

line management

confusion

overwhelmed

isolated

supported

use of practices which are no longer appropriate. Multidisciplinary work encourages a sharing of responsibility both within the team and with the family and this in turn encourages a more therapeutic relationship with them.

Often the problems of any one family are not confined to one team. The phenomenon of multiple multidisciplinary teams and the need for co-ordination between them is emerging. They may have different working practices and different goals and in theory if not coordinated could effectively cancel out one another's efforts.

Our approach to the problem of the integration of services has been the Community Paediatric Team. This consists of a medical team covering a defined geographical area of the city. The area is small enough for us to know and work closely with all other services in primary care, social services, education or other areas.

Community Paediatric team

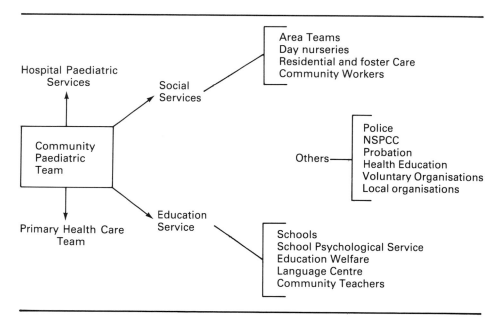

The roles of the team have been defined as follows:
— prevention through health education, parent counselling and immunisations
— screening procedures leading to early diagnosis of disorders of growth, disorders of development (motor, intellectual, speech, vision and hearing), somatic disorders, e.g. scoliosis, congenital dislocation of the hip, undescended testes, emotional problems, children experiencing emotional or physical deprivation or abuse, and children likely to have special education needs
— management of child rearing problems, handicapped preschool and school children with particular reference to their educational needs, problems related to groups of children within institutions like schools and day nur-

series, and paediatric problems in conjunction with the family doctor or hospital paediatric services

— advice to individual teachers, social workers and careers officers on children within the team's area

— evaluation of the health and other needs of children within the team's area and the implementation of new programmes where current facilities are lacking

— teaching doctors, medical students, community nursing staff.

Within the team, we acknowledge that health visitors and school nurses are highly effective in primary screening. We also acknowledge that parents are more effective than any professional for early identification of many problems. Given appropriate opportunities for acquiring information and easy access to the team, they are our and the children's most important resource.

2

Information

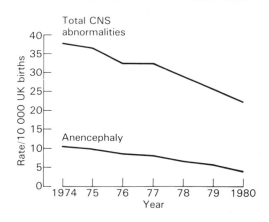

Epidemiology is the study of health and disease in relation to populations. It provides information on morbidity and mortality and enables their analysis in terms of causation, time trends, age distribution, geographical distribution and socioeconomic correlations. The value of epidemiological data rests with the accuracy of the clinical information collected and the precision with which this is applied to the population under scrutiny. Good data enables us to establish needs, plan and monitor services, determine causes and introduce preventive programmes logically.

WHY COLLECT DATA?

Measure and analyse problems

Data on mortality is readily available in countries where there is compulsory

Perinatal mortality in different countries compared with those in England and Wales. E.W. (from Social Services Committee on Perinatal and Neonatal Mortality, 1979–80), and the outcome of infants with birthweights 1500 g and under, collated published data by Stewart et al (1981)

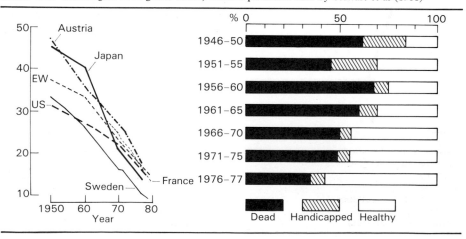

Major causes of death in childhood

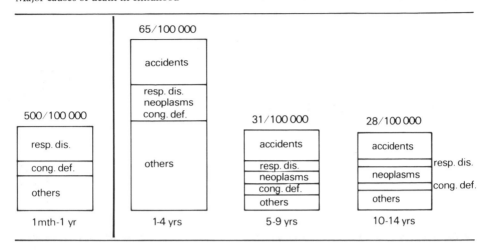

notification and certification of the cause of death. It provides information on the relative importance of inherited and acquired factors in mortality, the importance of environmental factors (accident statistics) and trends with time to reflect improved health care.

Look for causes

Examination of data, such as crude mortality statistics, gives us a direct cause of death but they do not answer questions such as 'why did this person get disease X in the first place?' Was it bad luck, poor housing, inherited predisposition, or 'why did he die when others with the same condition survived intact?'

Plan services and predict needs

We need to know the number of children in the population in each age group to determine, for example, the number of staff needed for health surveillance, the number of places needed in primary schools, the quantity of vaccine required for the population or the areas of greatest need. Short term planning of this type based on current data is comparatively simple compared with 'long term forecasting' where it is notoriously easy to get the answer wrong. We can respond quite quickly to a request for 'more vaccine', but a request for more doctors or more teachers implies a gap of at least 4 to 7 years for training. Similarly a request for a new health centre in an area of high need also means a slow response and the

Prevalence of physical disorder in 10–12 year olds (from Rutter et al 1970 Education Health and Behaviour)

Disorder	Rate per 1000	Disorders	Rate per 1000
All physical disorders	56.9	Orthopaedic conditions	3.4
Asthma	23.2	Heart disease	2.4
Eczema	10.4	Deafness	1.8
Uncomplicated epilepsy	6.4	Diabetes Mellitus	1.2
Cerebral palsy	4.6	Neuromuscular disorder	1.2
Other brain disorders	3.7	Miscellaneous	1.7

possibility that the need will have changed by the time the project is completed. One illustration of changing needs is the falling requirement for school places for children with physical handicap. One factor is the fall in incidence of children with spina bifida as a consequence of a change in the natural incidence of the disorder as well as antenatal detection and abortion of affected fetuses, genetic counselling and selective treatment of infants.

Monitor services

Information is also required to assess the effectiveness of the various therapeutic and preventive programmes that are set up. In the case of an immunisation programme, the data required is the uptake of the immunising procedure among the target population and the effect of this upon the incidence of the disease that it is designed to prevent.

Not all useful data is collected by official bodies such as the Office of Population Censuses and Surveys. This data comes from a single general practitioner, monitoring aspects of his own work (Jenkinson, 1978)

Year of birth	1972	1973		1974		1975		1976	
Acceptance %	95	75		54		55		30	
Whooping cough immunisation		+	—	+	—	+	—	+	—
No. affected by whooping cough		9	17	7	35	2	23	0	24
No. not affected by whooping cough		96	18	84	41	74	39	43	74
Vaccine protection		90		90.2		96.4		100	

To compare the costs and benefits of programmes

There are economic as well as social and ethical considerations in health care. Which is the best way of using the resources available? Thus proposals for programmes to prevent conditions such as Down's syndrome, hypothyroidism, spina bifida or tuberculosis must attempt to assess the cost of the preventive programme with that of the therapeutic/management programmes.

A cost benefit analysis of a prenatal diagnostic programme for Down's syndrome for women aged 40 years and over in the West of Scotland (from Hagard and Curtis, 1976)

Cost of programme 20 years	£311 855
would prevent 8.1 cases of Down's syndrome	
1.0 cases of meningomyelocele per year	
Cost per year for care	
Down's syndrome	£4150
Meningomyelocele	£3980
Annual economic benefit (8.1 × 4150)+ (1.0 × 3940) = £37 535	
20 year cost economic benefit (based on survival of children)	£351 699

In France many cost benefit studies have been done, for example the cost of discovering and treating one case of PKU is £12 000; the cost of one case of severe mental handicap is £80 000. They have applied this approach to the prevention of congenital rubella by immunisation, screening for dislocation of the hip, early diagnosis of deafness, the BCG programme.

WHAT DATA CAN WE COLLECT?

Most epidemiological data consists of rates related to a particular event in a defined population.

$$\text{Rate} = \frac{\text{Frequency of observed event}}{\text{total size of population}}$$

Both numerator and denominator must refer to the same population. *Incidence* rates refer to the number of new cases of the illness, *prevalence* to the total number of cases, new and old. Both must be confined not only to the particular event to be measured in a particular population, but also to a point or defined period of time during which measurements are made, for example:

Event: deaths by accident

Population: children aged 10–14 in England and Wales

Time: 1978

is a valid measurement which can be compared with other rates which we can obtain for the same population over the same period of time.

The population must be the population at risk. It is not a worthwhile measurement to obtain figures for

Event: admissions for severe sunburn

Population: children age 5–9 in Nottingham

Time: January 1980

and we cannot compare these with

Event: Casualty attendances for sunburn

Population: Tenerife

Time: August 1980

Commonly measured rates are:

Stillbirth rate: Babies born dead with a gestational age of at least 28 weeks per 1000 *total* births.

Neonatal mortality rate: Babies dying in the first 28 days of life per 1000 *live* births.

Perinatal mortality rate: Stillbirths and babies dying in the first 7 days of life per 1000 *total* births.

Infant mortality rate: Babies dying in the first 12 months of life per 1000 live births.

Post neonatal mortality rate: Babies dying between the ages of 1 month and 1 year per 1000 live births.

Infant deaths by month of birth 1969–76. England and Wales (from Studies in Sudden Infant Death, OPCS No. 45)

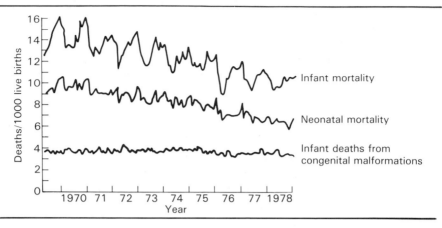

HOW CAN WE COLLECT DATA?

The event

The event must be clearly defined. There is unlikely to be trouble with mortality statistics, but measurements such as prevalence of visual impairment in school children could give problems. Some doctors might record all those children who wear glasses and others any children whose uncorrected near or distant visual acuity is such that they cannot read ordinary size print. A visual acuity of 6/12 or less in the worse of two eyes has the merit of being more precise. It is important to ensure that a suitable test is available to identify affected individuals, and to assess the test with respect to reliability in the hands of those who will use it. The test must of course, be properly applied in a standard manner. For example a test of visual acuity at 19 instead of 20 feet in a dimly lit room under conditions with the possibility that the child might memorise the sequence of letters is not adequate!

Population

The ideal population is first defined, for example all children age 5–16 in a country, and a decision taken whether to test the whole population or a sample which would be representative of the population as a whole. Samples such as 16-year-old girls attending embroidery classes or 12-year-old boys in detention may be

Cohort studies

	Population
Maternity survey (1946)	14 000 confinements
1000 family study (1947–62)	1142 newborn infants in Newcastle
Perinatal Mortality Survey (1958)	17 204 births
National Child Development Study (1958)	11 000 children from perinatal survey at ages 7, 11, and 16
Isle of Wight Survey (1964)	9–12 year olds on the Isle of Wight
Child Health and Education Study (1970)	15 000 children born 5–11 April 1970 and now followed up as far as age 11 years

suitable subjects for some studies but they are not a representative sample. A sample should be chosen at random. Its size depends on the prevalence of the event to be measured. If the event occurs frequently then a small sample will be sufficient; if it is rare a very large sample is required. Once a sample has been selected it is important that as many as possible within the sample are seen. It cannot be assumed that the prevalence is the same in attenders and non-attenders. Children who fail to arrive for an eye test may be afraid of being given glasses!

Time

Time may be expressed as a single point, 11 June 1983, or a period prevalence, January – March 1980, 1975–1985. Another approach which may be used especially if numbers are lost during the time of study, e.g. by death, leaving school, changing schools, is to use the exact number of person — years at risk. Comparisons of contraceptive effectiveness are usually given as number of pregnancies per 100 woman — years of use.

DRAWING CONCLUSIONS FROM DATA

The following questions should be asked: are the clinical data accurate? Is the population size adequate and representative? Is the time of data collection representative, for instance if we are looking at clinic attendances are the data distorted by bad weather, public transport strikes or staff shortages? Do the differences matter? Where we want to establish a causal relationship, for example between low birth weight and low educational achievement we need to compare the results for low birth weight children with a control group who are similar in every way except in the factors under analysis — birth weight.

Educational scores for low birth weight (under 2000 G) and matched controls in 1946 cohort (Douglas & Gear, 1976)

Age	LBW group	Matched controls	Difference	No. of pairs	P ('t' test)
15	45.1	47.5	—2.4	52	0.13
11	45.4	47.7	—2.3	58	0.14
8	44.5	49.4	—2.9	60	0.01

The final column shows the statistical analysis of the differences between the pairs. They are only significant $p < 0.05$ in the eight year olds tested. We do not always find what we expect to find. There were no differences between low birth weight and control babies in terms of severe physical, mental or behavioural handicaps. Opposite results were reported from other surveys done at different times, on different populations and with different perinatal and obstetric care.

When providing test results on two groups, it is advisable that the tester does not know which group the patients belong to, to avoid 'anticipation of results'.

Finding a relationship between two sets of reliable data serves to provide a hypothesis, it is not proof. Spina bifida has been related to the consumption of mouldy potatoes in pregnancy, though this theory, like many others has been discarded after closer scrutiny. Likewise is the proposed association between whooping cough immunisation and encephalopathy a causal one or a temporal one; both events taking place independently in the first years?

Ready made data

Much data is routinely collected by bodies such as the Office of Population Censuses and Surveys (OPCS). The accompanying diagram shows some of the information that is published in Great Britian. In addition, several cohort studies provide important information (see p. 18).

Some examples of 'ready-made data'

Morbidity	Infectious disease: Registrar General's weekly and quarterly returns Sickness benefit: Health and Personal social service statistics Chronic and acute illness: General household survey Hospital discharges: Hospital in-patient enquiry
Mortality	Mortality statistics in childhood: published by Office of Population Censuses and Surveys (OPCS) Analysis by age and cause On the State of the Public Health
Births	Births: OPCS (Annual Report) Population trends: OPCS (Quarterly analysis) Congenital malformations: OPCS Monitor Health and Personal Service Statistics
Abortion	Abortion: OPCS Monitor
Education	General Household Survey
Manpower (Health)	Health and personal social service statistics
Census (Most recent 1981)	Age, sex, marital status Country of birth Education Occupation/social class Age at marriage Size of family Size of household Household amenities e.g. bath Possession of a car Single parent households Tenure of household Analysis available at levels down to individual electoral wards

REFERENCES AND FURTHER READING

Alderson M 1974 Central Government Routine Health Statistics in Review of United Kingdom Statistical Resources (Ed. L L Maunden). Heinemann, London

Butler N R, Alberman E 1969 Perinatal problems: second report of 1958. British Perinatal Mortality Survey. E & S Livingstone, Edinburgh

Butler N R, Bonham D G 1963 Perinatal mortality: first report 1958. British Perinatal Mortality Survey. E & S Livingstone, Edinburgh

Central Statistical Office 1976 Guide to Official Statistics. HMSO, London

Chamberlain R N, Simpson R N 1979 The Prevalence of Illness in Childhood. A report of the British Births Child Study into Illnesses and Hospital Experiences of Children during the first three and a half years of life. Pitman Medical Books, London

Davie R, Butler N, Goldstein H From Birth to Seven. A report of the National Child Development Study (1958 cohort) National Children's Bureau. Longman, London

Douglas J 1948 Maternity in Great Britain. Oxford University Press, Oxford

Douglas J 1964 The Home and the School. MacGibbon and Kee, Hertfordshire

Douglas J, Blomfield 1958 Children Under Five. George Allen and Unwin, London

Douglas J, Gear R 1976 Children of low birthweight in the 1946 national cohort. Behavioural and educational achievements in adolescence. Archives of Disease in Childhood 51: 820–827

Douglas J, Ross J, Simpson H 1968 All our Future. Peter Davis

Hagard S, Carter F A 1976 Preventing the birth of infants with Down's syndrome: a cost-benefit analysis. British Medical Journal 1: 753–756

Jenkinson D 1978 Outbreak of whooping cough in general practice. British Medical Journal 577–579

Rutter M, Tizard J, Whitmore K 1974 Health Education and Behaviour. Longman, London

Spence J C, Walton W S, Miller F J W, Court S D M 1954 A thousand families in Newcastle Upon Tyne. Oxford University Press, Oxford

Steward A L, Reynolds E O R, Lipscombe A 1981 Outcome for infants of very low birthweight: survey of world literature. Lancet 1038–1041

Swinscow T D U 1981 Statistics at Square One. British Medical Association, London

3
Screening

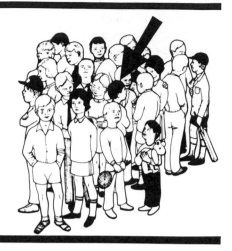

'Prevention is better than *no* cure' underlines much of the approach to child health in the community. Primary prevention aims to prevent a particular problem from occurring. Examples are prevention of infectious disease through immunisation or prevention of smoking related disease by health education. Secondary prevention is early or asymptomatic detection and prompt treatment, such as the screening programmes for phenylketonuria or hypothyroidism in the newborn period. Tertiary prevention is the process whereby once a condition is established, further deterioration is prevented and the best use is made of available assets. An example would be the appropriate treatment of a physically handicapped child to prevent contractures developing.

This chapter is largely concerned with secondary prevention, i.e. screening. Primary prevention is taken up in the chapters on health education, genetics, infectious disease and in the chapters related to handicap. Tertiary prevention is also covered in the chapters on handicaps.

Screening procedures are a major component of child health practice in the community. In contrast to the process of providing medical care for those who ask, screening investigates an apparently healthy population for occult disease. On these criteria examination of the newborn, well baby clinics and school medical examinations are all screening procedures. Screening is not examining a child 'to see what is wrong with him' but the seeking of named conditions.

A screening procedure, should fulfill the following criteria (WHO):
— the condition sought should be an important problem
— there should be an accepted treatment for patients with recognised disease
— facilities for diagnosis and treatment should be available
— there should be a recognized latent or early symptomatic stage
— there should be a suitable test or examination
— the test or examination should be acceptable to the population
— the natural history of the condition, including its development from latent to declared disease, should be adequately understood
— there should be an agreed policy on whom to treat as patients

— the cost of case-finding (including diagnosis and subsequent treatment of patients) should be economically balanced in relation to the possible expenditure on medical care as a whole

— case-finding should be a continuing process and not a 'once for all' project.

Early or asymptomatic diagnosis, such as in phenylketonuria by way of the Guthrie Test, enables treatment to be carried out before irreversible damage has occurred. There are strong economic arguments also in favour of the strategy of screening. To provide better medical care at less cost and without the need for human suffering as an initiating feature is an attractive proposition. Some of the economics of this approach are described in the Chapter on 'Information'.

Examination and validation of screening tests

The ideal screening test should be rapid and simple to apply and should reliably distinguish between those who have the *condition sought* and those who do not. Screening tests are not diagnostic. A person who is unable to read a car number plate at 25 yards has poor vision, but the test does not measure the extent of the visual impairment or the underlying cause. The breathalyser is a screening test for drunkenness; measurement of blood alcohol levels is a diagnostic test. These examples illustrate the necessary simplicity of screening tests if they are to be useful. A 'performance test for drunkenness' depending upon the ability to complete a defined obstacle course or equipping driving test examiners with Snellen charts are less valuable procedures.

Precision

This is the reliability or representability of the test. A test must give consistent results when performed more than once on the same individual. The main following factors should be considered.

Variation caused by the observer. This may be due to differences between observers, or variation in the performance of the same observer, for example in recording positive and negative responses of infants to test sounds.

Variation within the subject. The child's response to test sounds depends upon his level of interest and arousal. A hearing loss may fluctuate from day to day. Most physiological measurements — height, weight, blood sugar, blood pressure — vary in this way.

Variation in the method itself. The equipment may be faulty or incorrectly calibrated. Test conditions such as levels of background noise during hearing tests may vary.

All these variations can be reduced or eliminated by standardisation of equipment and procedures and intensive training and evaluation of observers.

Sensitivity and specificity

Sensitivity is the ability of a test to identify correctly those who have the disease. *Specificity* is the ability of a test to identify correctly those who do not have the disease.

An ideal test would reach 100% sensitivity and 100% specificity. In practice this combination is virtually unobtainable. An improvement in one criterion is often associated with a deterioration in the other. Sensitivity and specificity vary according to the level which is chosen to separate normal from abnormal results. This is shown in the diagram plotting the frequency distribution of the attribute and the results obtained when the cut-off point between 'normal and abnormal' is changed. Sensitivity and specificity are not of equal value. A test which is 40% sensitive and 90% specific could not be compared with one which is 90% sensitive and 40% specific. In the first case 60% of those with the disease would not be detected. In the second case 10% of the diseased group would be missed, but 60% false positives would be generated. Specificity is made with reference to the non-diseased group only, sensitivity with reference to the diseased group only.

Illustration of how the screening level selected may influence sensitivity and specificity

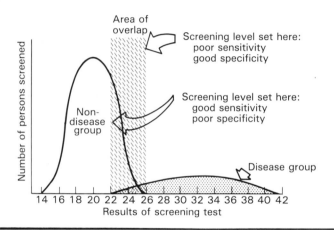

Calculation of sensitivity and specificity

Screening test result	'True' result		
	Present	Absent	Total
Positive	a	b	a + b
Negative	c	d	c + d
Total	a + c	b + d	a + b + c + d

a = true positives; b = false positives; c = false negatives; d = true negatives; a + c = prevalence; a + b, c + d = populations at risk. Sensitivity = $\frac{a}{a + c}$ Specificity = $\frac{d}{b + d}$

Predictive value

In assessing the acceptability of the levels of sensitivity and specificity, the prevalence of the disease which is being sought should be taken into account. When prevalence is low even a test with a high specificity will give rise to a relatively large number of false positives because of the large number of non-diseased subjects in the population. This phenomenon can be expressed as the predictive value of the test. The predictive value of a positive test is $\frac{a}{a + b}$ and the value of a negative test is $\frac{d}{c + d}$ The diagram (p. 30) shows the relationship between predictive value and prevalence when the test used has a high sensitivity 95% and high specificity 95%.

Screening programmes or checks?
Most countries have a series of recommended 'checks' for pre-school and school children. Only some elements of the checks are true screening procedures as defined in the first section of this chapter. This does not mean that the checks lack value, but indicates the need to examine closely their content and yield.

Some checks are true screening procedures. These may be either biochemical or clinical. Clinical screening procedures can involve history (e.g. of developmental achievement), examination (e.g. Barlow's test for dislocation of the hip) or special tests or measurements (e.g. height and weight or audiometry for hearing losses). History alone, unless by a highly structured questionnaire, can be a quite unreliable screening method.

Others are open ended interviews that allow parents or children the opportunity to ask questions or voice problems. The former permits the exchange of information which may be important in influencing behaviour or decisions, the latter may lead to a new diagnosis being made resulting from the parent's observations. This process is surveillance rather than screening. Both procedures are important but distinct. Asking the right questions of the doctor can be instrumental in making many new diagnoses for which history taking (the reverse process) claims credit.

Because the patient is the centre point of the services, he will have information about his health derived from agencies other than the one which he is currently seeing. Therefore, within a check, we discover problems identified by others, e.g. a hospital clinic, the general practitioner, optician, dentist, social worker, or psychologist. There is a strong argument for a parent-held record card.

In attempting to establish a successful programme of checks, a series of practical decisions need to be made.

1. What is the population to be seen? We need to be able to identify each individual to be seen and record the completion and result of the procedure. Some procedures may need to be applied to the total population, such as measurement of height and weight in order to identify growth disorders. Others may concentrate on the identification of high risk groups which will contain a much higher incidence of the problem being sought in the general population. Using this argument, selective screening of disadvantaged children will produce a high incidence of language problems, selective follow-up of certain neonates will yield a group of 6% which will contain 60% of all the sensori-neural hearing losses.

2. Knowledge of the natural history of the disorder sought will determine the appropriate age for applying the screening procedure and the need for repetition. For example, screening for colour blindness is undertaken on a once only basis whereas measurement of visual acuity needs to be repeated at intervals since changes occur with age.

3. Who is responsible for carrying out the procedure on any individual? Neglect of this essential aspect may cause a child not to be seen at all or result in a chaotic overlap and waste of effort between groups such as health visitors, school nurses, clinic doctors and family practitioners. Confusion can result from

Condition sought	Test to be applied	Agreed treatment	Justification for screening
Antenatal screening — examples			
Spina bifida Anencephaly	Serum alpha-fetoprotein	Termination of pregnancy if confirmed by raised amniotic fluid level	Prevention of severe handicap
Down's syndrome	Chromosomal analysis of amniotic fluid	Termination of pregnancy if agreed after counselling	Prevention of severe mental handicap
Duchenne muscular dystrophy	Chromosomal analysis of amniotic fluid	Counselling and termination offered	50% chance of an affected male infant
Neonatal Screening — examples			
Phenylketonuria	Guthrie test — heel prick blood	Low phenylalanine diet	Prevention of mental handicap
Hypothyroidism	Blood T4/TSH — heel prick blood	Thyroxine	Prevention of mental handicap
Congenital dislocation of the hip	Barlow's and Ortolani's test. Hip must abduct fully and is non-dislocatable	Splinting and observation	Poor results and need for surgery in late diagnosed cases
Undescended testes	Clinical examination	Orchidopexy	Risk of infertility, malignancy, psychological problems
Hypospadias	Clinical examination	Surgery	Psychological effects of untreated condition
Cleft palate	Clinical examination	Referred to plastic surgeon	Development of normal speech
Talipes	Clinical examination	Orthopaedic referral	Prevention of handicap
Hydrocephalus	Measurement of head circumference	Insertion of ventriculo-atrial shunt	Prevention of handicap
Congenital heart disease	Clinical examination	Paediatric or paediatric cardiology clinic	Correction of defect. Prevention of SBE

Condition sought	Test to be applied	Agreed treatment	Justification for screening
Pre-school screening — examples			
Squint	Cover test	Patching, orthoptic exercises or surgery	Prevention of amblyopia
Visual handicap	Detection of abnormal visual behaviour in infant — standardised test usually matching letters (Stycar) from age 2½–3 years	Correction of refractive error — educational and developmental guidance	Early intervention to reduce effect of possible handicap
Deafness	Distraction test Cooperation test Performance test or speech discrimination test Sweep test Tympanometry	To audiological centre — depends on severity and cause	Minimise handicap and promote normal language development
Growth disorders	Accurate measurement of length	Referral to a specialist growth clinic	Discovery of conditions where treatment is available, e.g. Growth hormone deficiency, Coeliac disease, Hypothyroidism
Child abuse or potentially abuse situations	History (PMH, FH or SH) Clinical examination	Agreed procedures generally laid down at local level	Prevention of injury. Help for parents and child
Dental caries	Clinical examination	Dental treatment and health education	Prevention of pain and need for dental extraction
School age screening — examples			
Scoliosis (11–14 years)	Clinical examination	Orthopaedic clinic	Prevention of severe deformity
Colour blindness	Ishihara colour test	Discussion of possible career limitations. No treatment	Minimal
Infestation	Clinical examination by school nurse	School treatment centre or GP	Prevent spread
Depression	Interview. The quiet, isolated, withdrawn child is frequently missed	Discussion and referral	? prevention of adult psychopathology

differing results or different decisions on future management.

4. Where is the procedure going to be carried out? The programme will fail if the centre is inaccessible and distant from the patient's home or if appointments are offered at inconvenient times.

5. How do we contact the parents and ensure their cooperation by persuading them of the value of the service that we intend to provide? This raises issues of effective communication, appropriate health education and the delivery of services in such a way that they are acceptable to the consumer. They need to be as convinced of the benefits as those providing the service are.

Within the context of 'checks', a series of poorly defined but important variables come into play. Parents, teachers, nurses and doctors have 'instincts' that 'something does not feel right' in spite of a failure to identify a specific abnormality. Such instincts are frequently correct and should not be overruled by the results of relatively crude examinations or tests.

Problems do not conveniently pop up at the time that checks are arranged. Some may be shy to show up at the appropriate time, like the TV set that works perfectly only when the repair man comes. This heavy reliance on infrequent checks is like sampling the water in a fast running stream once a year with a bucket and attempting through this to capture the 'problem fish'. This approach may work for some types of problem that can be reliably picked up at any time, but not others. Routine checks therefore need to be supplemented by unscheduled visits, usually at the prompting of teachers, parents or community nurses. They are our most valuable resource because of their extended contact with and observation of the child.

Within the context of screening or surveillance arises the question of decision making. However good the quality of the observations or recording, a decision needs to be made as a result of the consultation and any necessary action instituted. To leave this part open and let the process roll on to the next routine check is totally ineffective. The timing of the next check is not a 'routine', but is decided by the past history, risk factors and results of the present consultation. The place and person responsible for seeing the child next can also be decided.

Schedule for surveillance recommended by the Committee on Child Health Services (Court Report, 1976) with slight modification

Age (approx)	Aims and Comments
At birth	Immediate evaluation to assess need for resuscitation and special care, and identify obvious disorders.
Between 6–10 days	Full post-natal examination: start of ongoing child health record (including relevant pre- and perinatal data). Arrangements for achieving this examination in association with policies of early discharge from hospital need to take into account the time factor and the later onset of cardiac and other important physical signs.
	These examinations should ensure prompt recognition and explanation of apparent defects, and reassurance to mother of a normal infant. Mothers require positive advice, and mere absence of adverse comment is always insufficient.

6 weeks	Introduction to the 'clinic' premises, facilities and staff: opportunity for professionals to listen and advise on infant management and family problems and to give sympathetic support (and, where necessary, to initiate treatment or referral) to mothers experiencing fatigue, isolation and possibly depression.
	Unless for any reason the neonatal examination was not carried out, there will be a relatively low emphasis at this stage upon detection of handicaps.
7–8 months	Review of development, especially hearing and vision. The timing of this contact is important; 6 months is not a rewarding age to check motor development, while 9–10 months is often too late for the first routine hearing test.
18 months	Review of development, eg mobility, manipulative skills, hearing and early language, social relationships: opportunity to discuss the range of normal in growth and behaviour.
2½–3 years	Review of development: opportunity to discuss behaviour: language: appropriate vision testing and cover test for squint.
4½–5 years	Summing up of early health and development in relation to entry to school: early warning to teachers of potential or established difficulties (eg speech, behaviour) which could affect child's response to school: appropriate testing of vision (including cover test for squint) and hearing. Exchange of information with teachers, school nurse and parents.
	This examination, which should apply to all children should form the basis of a subsequent selective (ie non-routine) approach to ongoing oversight of the health and behaviour of children in school.
During school years Annually up to the age of 13–14 years	Health care interview with a school nurse, including a vision test and measurement of height and weight; dental examination by a dentist.
Twice during primary education	Hearing test by school nurse.
At approximately 13 years	Interview with the school doctor.

There are two crucial periods in relation to education when every child would be seen by a doctor; on entering school and at about the period of puberty.

SPECIFIC CLINICAL SCREENING PROCEDURES

This section covers the series of screening procedures within a framework that enables us to justify the programme as a whole and within which we are able to verify the nature of test, and criteria for referral and have an agreed policy on treatment.

Developmental screening

The identification of children who are delayed or deviant in their development is an important activity of community child health services. In order to do this it is necessary to know how to analyse developmental progress, to know the sequence of developmental progress and the normal variations of it, to have a theoretical framework on which to understand the process of the observed progress from one stage of development to another (for example theories of Piaget, Erikson, Watson), and to recognise both the limits of tests and those due to observer and subject variation.

The concepts of *initial age, median age* and *limit age* are useful in analysing developmental progress. These are illustrated in the diagrams. The initial age is when the first few children develop a particular ability, the median age is when 50% of children show the ability and the limit age when most children show the ability. Initial age provides a useful assessment of a minimal level for a handicapped child who has attained the ability. Children who have not attained a number of abilities by the limit age should be referred for further assessment.

Even with a screening test which has a high sensitivity and specificity (95%) the predictive value will be low if the condition is rare (left). In any screening test of development it is important to appreciate the age variation and to decide whether it is aimed at the initial, median or limit age of the ability

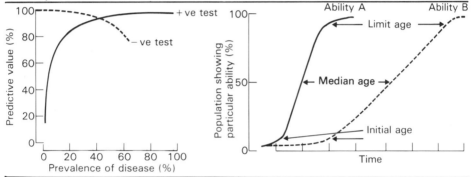

Developmental screening programmes
These are generally established as the backbone of the screening programmes for pre-school children. However, when viewed critically large areas of doubt emerge as to the effectiveness of such programmes.

Do the programmes identify previously unsuspected handicap?
Published accounts indicate that 'x' screening procedure identified 'y' children with handicap. They do not indicate whether the 'discovery' was unsuspected or whether it was previously known to the hospital paediatrician during follow-up, by the family doctor due to his frequency of contacts with young children, by the health visitor, or by the parents themselves. Screening often only adds precision of diagnosis to a suspicion voiced elsewhere, usually by parents.

Those at greatest risk of developmental problems are those least likely to attend clinics (the 'inverse care' law) and they also have parents least likely to express concern. Some programmes such as that for the identification of hearing loss are of undoubted value, but the development of parents as a resource in diagnosis might be more rewarding than the increasing professionalisation of the screening process.

How effective are developmental screening programmes?
The following data relate the results of early developmental screening to later diagnosis of handicap in three separate series.

Ellenberg & Nelson (1981) compared examination at 4 months with diagnosis of cerebral palsy at 7 years.

Sensitivity   67%
Specificity   89%
Predictive value of normal result   99.9%
Predictive value of abnormal result   2%

Bieman-von Eedenberg et al (1981) compared predictive value of neonatal neurological examination with finding at 18 months.

Sensitivity   87.5%
Specificity   54%
Predictive value of normal results   97.5%
Predictive value of abnormal results   17.5%

Boothman et al (1976) compared results of developmental examination at 8 weeks, 16 weeks, 28 weeks, 40 weeks, 52 weeks and 3 years.

Of 12 children abnormal at 4/52 — 3 remained so at 3 years
Of 12 children abnormal at 1 year — 3 remained so at 3 years
Of 10 children abnormal at 3 years — 2 identified at 4/52.
                                   — 4 identified at 1 year.

This sample of results demonstrates the unreliable nature of early developmental findings. The predictive value of normal tests is very good, but *most* children are normal and the normal group is likely to be five or ten times larger than the abnormal group. On the latter assumption an abnormal group of 100 children with a predictive value for the test of 10% will yield 10 abnormalities at follow-up, a normal group of 1000 children with a predictive value for the test of 99% would also yield 10 children.

The importance of establishing normality, of reassuring parents and congratulating them on their child's success is a process that might be more worthwhile than identifying the abnormal.

What is the value of early diagnosis?
Where developmental delay is due to environmental rather than to neurological causes, the results of early intervention studies show excellent results. These children may however be identified by examination of social rather than developmental data. In the case of mental or physical handicap, there is little evidence to support such a conclusion, though it must be admitted that research is difficult to carry out from ethical, practical and diagnostic reasons. There are difficulties with matched controls because of the diversity of handicap and ethical problems of denying control children what is regarded as standard treatment. Although it is hard, because of lack of evidence, to prove the value of early diagnosis for the individual child, other benefits do exist. It enables appropriate support for the family to be arranged as early as possible. It may permit a precise diagnosis and a prognosis to be given to parents whose anxieties may not be fully explained. Most importantly, a precise diagnosis can enable genetic counselling to be given where appropriate.

Developmental screening applied rigidly at fixed intervals to all children is a concept that does not stand up to close scrutiny. However, applied flexibly as a tool to be used to answer parents' queries, to examine high risk groups and for the application of selective areas of testing of proven value such as the detection of deafness, then it may be used to advantage.

REFERENCES AND FURTHER READING

Cochrane A L, Holland L L 1971 Validation of screening procedures. British Medical Bulletin 27:3
Cuckloe H S, Wald N J 1983 Principles of Screening in Antenatal and Neonatal Screening. Oxford University Press, Oxford
Court S D M 1976 Chairman. Fit for the Future. The Report of the Committee on Child Health Services
Rose G 1978 Epidemiology for the uninitiated: screening. British Medical Journal 2: 1417–1418

4
Families and Homes

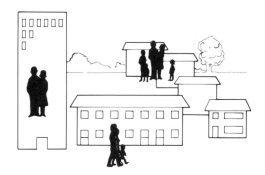

It is well established that there is a strong relationship between ill health and social deprivation and between social deprivation and educational failure.

Children in social classes IV and V have an increased morbidity and mortality, their parents are less likely to bring them for available preventive and screening services and their mothers are more likely to have received inadequate ante-natal care. Children disadvantaged in one area tend to be disadvantaged in others (Wedge & Prosser, 1973) and the pattern of disadvantage continues from one generation to the next (Rutter & Madge, 1976). The children are unable to learn from their parents the necessary skills and social behaviour to foster good health, educational attainment and social adjustment. They copy the mal-adaptive pattern of the previous generation.

SOME SOCIAL VARIABLES

Housing
There is an excess morbidity and mortality in children living in slums and also in the high rise flats in estates that replace slums. Younger children living in flats

Neonatal and post-natal mortality rates by social class, Scotland 1940, 1960 and 1975 (from Black report, Inequalities in Health, 1982)

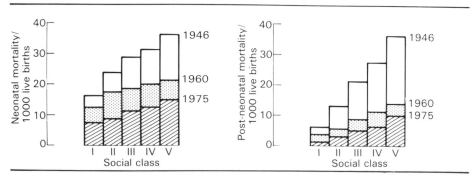

Height and weight by Social Class, Newcastle Upon Tyne, 1947–62 (from Miller et al, 1974)

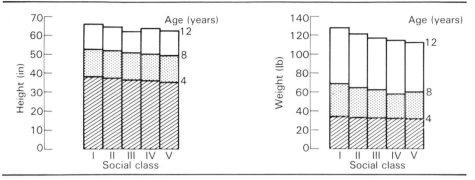

Morbidity rates by social class. On the left, the percentage of pre-school children suffering from staphylococcal infections and running ears (from Miller et al, 1960, *Growing up in Newcastle Upon Tyne*). On the right, the percentage of children at 7 years who were immunised against polio and who had visited a dentist (from Davie et al 1972, National Child Development Study, Age 7). N-m = Non-manual; M = Manual

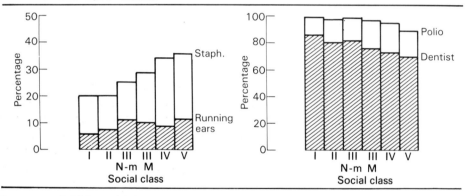

Percentage of children with 'poor' Southgate reading test score, 'poor' problem arithmetic test score and needing special educational treatment by social class (from Davie et al, 1972, National Child Development Study, Age 7). N-m = Non-manual; M = Manual

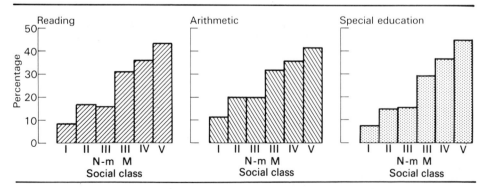

play outside less than those who live in houses; older children spend more time away from adult supervision. Play space and amenities are often lacking and anti-social activities replace more acceptable ones. Mothers living in flats more often feel isolated, lonely and depressed, which acts to reduce further the opportunities for the children to explore their environment — to learn. Paradoxically, with the loneliness and isolation, there is also a loss of privacy. Noise in one flat is heard in another which may lead to the infant's liveliness and curiosity being restricted for fear of complaints from neighbours.

Inner cities
Inner city life is often associated with added stress on families and their children. Closely knit communities which rely on one another for support may be broken up by property developments or rehousing policies. Housing shortages lead to homelessness (especially among the young adults) and high mobility. Inevitably sickness receives less attention and educational attainments are lower. In the relatively stable population in the Isle of Wight the incidence of reading retardation was 7.9% compared to 19% in an Inner London Borough.

Sanitation
Overcrowding, inadequate sanitation and dilapidated buildings encourage the spread of infectious diseases. Lack of refrigeration, clean storage space for food, adequate kitchen facilities and infestation of houses provide additional food borne hazards.

Safety
A child in an overcrowded house has less space to move and explore. Often for safety's sake he is left in the cot. Lack of personal space and privacy tends to increase aggressive behaviour. Families living in a single room cannot escape from the noise of their crying baby. In limited space, different family members wanting simultaneously to carry out different activities such as cooking, eating, sleeping, housework, dressing, watching TV are more likely to come in conflict. Slum housing also provides physical hazards such as increased fire risks. Inadequate heating in winter months may well be related to the rise in deaths during this period. Unsafe windows and stairs, poor lighting, dampness and poor ventilation, noise and air pollution provide additional hazards.

The members of a family at disadvantage are more likely to fall ill, they have fewer personal and material resources to cope with illness, and there are fewer medical resources available to them

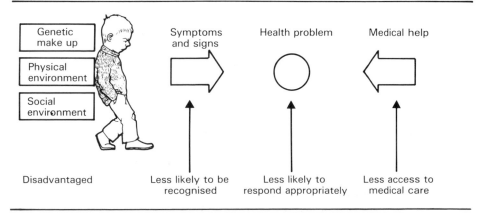

Immigrant families

Immigrant families are more likely to fall into the disadvantaged group. They tend to live together in poor and crowded accommodation in city centres where they can carry on their own traditions and use their own language. Limited knowledge of the local language and culture results in high levels of unemployment. Poor health of mothers provides extra obstetric hazards. Likewise lack of knowledge, differing religious and cultural beliefs may restrict access to medical help. Diseases may be imported such as tuberculosis and intestinal infestations. Dietary habits may result in nutritional deficiency such as rickets and anaemia.

The problems of immigrant families are increased by the inability of the professionals in the health services to understand their patterns of life. Advice on treatment must be offered within this context and doctors and nurses must appreciate that the patient's attitude to health and disease, birth and death, may not be the same as their own. *Asian Patients in Hospital and at Home* by Alix Henley (1979) provides a good review of the problems of Asian families in the UK. The immigrant child not speaking the language of the country is at a disadvantage in school. They have first to acquire a new language and adjust to a new society, a new physical environment and climate before being able to compete equally with their peer group in education. Schools in areas with large numbers of immigrant children tend to have a high pupil and staff turnover. Racial discrimination among school children and the conflicting patterns of home and school life may provide additional problems. Differences in religion, diet, dress, modesty, self-image, expectations, languages, marriage and discipline have to be appreciated by those concerned with the immigrant child especially his peer group at school. Different cultures have different child rearing practices and expectations. Children of parents born in the West Indies but living in Brixton were found to fare particularly poorly in development and later in education. The parents expected their children to become independent from an early age. The practice of slavery interrupted African child rearing practices and these have not been adequately replaced. Toys are often few. Working mothers leave their babies with illegal and inadequate minders who merely act as caretakers and provide very little stimulation. In the event the children grow up, like their parents, to have low expectations and self-esteem in the learning situation which results in underachievement.

Social conditions in U.K. (from Wedge &Essen, 1982)

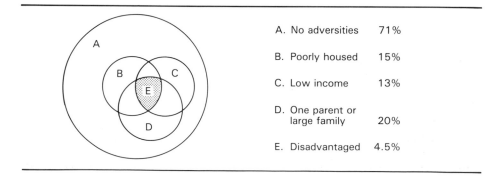

A. No adversities   71%

B. Poorly housed   15%

C. Low income   13%

D. One parent or large family   20%

E. Disadvantaged   4.5%

Factors associated with disadvantage defined by low income, poor housing, and large or single parent family (from Wedge & Prosser, 1973)

	Disadvantaged group (%)	No disadvantage (%)
Less than 5 antenatal visits	10.2	2.9
Teenage mother	7.2	3.9
Mother less than 5 feet	5	1.8
No bathroom	17.4	2.3
No indoor toilet	24.3	3.8
11-year-old sharing bed*	*32.8	9.3
In care before age 11	10.7	0.9
Father off work due to illness all year	9.5	0.2
Height over 4' 11''	9.7	22.2
Child Health Clinic non-attenders	33	25
regular attenders	23	66
Absent from school 3 months/year	2	0.4
Unprotected against polio	12.5	2.5
History of burns	14	9
10+ sutures	4	1
Hearing loss	2.8	0.7
Need for special education	7	1.25
Educationally subnormal	5	0.6
Maladjusted	25.9	9.2
Poor reading ability	58.2	20.7
Poor maths ability	56.4	21.7
Neither parent contacting school	61.4	34.7

* One in 22 of these children shared and wet the bed.

The disadvantages of children born in an inner city area compared with the community as a whole (from the Nottingham Deprivation Survey, 1983)

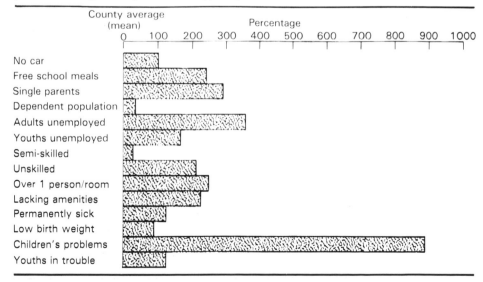

THE CONCEPT OF CHILDHOOD DEPRIVATION

The consequences of early sensory, social and emotional deprivation have been extensively studied. Children raised in institutions or who pass through a series of foster homes have poor language development, school attainment and have an impaired ability to form emotional attachments. This inability to form deep and lasting relationships leads to inadequate parenting for their offspring. An animal model of maternal deprivation shows similar patterns of behaviour: monkeys separated from their mothers at birth were solitary and aggressive and failed to fit in with the established social hierarchy. They failed to exhibit normal sexual behaviour and did not exhibit normal protective instincts towards their offspring. Sensory stimulation is needed for normal development. Denying sensory input in early life may lead to underdevelopment of the brain. This has been most clearly demonstrated with respect to visual stimuli and the development of the occipital cortex. The newborn infant fixes on a human face, and under normal circumstances this will be reinforced by the mother and thus the child is encouraged to take greater and greater interest. The deprived child becomes apathetic and does not learn the value of taking an interest in his surroundings. Likewise lack of early linguistic stimulation can impair the development of language. Restricted language in turn delays the development of basic reading and writing skills. Such children often become more aggressive and impulsive and are less able to rationalise and think through conflicts because of a lack of inner language. Knowledge of shape, colour, size, texture is needed as a basis for early education and these needs may not be met if the child is reared in dull surroundings. Neglected, suppressed children may, at school entry, have no real understanding about the sea, mountains, farms, animals which is assumed in much of the teaching material designed for children of this age.

Emotional attachments are important for normal development. Children make multiple attachments and it is the intensity of the reaction rather than the essential caretaking functions that seems most important. The bonding process between parent and child generates the security needed to explore strange situations. Total separation in a strange environment for young children, such as admission to institutions leads to the sequence of responses of protest, despair and detachment. In the final stage, the child treats his mother like a stranger and needs time to regain attachment. The effects of separation are greater when bonding is insecure. Emo-

Some consequences of disadvantage (from Wedge & Prosser, 1973; Wedge & Essen, 1982)

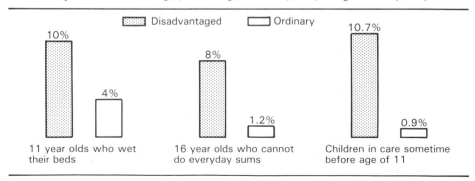

Road to educational failure

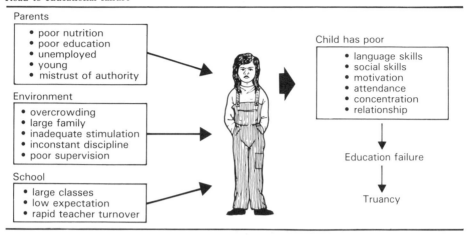

Parents
- poor nutrition
- poor education
- unemployed
- young
- mistrust of authority

Environment
- overcrowding
- large family
- inadequate stimulation
- inconstant discipline
- poor supervision

School
- large classes
- low expectation
- rapid teacher turnover

Child has poor
- language skills
- social skills
- motivation
- attendance
- concentration
- relationship

Education failure

Truancy

tional deprivation implies not only an absence of normal emotional links with parents but also strangeness and inconsistencies in those that do develop. Children distressed by virtue of 'broken homes' and marital discord seem at a greater disadvantage than those deprived through the death of a parent.

Emotionally deprived children in the pre-school years tend to be passive and apathetic. They form non-specific bonds to strangers and will greet or cling to anyone, being unperturbed for instance by a change in nursery staff. They are frequently investigated for failure to thrive: they grow poorly at home but have an accelerated rate of growth and development when admitted to hospital. The children characteristically have cold extremities. As the children grow up they show poor attainment in school with establishment of a pattern of truanting and antisocial behaviour. Their search for a satisfactory relationship which they are unable to sustain leads to teenage pregnancy, extra-marital conception or marital breakdown and poor care of their newborn infants.

Happily not all children follow the paths that might be predicted for them, some survive appalling childhoods with their abilities and personalities intact.

REFERENCES AND FURTHER READING.

Davie R, Butler N, Goldstein H 1972 From Birth to Seven. A report of the National Child Development Study. Longman, Harlow

Crellin E, Pringle M L, West P 1971 Born Illegitimate. Social and Educational Implications. NFER

Henley A 1979 Asian Patients in Hospital and at Home. Pitman, London

Miller F, Court S D M, Knox E, Brandon S 1974 The School Years in Newcastle Upon Tyne 1955–62. Oxford University Press, Oxford

Pollak M 1972 Todays Three-year-olds in London. Heinemann, London

Pollak M 1979 Nine Year Olds. MTP Press, Lancaster

Rutter M 1972 Maternal Deprivation Reassessed. Penguin, Harmondsworth

Rutter M, Madge N 1976 Cycles of Disadvantage. Heinemann, London

Seglow J, Pringle M L, Wedge P 1972 Growing up Adopted. NFER

Wedge P, Essen J 1982 Children in Adversity. Pan Books, London

Wedge P, Prosser H 1973 Born to Fail. Arrow Books

Wynne J, Hull D 1979 Why are children admitted to hospital? British Medical Journal 2: 1140–1142

5
Health
Education

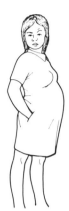

smoke?

drink?

drugs?

Health education is an integral part of the doctor's work with parents, and with children themselves as they become old enough to participate in their own health care. The essence of the work of child health services is helping parents to care for their young children adequately and to keep them healthy, working in co-operation with parents to detect signs of abnormality or illness early, and co-operating with parents and children in the management of chronic illness. This means defining problems, and then communicating the definition and giving advice on these problems. *Basic health education* is used here to describe what every doctor can and should be doing in each consultation; explaining and advising. *Second level health education* is a more sophisticated activity. It involves altering the shape of the problem, either through changing family attitudes or through changing the social situation in which the family finds itself. Most of us do not have the time, skills or contacts with other agencies which are required to tackle this kind of health education.

BASIC HEALTH EDUCATION — THE CONSULTATION

Giving advice in a one to one communication is the simplest form of health education, though it is not simple to do it well. There is the need to adapt advice and explanation to the situation of the child or parent concerned, which means listening to parents' and children's own account of the symptoms, their own understanding of the problem, and their own description of the social situations in which they find themselves. Listening with empathy and intelligence is, again, not a simple matter; yet without this skill, apparently clear explanations may fail in their purpose. Parents and children will not carry out advice which they feel is impractical or does not solve the problem as they see it. Basic health education in paediatric practice, therefore, involves cultivating the skills of listening, explanation and advice giving.

There is a considerable literature documenting patients' difficulties in obtaining adequate explanations from doctors and other health service staff. It is, of course, possible that in some of these cases explanations were simply not forth-coming, but few paediatricians will need convincing that parents (and children, according to their age and stage of development) should be given explanations of what is wrong and what is to be done about it. Indeed, management of much childhood illness or disability is impossible without this process. It is valuable to examine the techniques being used for explanations. 'But we do communicate with patients — it is just that they don't understand us!' is the cry of someone with poor technique.

It is easy to blame the parent. If any progress is to take place we must seek weaknesses in our communication techniques and try and improve them.

Listen to the parent

Listening to the parent (and/or child) not only provides material for a diagnosis of the problem; it also provides clues to the family's own understanding of the problem. Normal educational practice is to work from the known to the unknown, and the family's ideas are what they 'know', however shakily. If they are correct, we can reinforce their interpretation 'Yes you're right, it's . . .' before moving on to say what now needs to be done. If they are wrong, then we should make that clear before offering our own interpretation and suggestions for action. 'Well, you can stop worrying, Mrs X, it isn't heart trouble — there would be a lot of other signs if it were. What the problem really is . . .' If the family's definition of the problem does not emerge naturally, it may well be worth asking for it. Otherwise parents may carry on worrying throughout a beautifully constructed explanation, and take in very little.

Explanations and advice

Explanations need to be constructed with that particular parent or child in mind. However, some general principles can be identified:
— Whatever the intellectual level of the parents, complicated medical termin-ology is best avoided unless we are prepared to explain it as we use it. This may be necessary during the management of chronic illness, when a familiarity with medical vocabulary may be a help to parents in coping with the strain of their child's condition.
— Whatever the intellectual level of the parents, patronage is to be avoided like the plague. Parents have the main responsibility for the care of all but very sick children; we should convey our respect for this status by provid-ing them with more than perfunctory explanations. Speaking simply is not the equivalent of talking down to people.
— Physical discomfort, tiredness or anxiety impairs understanding. Parents or children may need several explanations, spaced at judicious intervals, before they can properly take in an explanation of a serious condition. The same may apply when the condition is not so serious but has strong emo-tional overtones for the parents or child concerned; for example, they may associate epilepsy with madness, eczema with infection, or head lice with social disgrace. Parents struggling with this kind of fear are unlikely to retain much of what is said to them about the management of the condition, until they have recovered their balance.

— Reviews of doctor–patient communication studies have until recently recorded patient dissatisfaction with medical explanation. They forget around 50% of the material conveyed. Philip Ley and his colleagues (1971) have made several suggestions for improving recall, for example — categorising the material to be presented, and teaching the categories first. So, the patient could be told:

I am going to tell you:
>   What is wrong with you
>   What treatment you will need
>   What you must do to help yourself

>   Firstly, what is wrong with you is . . .
>   Secondly, the treatment you will need is . . .
>   Thirdly, what you must do is . . .

Working along these lines gives parents an idea of what is coming, and may also, if pauses are made at the right time, give them the chance to ask questions to check their understanding of the first part before the second part starts.

When the diagnosis is presented first, it is usually remembered. Subsequent advice needs to be presented clearly and succinctly. (Patients recall proportionately less the more information is given. It must also be specific, for example, 'you must lose weight' is found less memorable than 'you must lose 7 lbs in weight'.

A recent research project on doctor–patient communication, funded by the Health Education Council, is rather more optimistic about doctor patient communication. It does, however, note that virtually no consultation contained any attempt by the doctor to check on the patient's understanding of what had been said. This is a basic educational technique which could well be used, tactfully, of course, to see that incorrect understanding does not survive the consultation and become the basis for incorrect action.

Self-assessment

We may feel that most of the above is obvious. It is always a challenge to see how far we achieve our own expectations about good communication. Video recordings of staged or live consultations, are useful ways of learning about one's own performance. Tape recordings of consultations, with the parents' permission of course, are more easily arranged, cheaper and less obtrusive. Listening to and analysing one's own performance may confirm one's existing high opinion of one's own technique! It is more likely, however, to reveal a mixture of strengths and weaknesses, and provide material to work on the weaknesses.

SECOND LEVEL HEALTH EDUCATION — BRINGING ABOUT CHANGE

Second level health education is considerably more complex, and may be beyond the resources in terms of time and skills of most of us, either within a consultation or in a wider context. It is desirable, however, that we should know something of the strategies and the chance of success and be able to co-operate with and encourage colleagues in other professions who do have the skills and time to engage in more sophisticated activities. We must avoid the error of believing that because our efforts as health educators have failed with a particular family, health education will not work. It may simply be that an alternative approach is needed.

Personal barriers to behaviour change

Basic health education depends on understanding the patient's ideas and situation well enough to provide appropriate advice framed in such a way that it is likely to be understood and remembered. With many families this will be enough. However, with a proportion there are emotional issues which can block action on the lines we want. This means that attention has to be paid to exploring underlying attitudes, increasing motivation, or to raising parental self-confidence in their own skills so that they feel able to handle the situation in accordance with medical advice.

One way of tackling motivation may be to help the parents to use behaviour modification techniques on their children or themselves. For example, if parental smoking is affecting a severely asthmatic child, parents could be helped to give up by organising a system of rewards for themselves for cigarette free days and weeks, and by planning alternative activities for times previously associated with cigarettes. An alternative approach which has been used in the past, perhaps particularly with smoking, is the deliberate arousal of fear. Research results suggest, however, that it is very difficult to gauge the appropriate amount of anxiety which for any one individual is likely to produce action; however an attempt to arouse fear may overshoot, causing the subject to block out the whole problem to stop the anxiety. It is as well to steer clear of this approach.

Raising parental confidence is a long-term project which doctors on their own may be unable to tackle. We can certainly contribute to it, or at least not depress confidence still further by the way in which we manage the consultation. If we assume that parents have an important contribution to make to the assessment and planning of care, as well as its execution, and conduct the consultation so as to bring them into partnership, this is likely to have a helpful effect; it will not, however, transform the situation overnight. Group work with parents may be helpful provided it can be managed so that parents learn and share skills and knowledge rather than depress one another still further.

Parents who suffer most severely from lack of confidence and general fatalism are often those embedded in 'cycles of disadvantage'. Attempts have been made to organise early intervention programmes on a multidisciplinary basis; concentrating resources on parents and young children in an attempt to help them to break out of the cycle. Isolating a specifically health education component in these programmes may be difficult and is probably futile, given the intertwined problems which the programmes are attempting to tackle. One pattern observed in some is a clear improvement in children's development during the programme, but there is a tendency for the benefits to fade after the programme ends or the child grows too old to participate. Two American studies, however, suggest that this need not always be the case. The Washington programme reported by Gutelius et al (1977) provided for the first 3 years of life, showed the persistence of behavioural effects in the children and educational efforts by the mothers at 5 and

6 years of age. In the Perry pre-school programme reported by Schweinhart & Weikart (1980), follow-up studies showed that participants had better educational achievements, were less likely to be involved in criminal activities, and were more likely to be employed on leaving school. If these results can be confirmed in other studies, there may well be ways of breaking into cycles of disadvantage to lasting effect.

Social barriers to child health

Some illnesses or accidents are not really preventable by personal actions but might be prevented by action on the part of the social unit in which the child lives. Pedestrian crossings, for example, may be more effective than the Green Cross Code alone. Better packaging and labelling of dangerous substances, safer construction of windows and doors, safer driving and the control of access to dangerous sites would all help to keep down the accident rate. Damp housing is unsuitable for most people; it is particularly unsuitable for children with lung complaints. There are plenty of other examples; doctors may be able to have some effect in individual cases. So, health education should also be directed at those who make housing and planning decisions, and here the medical view-point can carry useful weight.

THE PRACTICAL CONTEXT

So far this chapter has concentrated mainly on health education within the consultation. Consultations, however, take place in particular clinics, in particular buildings, in particular communities. Parents come with different expectations to a child health clinic or school medical examination, and may or may not be open to new approaches. It is as well to find out what our colleagues think and are doing. They may well have their own conceptions of what health education is about, and may well have their own programmes in existence, tackling their own professional priorities.

The environment of the clinic itself may well determine the success or failure of an education exercise within a consultation. How many tense women and screaming babies does a mother have behind her when she goes in to the consulting room? A long wait and a crowded waiting room is likely to make her feel she cannot talk at length, whatever the doctor's intentions. How much privacy do school children have to have to talk to the doctor?

The environment in many clinics whether in health premises, church halls, or schools, can be improved. If reform is impossible, we may have to refer parents and children whose needs the system cannot meet to an opportunity or a structure which is more flexible. Special appointments may be one answer; referral to health visitors or to other medical colleagues or to teachers may be another. Inherent in this referral, however, is an estimate of the skills and priorities of colleagues!

HEALTH VISITORS

Health visitors are nurses with a one year specialist training in health visiting. One of their primary responsibilities is health education. They struggle with a job description which potentially involves them in ministering to the health education needs of the whole population. Many, though not all, reduce this to manageable proportions by concentrating on a caseload of families with children under 5, together with a responsibility to share in the running of antenatal classes and a link with schools which may involve some school health education. The tradition of home visiting may give the health visitor the opportunity to try to build parental confidence; it has to be said, however, that the capacity to build confidence is a personal attribute as well as a professionally desirable skill, and it cannot simply be assumed that health visitor training equips every health visitor to do this. Health visitors have some training in work with groups, and may well be the appropriate people to experiment with a mothers' group in the health centre as an alternative approach to health education.

HEALTH EDUCATION IN SCHOOLS

Health education in schools needs to be approached from a rather different angle. Health visitors have traditionally worked with doctors on the health of individuals and families; schools represent a structure set up to do a different job, to teach children from the basis of established knowledge. A considerable amount of attention has been paid to the definition and development of strategies and materials for health education in classrooms with children at different ages and stages of development. The following is only an outline of the main developments and interested readers are referred to the bibliography at the end. Notwithstanding, it is essential that all are aware of the main lines of the work in school health education, particularly if we are directly involved in the health education of school children.

In the 1970s in the UK there was a considerable expansion of interest in health education in schools both at local and national level. Between 1973 and 1978 a series of DHSS reports on health and social problems recommended that part of the solution was more health education in schools. Department of Education and Science (DES) reports increasingly paid attention to the organisation of the subject as well as to suggestions for appropriate content. The Schools Council, the governing body concerned with examinations and the curriculum, funded a series of curriculum projects to produce materials for use in schools, and rationales and

Two of the many line drawings in the Schools Council Project: Health Education 5–13 on Deadly Decisions

strategies to promote a co-ordinated and structured approach to the subject in primary, secondary and special schools. The results have been an impressive series of curriculum packages, usually in the form of teachers' guides with pupil material incorporated: 'All About Me', for 5–8 year olds, 'Think Well', for 8–13 year olds, 'Health Education 13–18' for secondary schools, and 'Fit for Life', for special schools. In addition, dissemination projects have been funded by the Health Education Council; these have produced an in-service course aimed at teachers in primary and middle schools, and 'The Co-ordinators Guide', in-service course material aimed at those responsible for co-ordinating health education in secondary schools. There has been support for the appointment of such co-ordinators; because health education involves so many different subjects in the secondary curriculum, some form of central organisation within the school is highly desirable, if not essential.

The materials follow a developmental approach, relying on findings that children develop attitudes to such obvious health issues as sex, smoking and alcohol well before they start to experiment, and that teaching input should not be delayed until, say, the later years of the secondary school when habits may well be established and attitudes will almost certainly be difficult to change. They also lay great stress on the need to help children to develop a positive and realistic self concept, enabling them more easily to value themselves and their own abilities, and to resist pressures to get involved in unhealthy or damaging activities.

There are numerous other curriculum projects available for use with teachers or in schools; the Health Education Council has recently found it necessary to produce a guide for enquirers. The projects work from different rationales, but they all have in common the belief that if health education in schools is to have any useful effect, it needs to be planned and developed within schools by teachers to suit their particular area and requirements. The days of the visiting lecturer who 'did health education' with the fourth form on six Friday afternoons are numbered, if not already at an end.

Actual practice in schools does, of course, vary. Secondary schools tend to be more aware of problems to which health education might be an answer; schoolgirl pregnancy, smoking in the lavatories, and alcohol, solvent or drug abuse all look like reasons for doing something, and schools who receive good professional advice will be able to plan programmes which move beyond crisis prevention to a more thoughtful and structured development of one strand in the education of children. Primary schools are likely to be concerned at least about hygiene, dental health, road safety, and menstruation; again, with good professional advice they can start to recognise scope for, and develop, a greater volume of work and to structure it appropriately. Some local education authorities give considerable impetus to this development by issuing guidelines and providing advisory support within the local educational authority. Others leave much of the advisory work to be done by the local Health Education Unit.

What role can the doctor play in this development? From the foregoing account it will be obvious that doctors cannot be expected to be familiar with the latest new material and strategies, nor can we be expected to contribute to the teaching of health education in schools, except, perhaps, and very occasionally, as an outside speaker on a topic on which we are particularly knowledgeable. We can, however, take an interest in what is happening in the schools in which we work, and enquire about relationships with the local Health Education Unit. We can also see that the school is aware of any common health problems which might profitably be tackled through health education — though it will, of course, be up to the teachers to decide whether a teaching approach is the best one to take. Sometimes individual counselling is all that is needed, or the teaching may be better directed at a younger age group than that which actually manifests the problem. A school doctor with a good relationship with his school can enquire, pass on relevant information, and suggest sources of help; trying to do more will probably be unproductive, and may even be counter-productive.

SUPPLEMENTS TO THE CONSULTATION

Leaflets and posters

A very wide range of leaflets is currently available for parents; in Nottingham-shire, for example, over 100 000 of these are issued every year. However, leaflets vary in their suitability for particular parents and particular purposes, and leaving a selection on a rack in the clinic waiting room is not a particularly effective way of carrying out health education: a cynic might note that their main use may seem to be in keeping small children amused. Posters, by analogy, cover the cracks in the plaster and give mothers something to stare at while they wait to see the doc-tor. Both leaflets and posters have far more chance of being effective if they are part of a planned, professionally directed effort aimed at a particular problem, rather than a branch of interior decoration delegated to the clerical staff.

Leaflets probably have their most important use as a means of reinforcing and amplifying advice given by a professional. We should therefore know the range available and read them critically before using them. There is little point in giving a mother with limited educational attainments a leaflet which uses complicated words and long sentences, for she will not understand it. There is no point at all in giving out leaflets which refer parents straight back to the doctor. Some skirt

There is no lack of information

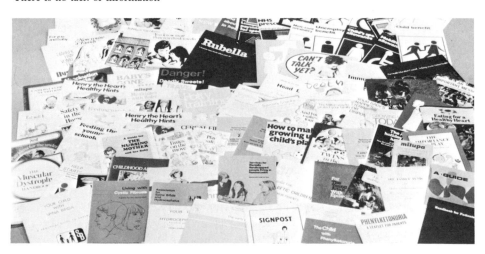

The 'readability' as indicated by the Flesch score comparing the daily newspapers with pamphlets related to health. The dot shows the mean and the vertical line the range. Only those who find the 'Times' light reading can understand the DHSS pamphlet on hospital complaint procedures! The interrupted line is the mean for the population (from A Nicoll)

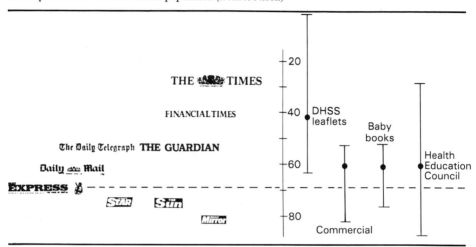

round controversial issues to such an extent that they provide little solid information for parents to use. Nor is there any point in using leaflets which have not been adequately revised to take account of recent developments; the British Medical Association pamphlets 'You and Your Baby, Parts I & II' in 1978 contained two contradictory statements on the value (or unimportance) of colostrum, and suggested that Rhesus incompatibility could be remedied during antenatal care. A BMA imprint is unfortunately no guarantee of accuracy. Leaflets may be very useful, but it is essential that doctors should read them first and thus be able to decide whether they are appropriate for the particular parent in front of them. They are an adjunct to the consultation, not a substitute for it.

Official documents can be difficult to read and understand

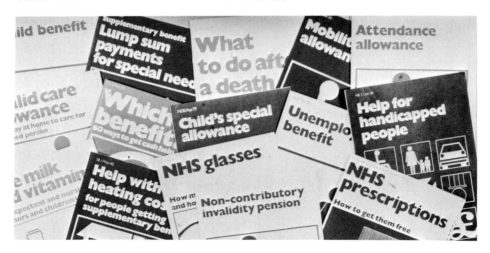

The leaflets should be assessed for tone as well as information. If the doctor wishes to build up parents' confidence in their own skills, or in their ability to have any impact on their child's health, it will help if leaflets handed out take the same general line. Note, for example, the exaltation of medical competence found in, for example, 'You and Your Baby' on antenatal care:

'You decide when to see your doctor and let him confirm the fact of your pregnancy. From then onwards you are going to have to answer a lot of questions and be the subject of a lot of examinations. Never worry your head about any of these. They are necessary, they are in the interests of your baby and yourself and none of them will ever hurt you'.

This approach is patronising; it is also hardly likely to promote an attitude of personal responsibility for the health of the baby. By contrast, Claire Rayner, in the Health Education Councils pamphlet 'You know more than you think you do' states 'This booklet sets out to help you discover and use the knowledge you don't know you have'; 'Play it Safe', produced by the Health Education Council and the Scottish Health Education Group in conjunction with a BBC television series; starts in similar vein

'This booklet is about the kind of accidents that happen to children and what *you* can do to prevent these accidents happening. Of course, the most important thing you can do is to *teach* children to recognise and cope with the dangers around them. And that isn't just a matter of telling children to be careful. It means setting a good example too. But it's just as important to prevent accidents by protecting children from danger — by using a fire-guard for example, or a car safety seat, or a child-resistant container for pills'.

Some leaflets and pamphlets may suit some doctors' purposes with some parents admirably. Where no suitable material exists, doctors may consider writing their own, either as individual assessments or management plans, or as general

There are many excellent baby books suited to different tastes

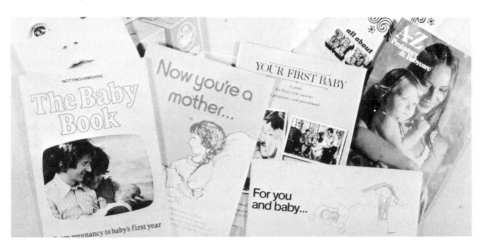

A page from a locally prepared booklet 'For You and Baby' designed with working class parents in mind (readability score 10.9 yrs)

HEARING TEST

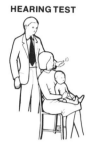

Babies need very good hearing to learn to talk. They must be able to hear very soft noises all the way from high squeaky ones to low rumbling ones. The test is best done when your baby is eight months. Two people are needed; one to make the sounds and the other to make sure that he does not cheat.

Test Date

Place

Test Done By

Result

---

advice leaflets on a particular condition or for a particular, neglected, social group. Individual assessments or plans may be very helpful to the parents and foster a sense of partnership; copies can usefully be sent to other professionals involved with the case, to show them what has been established and what advice and explanations parents have already been given. They do, of course, take time to produce.

General leaflets take far longer. All the tests of existing literature must be applied to one's own efforts. Doctors who are convinced that there is a need for another leaflet should seek collaborators, both from within and from outside the medical field. Those with educational and design skills would be particularly valuable; the local Health Education Unit is a good place to look for help.

Groups for parents

We may also be able to supplement our own efforts to inform and support parents, and to raise their confidence, by referring them to groups or courses concerned with their child's particular stage or condition. There is a considerable variety of these, and it can be difficult to discover the details of all the local groups. It is important, however, to have some idea of the range available, and where possible to gather information on the nature of the courses or groups — as with leaflets, some are more suitable for some parents than others, and there may be occasional groups which it would be unwise to recommend. This section can do no more than sketch a range of possibilities which could be investigated.

There is a wide range of self-help groups for parents of children with specific conditions. These can be immensely helpful to parents, both for the support they can offer and for the practical advice they can give from experience on the management of day to day problems. Many also accumulate considerable specialist knowledge of the condition, which will help parents to cope with the communication problems they are bound to encounter in repeated hospital visits with their child, and to take their share of the responsibility for care with greater ease. The numbers of these groups are themselves indicative of the need for them; a directory of self-help groups in one provincial town listed 29 relevant to paediatric practice. Doctors could usefully familiarise themselves with the range available in their locality, if they are not already aware of this from hospital practice.

For parents without specific and exceptional problems, an alternative range of groups exists. The NHS has a well established programme of antenatal classes; group work for parents after the baby has arrived is far more patchy and far more experimental. Some health visitors run mothers' groups; mother and toddler groups run by the parents themselves or by more organised parents' groups like the Pre-school Playgroup Association probably outnumber them. These unstructured groups may provide some opportunity for organised health education by a health worker, or even, on occasions, by a doctor; they are more likely to facilitate the exchange of information and skills between parents.

The Open University has produced short courses intended for parents of a wide range of ability, incorporating information booklets, and TV and radio programmes activities for parents involving their children and observing their behaviour. They are designed for individual use, but the material can readily be adapted to act as the basis for group discussions, or extracted for professionals to use with parents. 'The First Years of Life' and 'The Preschool Child' have now been followed by 'Childhood 5–10', and a further course for parents of teenagers will be published soon. There is also a course on adult health issues — 'Health Choices'. The material is bright, at times amusing, well written and well illustrated; it does, however, have limited value for parents of lower educational attainment. The Scottish Health Education Group have adapted some of this material to produce 'The Book of the Child', which requires lower reading ability and is more acceptable to working class parents.

Open University Courses for parents include programmes on the 'First Years of Life', 'The Pre-School Child' and 'Childhood 5–10'

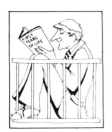 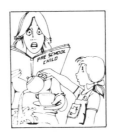 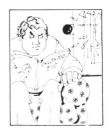

The Local Education Authority Adult Education Services frequently put on courses on child development, often in co-operation with the Preschool Playgroup Association; these may be very practical and suitable for almost any parent with a child of the right age, or they may be somewhat academic and cater mainly for middle class parents. Local practice varies widely; it would, however, be worth watching out for what is available in a particular area.

HELPING AGENCIES

Teachers, health visitors and midwives are only some of the more obvious professional staff who can be expected to recognise health education as a part of their job. However, at times it may be useful to ask for advice and support from an agency which has health education as its essential purpose. Reference has been made on several occasions in this chapter to the Health Education Council and to District Health Education Units. These bodies are the main agencies providing support for health education by the variety of professional groups who may be involved. The Health Education Council is the central agency; it has no direct relationship with District Health Education Units which are managed as part of the NHS, though the Council provides advice and support, and, of course, materials, to local units on request. Its main functions are to produce resources, to develop education and training materials for the various settings and professional groups concerned, and to provide a public image for health education in the media and through campaigns. Most people are only aware of the public image of the HEC; in fact much of its most valuable work is done more quietly, in developing and evaluating curriculum materials, liaising with the various professional bodies on design and dissemination, preparing and distributing resources, and liaising with the local District Health Education Units through which doctors are most likely to receive the fruits of the HEC's activities.

District Health Education Units exist in the majority of health authorities. District Health Education Officers (DHEO) head teams of varying sizes, depending on the priority given by the authority to this service; the Health Education Council recommended that each unit should have a minimum of five officers, including the DHEO and senior and basic grade officers, supported by technical and clerical staff. Larger districts than normal would, of course, require more staff. Despite this recommendation, in January, 1983, 50 of the 206 new districts had appointed a single officer without supporting staff. It is clear, therefore, that the level of service available to doctors will depend very considerably on the decisions made by their local District Health Authority.

Any health education unit, however poorly funded, can provide resources, though the range and quality of these will obviously depend on the money available. Beyond this the service provided will depend both on the staffing level and the quality of staff appointed. Most health education units aim to work through other professional groups, not directly with the general public; since the range of clients includes teachers, nurses, health visitors, occupational health staff, community groups, nursery nurses, playgroups, and the media, as well as doctors, it will be obvious that some units will be unable to do more than provide a resource service to some groups.

Assuming a reasonable staffing level, what kind of help can doctors expect? Health Education Officers come from a variety of backgrounds, but most have some previous professional experience, often as teachers or nurses. Many have completed the Diploma in Health Education — a postgraduate qualification concerned mainly with the theoretical background to health education in epidemiology, sociology and psychology, and the planning and evaluation of programmes; higher degrees in relevant disciplines are becoming increasingly common. Doctors can therefore hope to be dealing with professional staff with a broad academic background and often with considerable educational expertise. They will be able to seek advice on suitable resources for their particular needs, on the planning of teaching programmes, the construction of displays or exhibitions, and the evaluation of the work in hand. It may also be possible to arrange in-service training sessions on educational techniques. Doctors who seek such help will derive most benefit if they do some thinking themselves beforehand about what they want to achieve and what kind of parents or children they want to educate; the importance of suiting the approach to the client has been stressed earlier in this chapter, and the identification of the client group is obviously a decision doctors will make for themselves.

Basic health education in paediatric practice is about good two-way (or three-way) communication within the consultation, and advice presented appropriately. Help is available in developing this part of our work, both in the form of materials, groups and courses and in support from colleagues of various professions whose different training and experience can help to identify the needs and work on them. The first move, however, rests with us.

REFERENCES AND FURTHER READING

Anderson D C 1979 (Ed.) Health Education in Practice. Croom Helm. London. Chapters by Tones K, Davison L. Health Education in the National Health Service; Spencer N J Doctors and the Acquisition of Client's Health Knowledge

Bradshaw P W, Ley P, Kinley J A, Bradshaw J 1977 Recall of medical advice: comprehensibility and specificity. British Journal of Social and Clinical Psychology 14: 55–62

Cowley J, David K, Williams T 1981 (Ed) Health Education in Schools. Harper and Row, London. Chapters by Johnson V Health Education in Secondary Schools; McCafferty I The Role of visitors and Area Health Education Teams

Gutelius M F, Kirsch A D, McDonald S, Brooks M R, McErlean T 1977 Controlled study of child health supervision: Behavioural Results. Pediatrics 60: 294–304

Hull D Ed 1981 Recent Advances in Paediatrics. No. 6. Churchill Livingstone, Edinburgh. Chapter by Spencer N J, Perkins E R The Place of Health Education In Paediatric Practice

Janis I L 1967 Effects of fear arousal on attitude change: Recent developments in theory and experimental research. In: Berkowitz L (ed) Advances in Experimental Social Psychology. Vol. 3. Academic Press, New York.

Ley P, Bradshaw P W, Kincey J A 1971 Patients' compliance with medical advice. First Annual Report, Unit for Research into Doctor/Patient Communication

Ley P, Bradshaw P W, Eaves D E, Walker C M 1973 A method for increasing patients' recall of information presented to them. Psychological Medicine 3: 217–220

Ley P 1974 Communication in the Clinical Setting. British Journal of Orthodontics 1:173–177

Ley P, Spelman M S 1967 Communicating with the Patient. Staples Press, London

McCafferty I, Perkins E R, Spencer N J 1981 Planning In-Service Training for Health Visitors and Doctors, Nottingham Practical Papers in Health Education. No. 1. Nottingham University Department of Adult Education Nottinghamshire Health Education Unit

Perkins E R 1980 Education for Childbirth and Parenthood. Croom Helm, London. Chapters on Clinic Booklets (Perkins E R Spencer N J) and Child Health Clinics (Perkins E R, Anderson D C)

Perkins E R, Anderson D C 1981 Self-assessment in the NHS: techniques for monitoring and research. Nafferton Books. Driffield. Practical suggestions and examples of the use of audio-taping for self-assessment; written for health visitors, midwives and dieticians in particular, but readily adaptable to medical practice

Schweinhart L J, Weikart D P 1980 Young Children Grow Up. The effects of the Perry Preschool Programme on Youths through Age 15. High/Scope Monographs, No. 7, High/Scope Press

Spencer N J 1980 The identification and management of illness by parents of young children. Unpublished M. Phil Thesis, University of Nottingham

6
Growth and Development

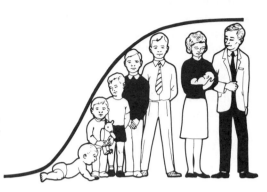

It is far more difficult to be confident about normality than it is to catalogue abnormal characteristics. The paediatrician working in the community must be an expert in 'normality' and the wide range of individual variations which it embraces. Failure to recognise the normal, be it growth, development, heart noises, tonsils or foreskin, may result in unnecessary investigation, treatment, follow-up and anxiety amongst parents and children. It is important to be able to observe, measure and record aspects of children's growth and development accurately and to appreciate the limitations of each observation or measurement. Standards of normal apply only to the population from which they were collected, so that data collected from children at one time and in one place can only be usefully applied to another population if that limitation is kept in mind.

PHYSICAL GROWTH

In a given population at a given age many human characteristics such as height, have a Gaussian distribution. The centiles are used to divide up the population. The 50th centile is not an 'ideal', it is that measure which separates the population into two equal groups. Three per cent of the normal population are below the 3rd

Normal distribution

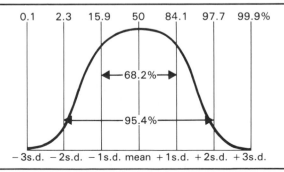

centile. The 3rd and 97th centile lines correspond roughly to plus or minus 2 SD from the mean. All the processes in growth and development are dynamic and a single point on a centile chart unless well outside the 3rd and 97th centiles should be interpreted with caution. Serial measurements showing changes along the given centile or towards or away from the 50th centile line are more valuable. For correct interpretation centiles for more than one parameter, such as height and weight, need to be available in order to make valid conclusions. Family body shapes (somatotypes) need to be taken into account.

Measurement of length and height

Supine length is usually measured until the age of 2, after which standing height is measured. A supine length may be up to 1 % greater than standing height in any one subject. Both measurements require training and skill if reproducible results are to be obtained. Accurate measurements cannot be obtained with a tape measure used freehand. A ruler or chart fixed to a wall may be the only equipment available. It is just adequate for screening but it is certainly not accurate enough for growth velocity assessment, monitoring therapy or medico-legal reports.

Length measurement. The Harpenden Infant Measuring Table can be used to measure length. The equipment consists of a table with a fixed head piece and a sliding foot piece. The infant lies supine with an assistant holding the head against the headboard. The measurement is made by the second observer who stretches the leg downwards so that head, body and legs are in line. The sliding footpiece is then brought into contact with the heels and soles and the measurement recorded. Accurate measurements cannot be made by a single observer.

Height. The Harpenden Stadiometer can be used to measure height accurately. Measurements should be made without shoes. The heels must be in contact with the ground and the back and heels in contact with the wall or stadiometer. Variation due to head tilt is avoided by ensuring that the outer canthus of the eye is at the same level as the external auditory meatus. Gentle upward pressure under the mastoid process is then exerted. The sliding headpiece is brought down to make the required measurement.

Weight

Measuring weight is easier than length or height, nevertheless large errors can creep in. Children are often weighed fully or partly clothed. It is important to record this with the weight. Small weight changes may merely be due to the fluctuations which occur over a normal day in normal children. Despite the benign nature of the procedure children may still 'hold on' to mother, or nearby chair or table, or they may be so distressed on the scales that the balance never comes to rest. In this situation it is perfectly permissible to obtain a child's weight by subtraction of the weight of the parent holding the child and the parent alone. Ages are often now expressed as decimal ages because of the ease of calculation of growth velocity when these are used. Decimal ages are easily calculated from the data given with the charts. The 1st January is .000 year, the 31st December is .997 of a year and the intervening decimal figures are given for each day.

Physical growth, height, height velocity and weight for girls (from Tanner & Whitehouse)

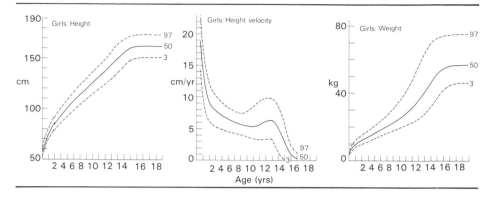

Velocity Charts

It is usual to record growth velocity over 1 year periods. Velocity may be calculated from the differences in measurements over the whole year or by using a shorter term by multiplying the figure by an appropriate time factor. The recording on the chart is made at the mid-point in time between the two measurements. Growth velocities stay much closer to the 50th centile than those for absolute measurements of height and weight. Variations above or below the 50th centile will cause deviations from the height centiles. An acceleration of growth occurs during the pubertal growth spurt though, as shown in the diagrams, the timing of the peak of this growth spurt shows wide variation from child to child. In any individual variations in growth velocity occur. They may be related to periods of illness or just seasonal variations. Growth is not a continuous linear process, there are seasonal variations. Over 2 years of age there is little to be gained by measuring height at periods shorter than 3 months.

Head circumference

The measure is of maximum circumference of the head. It is made in a horizontal plane just above the ears using a tape measure of non-stretch material. The results

Skull circumference illustrating the value of serial measurements (normal values mean ± 2 s.d. after Nellhaus, 1968)

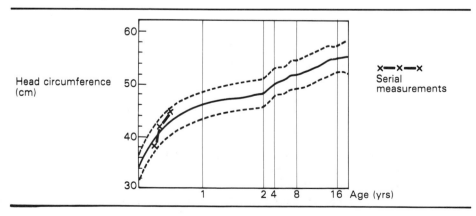

need to be corrected for gestational age before being plotted on 'normal' charts. Measurements at birth may be misleading as the effect of caput or a cephalhaematoma or other effects of the birth process on skull shape may cause difficulties in measurement. Serial measurements are most important. The head circumference must, of course, be related to overall body size in order for results to be correctly interpreted.

CHANGES ASSOCIATED WITH PUBERTY

In the process of normal pubertal development there is an enormous range of individual variation. Routine inspection to assess pubertal development is generally unnecessary and certainly is not a procedure that would obtain the cooperation of the average population of adolescents. If linear growth is normal, inspection of the genitalia is not likely to add much useful information except that an occasional case of Kleinfelter's syndrome might be diagnosed. Other clues that puberty is taking place such as breast enlargement, acne, and deepening of the voice in boys, are obvious without formal examination.

Girls

Peak height velocity. In girls this occurs before the 10th birthday in 3% and after the 14th birthday in a further 3%. The 50th centile for peak height velocity is age 12.

Menarche. In 3% this occurs before the 11th birthday and a further 3% after the 15th birthday. In 50% this is achieved by 13 years.

Breast development. The following five stages are described.
Stage I	Pre-adolescent with elevation of papilla only.
Stage II	Breast bud stage, elevation of the breast and papilla as a small mound. The areola enlarges in diameter. Fifty per cent have reached this stage by the age of 11.5 years but in 3% it will occur before 9 and in a further 3% not till after 13.5 years.
Stage III	Further enlargement and elevation of the breast and areola but without separation of their contours. This occurs on average at age 12.5 but 3% must wait till 14.5.
Stage IV	The areola and papilla form a secondary projection above the level of the breast. This occurs on average at age 13.5 but in 3% this does not occur until near the 16th birthday.
Stage V	Is the mature stage when the papilla only projects due to recession of the areola.

The enormous variation within the normal range, covering five years, must be emphasised. Children, parents, doctors and nurses may all become anxious if these differences are not properly appreciated.

Girls' pubic hair. The following five stages are distinguishable.
Stage I	Pre-adolescent, no pubic hair.
Stage II	Sparse growth of slightly pigmented downy hair along the labia. The mean age for this is 11.5 years though in 3% it occurs before

Stages of puberty in girls. The bars show the 3rd, 50th and 97th centile. Thus 3% of girls have started periods by 11 years, 50% by 13 years and 97% by 15 years of age (from Tanner & Whitehouse, 1965)

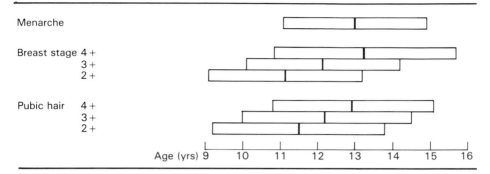

9 and in 3% not till just before the 14th birthday.

Stage III   Pubic hair becomes darker, coarser and more curled and although sparse has spread over a wider area. The mean age for this stage is 12 years though in 3% it will occur before 10 and in a further 3% after 14.5 years.

Stage IV   The hair is adult in type but covers a considerably smaller area and does not involve the medial surface of the thigh. The average age for Stage IV is 13 years with it occurring in 3% below 10.5 and 3% above 15 years.

Stage V   The adult pattern is established of wider distribution involving the medial surface of the thighs.

Changes in Boys

Peak height velocity. This occurs at an average age of 14 years though in 3% it occurs before the 12th birthday and in 3% after the 16th birthday.

Genital development. The following stages are noted:

Stage I   This is the pre-adolescent stage when the testes, scrotum and penis are the same size and proportions as in early childhood. The testes are about the size of a small olive.

Stage II   There is enlargement of the scrotum and testes and the skin of the scrotum reddens and changes in texture. There is no change in the penis at this stage. The mean age is 12 years old but with 3% having these changes before the age of 10 and 3% after the age of 14.

Stage III   Lengthening of the penis now occurs with further growth of the testes and scrotum. The mean age is 13 with 3% occurring before 11 and 3% after the age of 15.

Stage IV   This is followed by an increase in the breadth of the penis and development of the glans. The testes and scrotum are larger and the scrotum darkens. This occurs at a mean age just under 14 with 3% occurring before 12 and 3% after 16.

Stage V   This is the adult stage.

Boys' pubic hair. This follows a similar pattern to that in the girls, though with a different time span.

Stage I   Pre-adolescent. No pubic hair.

Stage II   Sparse growth of downy hair mainly at the base of the penis. This occurs at a mean age of 12.5 years though in 3% it occurs before the age of 11 and in 3% around the age of 15.

Stage III   The hair is darker and coarser and becomes curled spreading sparsely over the pubic region. This occurs at an average age of 13.5 years, 3% after the age of 15 and 3% before the age of 12.

Stage IV   The hair is adult in type but covers a considerably smaller area and does not involve the medial surface of the thighs. The mean age for this level is 14.5 years with 3% occurring around the age of 12 and 3% after the age of 16.

Stage V   This is the adult pattern with involvement of the medial surfaces of the thighs.

GENERAL DEVELOPMENT

This section is concerned with milestones as they are currently used in child health practice with respect to gross motor and fine motor skills, cognitive and social development. Development of speech, vision and hearing are described in the appropriate chapter. The ability to assess the development of a child cannot be obtained from written accounts alone and indeed a written account is only a very minor part of such training. Although charts, such as the Denver Developmental Screening Chart, acknowledge the enormous range of normal that exists, it is impossible within a single scale to record all the individual variations in the quality of response obtained. Obtaining rapport with the child and recognising for example the shy, nervous or withdrawn child who is not performing to his real level of ability, are important skills which only come with practice and experience. In a way, what is needed is observation of the subtleties and fine detail of behaviour rather than testing for the crude gross milestones of development which are used in screening. If we are particularly concerned about a child more detailed and graphic descriptions are certainly required in order to highlight areas of difficulty where particular help may be provided. Those using the standardised tests of developmental progress such as the Stanford Binet intelligence scale, the Wechsler intelligence scale for children, the Bailey scales of infant development and the Griffiths scales must ask themselves the reason for doing so. Is it to provide a clinical description of the child, his abilities and his difficulties which would aid diagnosis and management, or is it to provide a comparison of an individual child with his peer group?

Assessment of reflexes

Reflexes in the newborn are a useful way of studying motor development. Exaggeration of reflexes, diminished reflexes, asymmetry of reflexes, persistence of primitive reflexes or delay in the acquisition of secondary reflexes form a useful body of knowledge in the study of developmental progress.

Moro reflex. This is elicited in the supine position, with the head supported by one hand a little off the table. The head is then suddenly released, causing first abduction and extension of the arms with opening of the hands, followed by adduction of the arms and crying. This reflex is present very consistently at birth and disappears around 5 months. Persistence after 6 months of age must be considered abnormal. Because this reflex can be elicited so easily in its classical form, any variation from this should be considered with suspicion.

An asymmetrical Moro reflex may be due to a fractured limb as well as to neurological causes.

Galant's reflex. With the baby held in ventral suspension, sharp stimulation with the fingernails of the skin down each side of the back results in flexion of the spine to the stimulated side. The Gallants response is present in very preterm babies and its persistent absence in the newborn may well indicate a poor prognosis. Asymmetry is also important, as in the Moro reflex.

The stepping reflex. With the baby held vertically, contact of the soles of the feet on to a table causes reflex stepping movements of the legs. Persistence of the stepping reflex beyond the age of 6 months may indicate cerebral palsy.

The palmar grasp reflex. Insertion of an object or the examiner's finger into the palm of the hand or on to the sole of the foot, produces reflex flexion of the fingers or toes. This produces a strong grasp with the palm and secondary contraction of the arm muscles sufficient to raise the baby from the supine position when traction is exerted by the examiner's finger. This reflex needs to be lost before voluntary grasping can occur. Abnormal persistence may indicate cerebral damage as may absence or asymmetry in the newborn period.

The asymmetrical tonic neck reflex (ATNR). Turning of the head to one side leads to extension of the arm and leg on that side and flexion on the opposite side. This has been likened in boys to the position required to use a bow and arrow or in girls to the posture required to brush the hair holding a mirror in one hand and a brush in the other. In early life it may be useful in directing the hand towards objects in the visual field. However, it may prevent rolling over or the hands being brought to the face. Abnormal persistence of the ATNR, particularly in an exaggerated form, is very frequently found in infants with cerebral palsy.

Balance reactions. These are necessary in order for the child to develop ability

Primitive reflexes

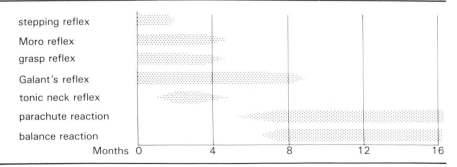

in the sitting position. The response consists of extension of the arm to prevent falling when the child's body is displaced to either side in the sitting position. Similar saving reactions occur in the standing position.

The parachute reaction. The child is held in a ventral position and is rapidly lowered head first towards the table. The arms extend in order to 'save' the child. Failure to appear is frequently seen in children with neurological abnormalities.

Normal patterns of development

The rate of development within an individual child varies depending upon his state of health, the degree of stimulation that he receives and such events as the arrival of a new baby, admission to hospital or a change of house. Allowance also needs to be made for prematurity. For this reason data related to a child's development cannot be taken in isolation from the environment in which he is living. Furthermore the child's personality and temperament may distort his response to the test procedure.

Posture and gross motor development

Children follow different patterns of events leading to walking including crawling, creeping and bottom shuffling. Those who bottom shuffle are usually late to walk because it is more difficult to get to the upright posture from the sitting position than from the crawling position. When assessing children who are slow to stand and walk it is obviously important to enquire about other methods of locomotion. Children who bottom shuffle tend to dislike lying in the prone position and thus do not develop crawling. Some children go straight from sitting to walking without an intervening stage. Negro babies are generally more advanced in early motor development than other babies.

At the age of 6 weeks when lying prone, the baby is just able to raise his chin momentarily. When he pulls to sit from the supine position the child still shows head lag but is able to show some ability to raise his head, particularly in the halfway position of this manoeuvre. When lying in the supine position the baby still adopts a pattern of flexion at the elbows, knees and hips. A pattern of extension at this age, may be an indication of spasticity. Held in ventral suspension he can hold his head in line with the rest of the body. A large discrepancy in the performance of the baby in the prone and supine position with superior performance when prone, may indicate a developmental abnormality such as cerebral palsy. However, some babies such as those who are bottom shufflers, greatly prefer one posture to another. Others are not given the opportunity to develop their motor skills in a wide variety of postures.

By the age of 3 months there are some most impressive changes in the child's motor abilities. In the prone position, the child is able to lift the head and upper chest clear and is able to sustain this posture supported by the forearms. When pulled to sitting there is only minimal head lag. In ventral suspension the head is now above the level of the body. When held sitting, the back is straight and the head only occasionally drops forward. When held standing the child sags at the knees.

Gross motor development

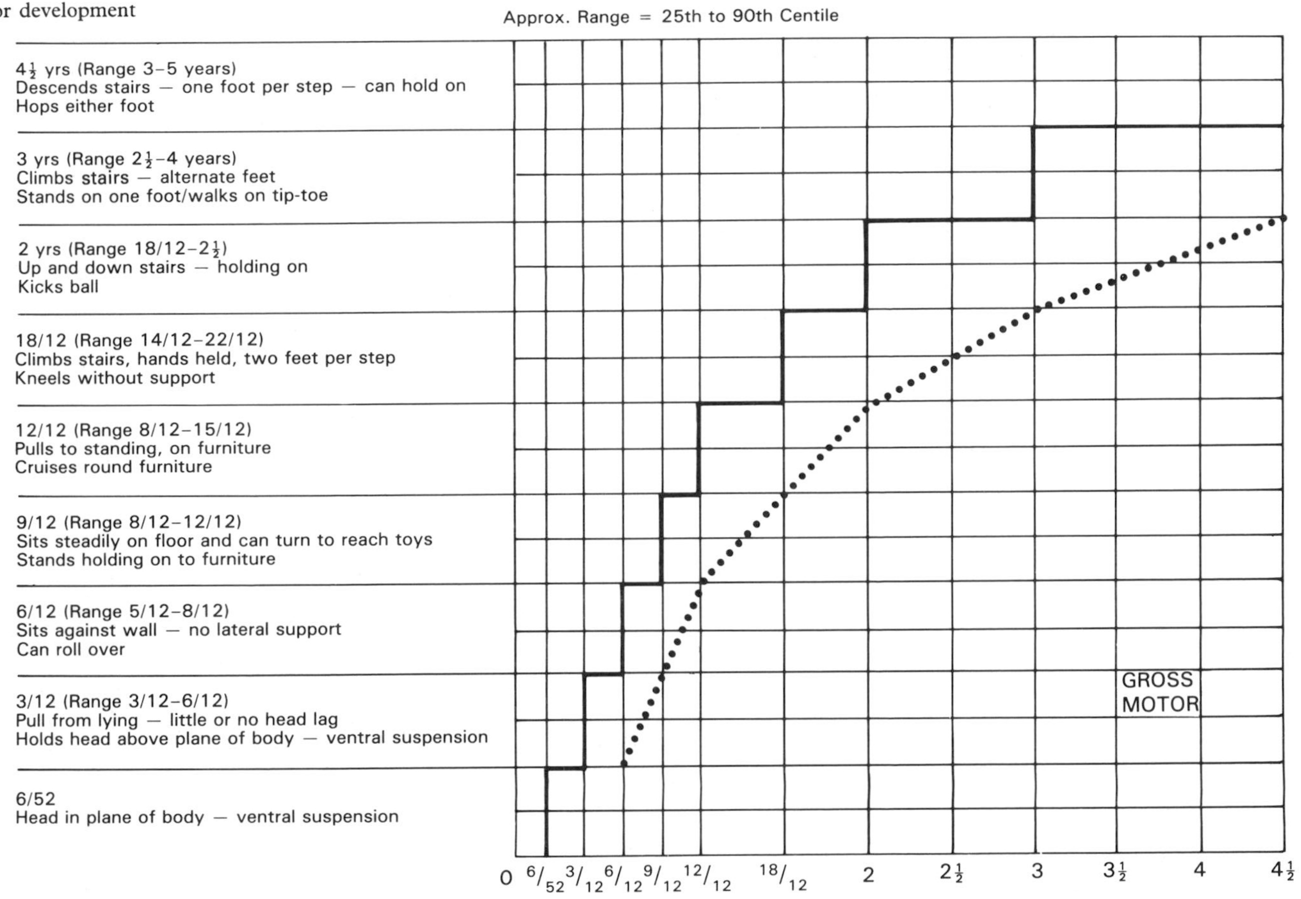

Approx. Range = 25th to 90th Centile
4½ yrs (Range 3–5 years)
Descends stairs — one foot per step — can hold on
Hops either foot
3 yrs (Range 2½–4 years)
Climbs stairs — alternate feet
Stands on one foot/walks on tip-toe
2 yrs (Range 18/12–2½)
Up and down stairs — holding on
Kicks ball
18/12 (Range 14/12–22/12)
Climbs stairs, hands held, two feet per step
Kneels without support
12/12 (Range 8/12–15/12)
Pulls to standing, on furniture
Cruises round furniture
9/12 (Range 8/12–12/12)
Sits steadily on floor and can turn to reach toys
Stands holding on to furniture
6/12 (Range 5/12–8/12)
Sits against wall — no lateral support
Can roll over
3/12 (Range 3/12–6/12)
Pull from lying — little or no head lag
Holds head above plane of body — ventral suspension
6/52
Head in plane of body — ventral suspension
GROSS MOTOR
0 6/52 3/12 6/12 9/12 12/12 18/12 2 2½ 3 3½ 4 4½

The boxes are filled in for each developmental item completed at the ages indicated on the horizontal axis. 10% of children falling below their 'developmental step' require further investigation. Those below the dotted line are severely delayed.

At 6 months of age, in the prone position, the baby can lift his head and chest clear, supporting his weight on extended arms and can roll over. Rolling is a very complex motor activity involving coordination of right and left sides, arms, legs, head and trunk. If the child is able to execute such a complicated manoeuvre it is most unlikely that any motor deficit exists. In the supine position he is able to lift his head from the pillow and in this posture grasp his foot. When pulled to sit the head is erect and the back is straight. He is able to sit against a wall requiring no lateral support. When held standing the baby is able to bear weight on his feet.

By the age of 9 months most children will be able to sit unsupported for 10–15 minutes. This posture will be stable and the baby is able to maintain balance as he reaches out to grasp nearby objects. By this age the child can also stand holding on and may attempt to take steps if supported. In the prone position some may be crawling and most should be making some attempt at this manoeuvre.

At the age of 1 year the child can sit well and for an indefinite period of time. He can rise independently from the lying position to the sitting position and from the sitting position is able to crawl effectively on all fours. Children get along by either hauling using the arms alone, or creeping on the hands and feet, or by bottom shuffling: some miss out these stages altogether. The child is now able to get up and down from the standing position and is able to walk around the furniture, a manoeuvre known as cruising. He may be able to stand alone for a few seconds.

At 15 months the child can get to the standing position without the aid of nearby objects. He is able to walk unsteadily on a wide base but frequently falls due to minor obstructions. Additional hazards to safety occur as the child learns to crawl upstairs but is unable to get down. He is also able to kneel with or without support.

By 18 months of age walking skills are well developed and falls are seldom though there is obviously wide individual variation. He is now sufficiently stable to stoop and pick up an object from the floor without overbalancing. He can run for short distances and can push or pull toys around the floor. Carrying a large object does not result in falling over. He is able to sit down without help in a small chair. Getting upstairs can now be accomplished in an upright posture with the hand held and downward progression may occur by creeping backwards or by proceeding downwards step by step on the buttocks.

By 2 years of age the child can go up and downstairs holding on in the upright position. This is done step by step and does not follow the adult pattern of alternating feet on each step. Running is now more skilled and the child is able to change course to avoid obstacles. He may play in a squatting position from which he can easily rise to his feet. Climbing on and off furniture is performed with ease but often not with the approval of his parents. He is beginning to be able to both throw and kick balls without falling over in the attempt.

By the age of $2\frac{1}{2}$ the child can walk upstairs without holding on but cannot yet do this downstairs. He has now developed the ability to jump with both feet together

Fine motor development

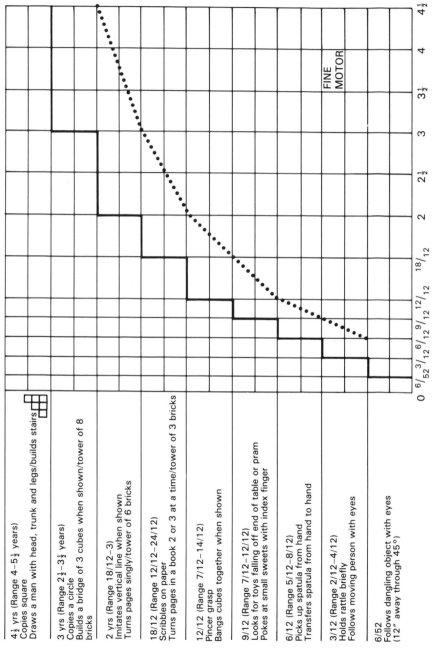

4½ yrs (Range 4–5½ years)
Copies square
Draws a man with head, trunk and legs/builds stairs

3 yrs (Range 2½–3½ years)
Copies a circle
Builds a bridge of 3 cubes when shown/tower of 8
bricks

2 yrs (Range 18/12–3)
Imitates vertical line when shown
Turns pages singly/tower of 6 bricks

18/12 (Range 12/12–24/12)
Scribbles on paper
Turns pages in a book 2 or 3 at a time/tower of 3 bricks

12/12 (Range 7/12–14/12)
Pincer grasp
Bangs cubes together when shown

9/12 (Range 7/12–12/12)
Looks for toys falling off end of table or pram
Pokes at small sweets with index finger

6/12 (Range 5/12–8/12)
Picks up spatula from hand
Transfers spatula from hand to hand

3/12 (Range 2/12–4/12)
Holds rattle briefly
Follows moving person with eyes

6/52
Follows dangling object with eyes
(12″ away through 45°)

The boxes are filled in for each developmental item completed at the ages indicated on the horizontal axis. 10% of children falling below their 'developmental step' require further investigation. Those below the dotted line are severely delayed.

and to stand on tiptoe following a demonstration of this.

At the age of 3 the child can walk upstairs with alternating feet but still has to use two feet on each step for descending. He can walk as well as stand on tiptoe and can also stand momentarily on one foot, a skill which many adults cannot demonstrate. The child can now pedal a tricycle as opposed to the previous manoeuvre of pushing it along with his feet on the ground. Increasing agility enables the child to climb nursery apparatus and to jump down one step. Others may attempt more than this but are not likely to succeed.

By the age of 4 years the child can walk both up and down stairs using alternating feet. He can stand on one foot for 3–5 seconds and can also hop on one foot, though there is wide variation depending upon the opportunities and encouragement to develop these skills.

By the age of 5 years the child is able to skip on alternate feet and to run lightly on his toes. His wide repertoire of motor skills will be illustrated by climbing, sliding, swinging, etc. There is increased skill in kicking, throwing and catching balls. He is able in 90% of cases to walk heel to toe. By the age of 5 the child has developed a basic repertoire of gross motor skills. Following this there are improvements related to greater strength, greater precision, greater speed and length of performance.

Fine motor skills

Development of fine motor skills depends on normal vision and appropriate opportunities for learning. Deprivation of either will result in delay of acquisition of such skills.

At 6 weeks the palmar grasp reflex operates but there are no voluntary fine motor movements.

At 3 months of age there is intense hand regard, in which the child stares continually at his own hand. This intense observation leads in the next few months to the development of voluntary use of the hand which is visually directed. At 3 months the child may reach out and hit objects such as pram beads.

By 6 months of age the child is able to pick up voluntarily an object such as a cube using a palmar grasp. Both the cube and his hand need to be within the same field of vision. At first this is only done with the greatest of difficulty and the cube is soon dropped. Lacking memory, the child does not look for the dropped object but seems to carry on unperturbed. Although voluntary grasp is established at this age, voluntary release is not seen for several months. At 6 months the child also begins to be able to transfer objects from one hand to another. However the child is not yet able to use this as part of a problem solving exercise. So, if the child is offered a second cube, he is likely either to ignore this cube or to drop the first one and use the same hand to retrieve the second object. Once the child has learned the ability to grasp objects he soon learns to be able to bring them to his mouth, and to add these sensations to his other means of exploring and understanding objects.

At 9 months of age the child has developed a mature grip between thumb and index finger and can also use his index finger to approach and poke at small objects. Toys that are dropped are now sought for. The child has a wide range of manipulative skills, objects can be shaken, bashed, pulled, pushed or held.

By 1 year of age the practice of fine motor skills has enabled the child to pick up small objects such as crumbs. The child is able to use his fine motor skills to feed himself with a biscuit or hold his own bottle. He has developed the phenomenon of casting, in which toys are deliberately dropped and watched as they fall to the ground. Given two objects he may bring them together in the midline and match them or imitate a simple action such as banging two bricks together. If offered a third object, most children seem unable to transfer in order to grasp the third object but may become quite upset by this apparent dilemma and drop both of the original objects.

At 15 months of age the index finger has developed as an organ for pointing to objects that he wants. Children are reported to be able to build a tower of two cubes though there is a wide variation between these abilities from various reports. This may well be highly dependent on the child's previous experience of bricks and his opportunity to practise. It cannot be assumed as perhaps some developmental tests do, that most children grow up surrounded by one inch cubes.

By 18 months of age the average tower builder has progressed to a somewhat precarious edifice of three bricks. If given a crayon this will be used for spontaneous scribble usually in a preferred hand. The index finger may be used to point at objects in the book and the child can usually turn the pages two or three at a time, inflicting a variable degree of damage.

At 2 years of age the average tower builder is up to a tower of six cubes, again bear in mind the wide variation in accomplishment in this task. Although performance with crayon and paper is still largely scribble this may begin to assume a circular form and the child might also be able to draw dots and imitate a vertical line. Page turning one at a time is now achieved though it must be remembered that many children do not have books and cannot therefore develop the skill. Between 18 months and 2 years most children are able to perform simple jigsaws involving fitting a circle, square, and triangle — initially by trial and error and only later by matching. Gains of skills and their level of development depend upon the availability of such toys as posting boxes, etc. Children may more readily demonstrate their fine motor skills in terms of manipulation of toys from activity centres up to small miniature toys, peg boards, jigsaws, dressing dolls, etc than in more standardised tasks which do not hold the same degree of interest.

At 2½ years of age the child is able to build a seven block tower. He is also able to construct a 'train' from three blocks placed horizontally in a row and one block placed on top for a chimney. With a pencil he is able to imitate a circle and a horizontal line if this is demonstrated. Only at the next stage are they able to copy the completed symbol without a previous demonstration.

By 3 years of age the child's tower has grown to nine bricks and using three

Simple and reliable tests of development

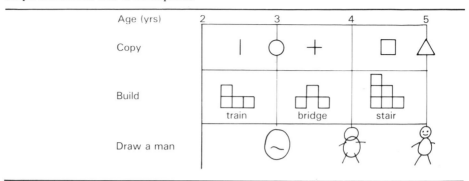

bricks the child can copy a bridge design. He can draw a circle from a copy and can now draw a cross if this is first demonstrated. The child is at this stage, beginning to produce recognisable pictures and will produce the first crude picture of a person plus a variety of assorted parts. The Goodenough draw a man test is a useful and reliable way of assessing development of children between ages 3 and 10. The child is asked to draw a man. He is left undisturbed and given as much time as he wants. The final drawing is scored using 51 criteria which record the degree of complexity and the anatomical details shown. The child is given a basal age of 3 years and is accorded an extra 3 months for each of the features recorded in his picture.

By the age of 4 years we have now reached the limits of tower building, bearing in mind the number of one-inch cubes the paediatrician can carry in his bag at any one time. The tower is now 10 or more cubes high. From about $4\frac{1}{2}$ the child is able to construct stairs with the one-inch cubes after an initial demonstration. He can now copy a cross without a previous demonstration and can also draw a square if the technique is shown first. The drawing of a man will now have a head and legs and the picture may or may not have a separate trunk. Most children will also be able to draw a very simple representation of a house. The child of 4 should be able to name the four primary colours in the one-inch bricks and is certainly able to match them. Some children may have been able to do this since the age of 3. A four year old can generally do buttons up, a useful practical skill which enables him to dress himself. However, absence of the skill probably indicates that the mother dresses the child because it is quicker.

The 5 year old can draw a square and a triangle from a copy. (He will need to be 7 to be able to copy a diamond and 9 to be able to copy a parallelogram.) He can also draw a house with door, windows, a roof and a chimney. Using one-inch cubes he can copy the step design without demonstration and also construct a 'gate'. Ideas of shape and copying ability have improved to the extent that the child can now learn to recognise and copy letters from the alphabet.

Social development and play
Although appropriate toys for each age group are inserted into the text it must

Social development

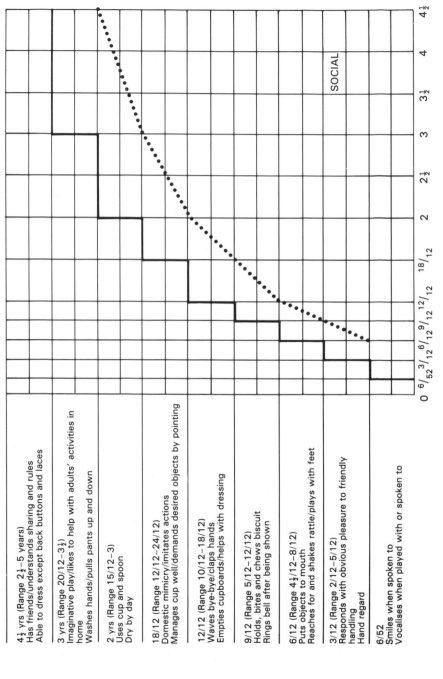

The boxes are filled in for each developmental item completed at the ages indicated on the horizontal axis. 10% of children falling below their 'developmental step' require further investigation. Those below the dotted line are severely delayed.

be recognised that to a large extent, the toys without the parent are useless. Also the importance of play such as peep-bo, round and round the garden, and nursery rhymes which do not require any toys are a very important aspect of stimulation.

At 6 weeks of age the child smiles in response to a friendly human face. The child is visually very alert and will fixate and stare at the mother's face for long periods. As well as crying they develop a whole range of sounds; coos, glugs, grunts and laughter, which indicate mood. An awake baby in a carrycot only receives the stimulation that is brought to him. This may be obtained from mobiles suspended above the cot, by carrying him around or by the use of a bouncing cradle in which the baby reclines.

At 3 months of age the child begins to react with excitement to familiar and pleasant situations such as feeding and bathing. Similar responses occur when he is played with. From 3 months the child may attempt to hit toys suspended on a string across the pram. Although the child can do very little with toys, things to listen to such as a musical box and things to look at such as mobiles, are very useful.

At 6 months of age the child can successfully grasp suitable toys and transfer them to the mouth. He is capable of grasping a rattle and shaking it and may apply this strategy to many other objects. He is also able to play with his feet and take these to the mouth too. The child is now able to play with a wider range of toys of many different shapes and colours; they appear to enjoy those they can grasp or which make a noise like rattles and bells.

At the age of 9 months the development of memory means that the child becomes much more wary of strangers and sensitive to separation from his mother. It also means that lost toys are looked for and he can play games such as peep-bo. He can feed himself with a biscuit, and attempts to hold his own cup or bottle. He may also try and grab the spoon. He can now handle toys which require a wider range of manipulative skills to make them work.

At 1 year of age children who have been given the opportunity are able to drink from a cup. However many parents feed their children as this is tidier so that they do not develop the skill until somewhat later. The same applies to spoon feeding which children can manage with help at this age but not all get the opportunity. At 12 months children understand how to cooperate in dressing, recognising that shoes go on feet and arms go in the sleeves. However, although many children do begin to cooperate with dressing at this stage, others who seem to dislike being dressed, develop the ability of doing the reverse of what is being required. The same can apply to nappy changing which can be a nightmare with a mobile uncooperative child. The child is now able to imitate gestures such as clapping hands and waving bye-bye. Some are able to produce this spontaneously in appropriate situations and others on demand. The child is also able to grasp quickly and imitate other actions such as ringing a bell or banging two bricks together. In play the child will often concentrate for long periods of time, putting objects in and out of boxes or quietly emptying mother's cupboards. Simple cooperative play is developing and the child will give a toy to the parent on request. Toys such as stacking beakers and pop-up men can be useful, though the child's skills are more directed towards taking apart than putting together. Rag books are also useful.

At 15 months the curiosity and exploratory behaviour becomes more intense aided by the improved mobility and manipulative skills developed over this time. The child grasps anything within reach and cannot distinguish safe from dangerous objects. He will begin to be frequently told 'no' and reacts adversely if removed from unsuitable situations.

The child of 18 months should be able to manage a cup without too much spillage and to be pretty adept at using a spoon independently. He may be able to take off shoes and socks, often in inappropriate circumstances. Negativism and the need for constant supervision are usually more marked than at 15 months. Domestic mimicry is seen in terms of the child copying mother sweeping. The beginnings of symbolic play are also seen, for example putting dolly to sleep or giving mother 'a cup of tea' in a toy cup. The child has progressed from toys that one pushes to trucks that he can sit astride and propel with his feet. The child can now manage the simpler kind of toys which involve fitting objects into shapes, e.g. 'men' into trucks or cars, or pieces into other types of shape fitting toys. Sand and water are most appreciated and the child will begin to be able to use drawing and painting materials in a chaotic uncoordinated and sometimes undesirable manner.

The 2 year old may be slightly less of a danger to himself than the child of 18 months. Greater awareness and knowledge and improved motor abilities may reduce some hazards but increase others. Negativism continues to be prominent and temper tantrums a common feature. The 2 year old should be pretty competent in eating and drinking. The 2 year old is also ready though frequently not willing to be toilet trained, however with greater or lesser difficulty, most children become dry during the day around this age. The child's play shows further development in domestic mimicry. He begins to want to join in and 'help' with adult activities. Simple make believe play is also developing. Children of 2 years are unable to share their belongings and play along side one another rather than with one another. Useful toys are replicas of adult materials such as tools, cups and saucers, toy cars, simple wooden trains and, of course, picture books and being told stories.

The 2½ year old is usually pretty reliable with using the toilet during the day. However many need help in that they are unable to pull down their pants or replace them. Make believe play is becoming increasingly elaborate with the child frequently talking to himself in play. Tray jigsaws may be very popular. Stories and picture books remain very popular. Scribbling with crayon and painting may just be beginning to emerge with some recognised form or pattern.

Three year olds should at last be fairly independent with toileting and accomplish all the subsidiary functions such as pulling pants up and down and washing hands. He is also able to play together with other children and understands concepts such as sharing or taking turns. Many 3 year olds, and quite a number of younger children too, are confident enough to separate from their parents at nursery school or play group. Recognisable drawings of a human body or

Activities of daily living

Age (yrs)	0	1	2	3	4	5	6
Feeding		uses spoon	fork		knife cutting		
Drinking		handles cup messily			carries cup no spills		
Undressing		offers limbs	removes lower clothes	unbuttons			
Dressing			assists dressing		buttons		bows
Toilet training			indicates needs	uses toilet	independent		
Washing			hand washes	dries		baths themselves	
Self-care			uses toothbrush	blows nose		combs hair	

a house begin to be made. The 3 year old can begin to make real constructions out of bricks or construction toys of various types and can make sensible layouts using things like miniature animals, people, etc. The 3 year old is able to remember nursery rhymes and also stories. He is constantly asking questions about things that he sees.

The 4 year old continues to ask questions though they are now of the 'why' or 'how' variety rather than the 'what' or 'who'. He can dress and undress except for difficult buttons and laces. Though the result may often be back to front or inside out. Imagination is shown strongly in play with such items as dressing up. He needs other children to play with and the idea of 'friends' becomes a well established need.

The 5 year old is able to play games with increasingly complicated sets of rules. A wider time perspective occurs in play. Particular themes either in play or within school can be carried on over a prolonged period in time. A 5 year old can, but not always, be protective and responsible towards his younger brothers and sisters. The 5 year old can play and build constructively and copy or produce increasingly complicated designs. He has the ability to tell the time, recognise letters and numbers, beginning the process of learning to read.

EMOTIONAL DEVELOPMENT

There are many profiles of childhood describing behaviour at different ages. Theories based on these observations give us a means of understanding the process of learning, the development of reasoning and of emotional responses. Such theories have contributed towards educational progress and in our understanding abnormal or difficult behaviour. They provide a view of the child's world as the child perceives it, as opposed to our description of what the child does. The theories are not only clinically useful but also provide a fascinating insight into the world of a developing child. They are not mutually exclusive for each examines different aspects of child development and each makes its separate contribution towards our understanding.

GESELL

Arnold Gesell at Yale University, first made detailed observations of normal child development which he classified into gross and fine motor, adaptive, language and personal/social.

On the basis of these observations, he drew three conclusions:
— that there is a defined sequence of development
— that development proceeds in a cephalo-caudal progression
— that development proceeds from gross undifferentiated skills to precise and refined ones.

The important implication of these findings for management in cases of developmental delay is that the child should be helped to acquire skills according to the sequence. Thus, it is inappropriate to teach a child to walk when he is yet unable to sit. Gesell thought that development reflected maturation of the central nervous system, rather than the results of learning. This theory was supported by observations that motor skills developed in a normal way in infants who were swaddled, however the quality of their performance was not studied.

Gesell also observed that it was not possible to induce the earlier development of particular skills by specific training and practice. He concluded from this again that central nervous system maturation was the dominant factor rather than training. It would be wrong to draw the conclusion from these relatively limited observations that nothing need be done or can be done for the young handicapped child on the argument that progress awaits brain maturation. This approach is too simplistic and although it must be accepted that damaged or delayed maturation will cause delay in development, it cannot be accepted that appropriate therapy and stimulation are not required. Some aspects of development are certainly dependent upon external stimulation; thus, the development of visual function depends on appropriate stimulation of the retina. Deprivation of this stimulation by opacities or gross uncorrected refractive errors results in the failure of development of visual function if these ophthalmic problems are corrected late. Similarly, cutting off the whiskers of mice results in defective development of the parts of the brain which control these sensitive organs. Others have developed the idea of critical periods for the acquisition of particular skills which suggests that optimum learning occurs only if the required stimulation is obtained at a particular time in development.

In spite of these criticisms, Gesell has contributed an enormous amount towards our understanding of normal development, particularly motor development, and its clinical application to developmental diagnosis.

LEARNING THEORY

Learning theory and behaviour modification practice has wide application in many areas including the management of mentally handicapped children. Learning theory is based upon the assumption that, with the exception of reflex responses, all behaviour is learned. It therefore stresses the role of experience in the environment rather than that of cerebral maturation. Certain responses are learned following specific stimuli and appropriate responses are reinforced. This has led to the therapeutic tool of behaviour modification whereby new responses may be learned and reinforcement withdrawn from inappropriate responses.

The theory on which behaviourism is based rests largely on animal experiments starting with Pavlov's classical experiments conditioning dogs to salivate when a bell was rung, through to the later experiments of Skinner and of Watson. The extreme point of view that all behaviour results from external learning cannot be accepted, but taken in conjunction with the other theories explaining child development, behaviour theory has an important application to our understanding of certain aspects of normal development and certain abnormalities in behaviour.

For example, children probably acquire their gender identification by means of the type of stimulation they receive. Thus boys are encouraged to model themselves on their father's behaviour and are given trains and guns to play with whilst little girls are encouraged to model themselves on maternal behaviour and are given dolls and pushchairs to play with.

Animal experiments have shown that there are critical times for acquiring certain types of behaviour, for instance monkeys reared entirely away from their own mothers do not exhibit normal maternal behaviour and are aggressive and not protective towards their offspring. This animal model parallels that of early childhood deprivation and the failure of those individuals to bond or take care of their children.

Behaviour theory has been very useful in that it has identified how certain types of normal social behaviour are developed. Some understanding of the genesis of disturbed behaviour is gained and why within some families they recur. However, all external influences act upon some substrate. It is clear that babies have particular personalities right from birth, and that these personalities are to some extent independent of external factors.

ERIKSON

Eric Erikson's psychoanalytical theory covers the whole of human life from birth to old age. He describes each stage in terms of conflicts between two opposing forces. These conflicts arouse anxiety. Failure to resolve the particular conflicts of each stage in development results in maladaptive behaviours which continue into adult life.

Phase I. Infancy (the first year of life)
— acquiring a sense of basic trust
— whilst overcoming a sense of basic mistrust
— realisation of hope

In this phase, the child is entirely dependent. His satisfactions are in being fed and in the process of bonding to his parents. Absence of these results in anxiety. It is easy to see how important it is for the child to acquire, early on, a sense of confidence in the world around him. If he fails to do this and the world is seen as a hostile, unpredictable place, then he is likely to be 'a difficult baby' and to have feeding and sleeping problems. As adults, those severely deprived in this early stage are likely to be emotionally detached and aggressive, being unable to form deep and lasting relationships with others.

Phase II. Early childhood. 1–3 years
— acquiring a sense of autonomy (own will)
— whilst combating a sense of doubt and shame
— a realisation of will

In this stage the child acquires confidence in his own ability as opposed to self doubt. He realises his own will and has the ability for independent action. He is, however, required to conform to certain behaviours and may feel guilty if he does not. Children of this age develop negativism, temper tantrums and toilet training difficulties. He needs to learn to balance his own wishes against those of others. If he is unable to realise the strength of his will then as an adult he may be lacking in confidence and initiative. On the other hand if he does not develop any form of censorship mechanism then he might have difficulty accepting the demands made by society.

Phase III. Nursery school age. 3–5 years
— acquiring a sense of initiation
— overcoming a sense of guilt
— realisation of purpose

From the self confidence acquired in phase II, a child goes on to initiate social behaviour which goes beyond himself into group situations. He must learn to share attention, affection and materials. In this phase conscience formation occurs and the child internalises previously external standards of behaviour. He may feel anxious that his separate autonomous behaviour is not always in accord with that of the group and guilt may result from this or from the fear of being found out.

With the greater sense of initiative the child begins to assume responsibility for himself as well. The child obtains his primary identification as male or female. Sexual curiosity and erotic feelings may arise and the Oedipus complex of attachment to the parent of the opposite sex is often seen. The child develops ideas of the future and can postpone satisfactions or pleasures till a later time.

Success in overcoming the conflicts of this stage result in a confident, outgoing person who is able to generalise his confidence into the group situation. Failure to do so at this stage may result in nightmares, fears of the dark, animals, or physical injury.

Phase IV. Primary school age (latency). 5–11 years
— acquiring a sense of industry
— whilst fending off a sense of inferiority
— realisation of competence.

In this age group children acquire the drive to achieve whilst attempting to overcome a feeling of failure. This drive and competitive spirit applies in intellectual activities, physical activities and in social relationships. Success at these results in increasing self-esteem (and esteem from others) whereas failure or a sense of failure, can result in difficulties in learning and impaired relationships. Those involved with school health will be very familiar with the child who finds himself isolated outside the competitive and energetic world of this age group.

Phase V. Adolescence
  — acquiring a sense of identity
  — whilst overcoming a sense of identity diffusion
  — a realisation of fidelity.

This description is perhaps best illustrated by Gauguin's picture 'Où venons nous où sommes nous où allons nous' — 'where have we come from, where are we, where are we going to?' The child needs to acquire a firm sense of who he is, what he wants from life and where he is going. Failure to do this is described by Erickson as role diffusion.

In this stage the child acquires a time perspective and is able to work towards distant goals such as examinations. There is anticipation of particular achievements in the future. The role of leadership is further developed in this age group and for the first time idealogical identification is seen in terms of political attitudes. Sexual identity develops further.

At this age the child should have acquired sufficient self-certainty in preparation for an independent life and decision making. The drive towards decision making is combated by a sense of doubt and uncertainty. Role experimentation in terms of jobs, ideology, and allegiances may cause added conflicts with parents as the adolescent seeks to acquire his own individual identity. Understanding adolescent problems is understanding the balance between acquiring the self certainty and anxiety about the ability to do so.

Phase VI
  — acquiring a sense of intimacy
  — avoiding a sense of isolation
  — a realisation of love
This is the phase of courtship and marriage.

Phase VII
  — acquiring a sense of generativity
  — avoiding a sense of self absorption
  — a realisation of care
This is Erickson's description of parenthood and the ability of parents to put the demands of their own child beyond that of their own.

Phase VIII
  — acquiring a sense of integrity
  — avoiding a sense of despair
  — a realisation of wisdom
This is maturity!

PIAGET
Jean Piaget, a Swiss Zoologist, based his explanations of child development upon precise observations particularly of his own children. His observations on cognitive development have been widely incorporated into teaching schemes in primary education.

The sensori-motor stage. 0–2 years. In this stage the child acquires a permanent image of himself and of the practical world about him. He learns to understand his separateness (dualism) from his mother.

1. Reflex action. 0–1 month. At this time Piaget describes all reactions as being simply reflex. For example, the child sucks in response to any object put into his mouth and he cannot distinguish between his own finger and the nipple.

2. Primary circular reactions. 1–4 months. By this time the child has formed motor habits which Piaget calls schema. Having developed these motor habits they can be wilfully repeated for their own sake, e.g. wilfully sucking the thumb.

3. Secondary circular reactions. 4–9 months. Now actions are produced not for the pleasure of their doing, but for the results they produce in the external world. Intentional acts are carried out. The child tries out all his various schemata on a new object until he finds one which produces the most satisfying results. Coordination of vision and movement develop although the child only grasps an object if the hand and the object are seen simultaneously.

4. Coordination of Schemata. 9–11 months. In this stage the child pursues a particular end rather than trying out all his various motor habits to look for a satisfying result. Therefore if the result is obtaining a particular object that he desires he might use his previous experience, such as tugging at the blanket on which the object is placed, to bring the object sufficiently near for it to be grasped.

Piaget describes memory developing at this time — the child realises that objects that have disappeared have not gone and that he should look to see where they have dropped or where they might reappear. A child will discover a block which has been hidden under a cup. He is able to imitate gesture and understand situational clues, for example preparations for a meal. With memory comes distress at separation from the parents. The child becomes much more discriminating in terms of adults and will not go willingly to a stranger. Children remember the Child Health Clinic and immunising injections. Anticipatory crying occurs in the expectation of receiving a further injection.

5. Tertiary circular reactions. 11–18 months. At this age, the infant seeks new results by active experimentation. Thus if he is dropping objects from a pram he may vary the position of dropping the objects to observe the variation in effect that can be obtained.

6. Invention of new means through mental combinations. 18–24 months. In this stage, the child may be seen to solve problems not by physical experimentation but through mentally working out the solution and then applying this knowledge. Thus if a chain is in a small box, which does not admit the child's fingers, his first action may be to invert the box so that the chain is expelled rather than make unfruitful attempts to get his fingers into it to grasp it.

These observations of Piaget can be readily repeated. They are a most worthwhile and rewarding part of a developmental assessment.

Infantile realism. 3–7 years. By 3 years of age, the child sees himself as the centre of the universe. He cannot conceive that others can have a different viewpoint (egocentrism). Animism describes the child's belief that everything is alive and has thoughts, feelings and wishes, just as he does. Dreams exist and thoughts and wishes are just as powerful as real events.

In his pre-causal logic, nothing happens by chance. There is always a cause and causes are motivational. For example, balloons go up into the air because they want to. The child's beliefs are based not on what he perceives but on an internal model of the world which may bear little relationship to what his senses tell him. For instance the child is insensible to the contradiction that babies come from a baby shop even though he has never seen one.

In the authoritarian morality of this age, the child believes that the punishment arises out of the crime. Bad events are explained as a punishment for something that he has done. It is easy for the child to feel responsible for events that have taken place, particularly in view of his egocentric standpoint.

It is during this period of infantile realism the child may suffer excessive anxiety if he feels that his bad thoughts and wishes may actually have come true or that having such thoughts may result in some punishment following automatically. The pre-causal child will see teaching about heaven or hell or stories of Father Christmas coming down the chimney as very concrete and real. Rules are rigid and unalterable. Thus the child in the back seat is happy to point out the red light the parents have just crossed or the double yellow line at the kerbside!

Although there is a rapid expansion of language ability, Piaget observed that children mainly talk to themselves and that their 'conversations' are really a collective monologue.

Concrete operations. 8–11 years. At the time of his move to junior school the child acquires the ability to think logically. He realises that words, thoughts and rules are separate from concrete objects and activities. He is able to learn to compare and to contrast, and to understand the relationship of parts to the whole, to be able to group objects in time and space, and to understand the principles of conservation of mass, weight and volume.

Formal operation. From age 12 years. From 12 years of age the child acquires the ability for abstract thinking. This involves a systematic approach to problems

Conservation of matter and volume. Reasoning ability (from Piaget)

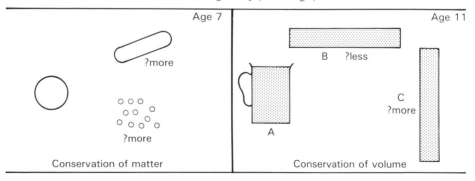

and the ability to understand hypotheses. There is a progressive ability to acquire an understanding of concepts of space, time, causation, number, definition, order, shape, size, motion, speed, force and energy. It is only within the secondary school that such concepts can be properly understood and taught within the syllabus.

REFERENCES AND FURTHER READING

Buckler J M H 1979 A Reference Manual of Growth and Development. Blackwell Scientific
    Publications, Oxford
Egan D, Illingworth R S, McKeith R 1971 Developmental screening 0–5. Clinics in
    Developmental Medicine No. 30. S.I.M.P. William Heinemann, London
Erikson E H 1967 Childhood and Society. Penguin Books, Harmondsworth
Gessell A 1948 Studies in Child Development. Harper and Row, London
Gessell A 1966 The First Five Years of Life. Methuen, London
Holt K S 1977 Developmental Paediatrics. Butterworths, London
Illingworth R S 1979 The Normal Child. Churchill Livingstone, Edinburgh
Maier H L 1969 Three Theories of Child Development. Harper and Row, London
Nellhaus L 1968 Head circumference from birth to eighteen years. Paediatrics 41: 106–114
Piaget J 1929 The Child's Conception of the World. Routledge and Kegan Paul, London
Piaget J, Inhelder D 1969 The Psychology of the Child. Routledge and Kegan Paul, London
Robson P 1970 Shuffling, scooting and sliding; some observations on 30 otherwise normal children.
    Developmental Medicine and Child Neurology 12: 608
Sheridan M 1973 Children's Developmental Progress. NFER.
Tanner J M, Whitehouse R H, Takaishi M 1963 Standards from birth to maturity for height,
    weight, height velocity and weight velocity. British Children. Archives of Disease in Childhood
    41: 613–635

7

Genetic Counselling

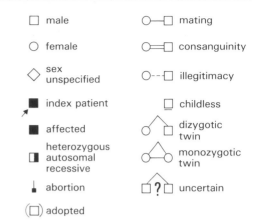

□ male	○—□ mating
○ female	○⊐ consanguinity
◇ sex unspecified	○--□ illegitimacy
■ index patient	□ childless
■ affected	dizygotic twin
◧ heterozygous autosomal recessive	monozygotic twin
↓ abortion	□?□ uncertain
(□) adopted	

Genetic disorders have assumed increasing importance over the years and now make a significant contribution to the total burden of community disease. At present congenital malformations, including those due to genetic factors, occur in 4–5% of all live births, are responsible for 30% of the admissions to paediatric hospitals and are the primary cause of 50% of all deaths under the age of 15. In 1975, congenital abnormalities accounted for almost 25% of the total stillbirths; 20% of deaths in the first week of life; and 1 in 4 deaths in the first year of life. It has been estimated that 1 in 10 of the total population, both adults and children, will suffer from genetic disease at some time in their lives (Alberman, 1982).

INHERITANCE PATTERNS

Although not all disorders present at birth have a genetic basis, the majority of serious defects are hereditary and the community paediatrician dealing with childhood handicap needs to have an understanding of basic genetic principles and

Common Congenital Abnormalities. Incidence of defects varies with age (25/1000 at birth to 30/1000 at 1 year) and with locality (neural tube defects 2/1000 East Anglia, 7–9/1000 South Wales)

	Approximate incidence /1000 births
Congenital heart disease	6
Severe mental retardation	4
Neural tube defects	3
Down's syndrome	1.5
Abnormality of limbs	2
Blindness	0.2
Deafness	0.8
Cerebral palsy	3
Cleft lip/palate	1.5
Talipes	1
Others including renal tract abnormalities	2
Total	25

their relevance to clinical medicine. Diseases in man thought to be genetic in origin may be divided into three major groups. Those resulting from the action of a single major gene, the Mendelian or unifactorial disorders; those due to abnormalities of the chromosomes and, therefore, due to the action of multiple genes; and those in which genes and environmental factors work in conjunction. Other developmental disorders may have a genetic basis which has not yet been identified.

Single gene inheritance

Autosomal dominant inheritance. A large number of conditions, over 1000, are transmitted in this way. Although they are individually rare — most have a frequency of less than 1 in 5000 — they are important because of their total number and because some present very striking clinical features. The prevalence of these conditions at birth has been estimated at about 7 per 1000, but not all cause problems early in life, for example Huntington's chorea. Dominantly inherited disorders likely to cause childhood handicap occur in approximately 1 per 1000 births.

Some dominantly inherited disorders

Achondroplasia	Hypochondroplasia	Retinal aplasia
Anorectal anomalies (some types)	Klippel-Feil deformity and deafness	Retinitis pigmentosa
Aperts syndrome	Marfan's syndrome	Retinoblastoma
Brachydactyly	Myotonic dystrophy	Spherocytosis
Cataracts	Nail-Patella syndrome	Split-hand deformity
Charcot-Marie Tooth disease	Neurofibromatosis	Stein-Levanthal syndrome
Ectodermal dysplasia	Noonan's syndrome	Syndactyly
Ehlers-Danlos syndrome	Optic atrophy (congenital)	Treacher-Collins syndrome
Freeman Sheldon syndrome	Osteogenesis imperfecta	Tuberose sclerosis
Haemangiomata	Polycystic kidneys	Van der Woudeś syndrome
Holt-Oram syndrome	Polydactyly	Von-Willebrands disease
Huntington's Chorea	Polyposis coli (Peutz syndrome)	Waardenburg's syndrome
Hyperlipidaemia Type II	Porphyria	

In this type of inheritance, males and females are affected and each offspring of an affected parent has a 50% or 1 in 2 chance of inheriting the abnormal gene and hence manifesting the disease. This risk remains the same for each successive pregnancy, irrespective of the outcome of the preceding one. As in other forms of disease, irrespective of their cause, the severity of the condition may vary considerably from one individual to another. In clinical genetics this variation is referred to as expressivity and some of those affected may have only minor physical manifestations, but by passing on the responsible gene, may produce a child with a more serious form of the disease. A good example is Waardenburg's syndrome which may be manifest by a blond forelock, heterochromia irides and lateral displacement of the inner canthi of the eyes, or may in addition be associated with profound congenital deafness. The importance of recognising this varying clinical expression cannot be over-stressed.

In some families, disease normally dominantly inherited may affect the off-

Waardenburg's syndrome — a dominant disorder

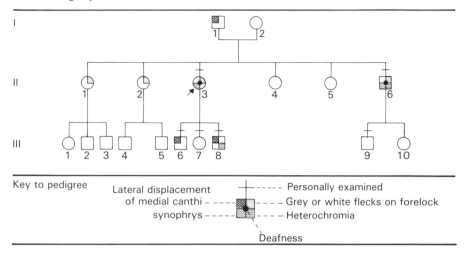

Key to pedigree

Lateral displacement
of medial canthi ----- ----- Personally examined
---- Grey or white flecks on forelock
synophrys ----- ---- Heterochromia

Deafness

Note:
— Each child, either sex, born to I1 has 50/50 or $\frac{1}{2}$ risk of inheriting the gene.
— Variation in clinical severity of affected offspring II1, II2, II3, II6.
— Individuals II1, II2, II3, II6 have 50/50 risk of affected offspring.
— II4 and II5 have no evidence of disease and cannot pass the abnormal gene to offspring.
— Deafness occurs in 1:6 (approx.) of those who inherit the gene; therefore, probability A of inheriting the gene is $\frac{1}{2}$; probability A (a) of inheriting the gene and being deaf is $\frac{1}{2} \times 1/6$; probability B of not inheriting the gene is $\frac{1}{2}$; probability B (b) of not inheriting the gene and having normal hearing is $\frac{1}{2} \times 1$. Therefore, the probability of being deaf and inheriting the gene is $\dfrac{\frac{1}{2}}{1/12 + 6/12} = 1/7.$

spring of parents who appear completely normal. In such situations the abnormal gene is absent in the somatic or body cells of the parents and hence does not produce disease. However, the mutated gene responsible for the condition is present in their gametes, either the ovum or sperm, and in this way can be passed to the offspring as a permanent change. The end result is the same as if one of the parents had the disease, and the affected child will have the same risk of passing on the abnormal gene as any other affected person. Achondroplasia is a good example of the inheritance of a new mutation; as many as 80% of all achondroplastics have normal parents. New mutations are more likely to be responsible for a dominantly inherited genetic disease if the condition is known to interfere with reproduction hence reducing genetic fitness or if there is advanced paternal age.

Finally, it does occasionally happen that a genetic disorder present in one generation fails to appear in the next but reappears in subsequent generations. In these circumstances the gene is said to lack penetrance; it has failed to produce any demonstrable evidence of the disease. This is not a common occurrence and may well only highlight our inability to detect minor clinical effects of the abnormal gene. Although the concept of single gene inheritance is a useful one and of practical value, gene action can obviously be modified by many factors, particularly the environment. Genes do not work in isolation.

Summary of characteristics of autosomal dominant inheritance

— Normally an affected person has an affected parent, with the exception of the new mutation.
— Affected persons have, on average, affected and normal offspring in equal proportion.
— Both sexes are affected and there may be considerable variation in the clinical severity of the disease.

Autosomal recessive inheritance. More than 500 disorders result from this type of inheritance and they occur in approximately 2.5 per 1000 live births. Recessively inherited disorders commonly result in a demonstrable biochemical disturbance, for example phenylketonuria and galactosaemia. However, in some conditions, including cystic fibrosis and a number of syndromes, for example Laurence-Moon-Biedl or Ellis-Van Creveld, the basic abnormality has not yet been identified.

Some recessively inherited conditions

Adrenogenital syndrome	Glycogen storage disease	Retinitis pigmentosa
Agammaglobulinaemia	Homocystinuria	Robert's syndrome
(some types)	Ichthyosis (collodion fetus)	Russell-Silver dwarfism
Albinism (complete form)	Krabbe leucodystrophy	Sickle cell disease
Ataxia — telangiectasia	Laurence-Moon-Biedl	Smith-Lemli-Opitz
Bloom syndrome	syndrome	syndrome
Cystic fibrosis	Letterer-Siwe disease	Spastic paraplegia
Dandy-Walker syndrome	Maple syrup urine disease	Tay-Sachs disease
Deafness (some types)	Microcephaly (some types)	Thalassaemia
Ellis-van Creveld syndrome	Microphthalmos	Thanatophoric dwarfism
Epidermolysis bullosa	Mucopolysaccharidoses	Werdnig-Hoffman disease
dystrophica	(some types)	
Galactosaemia	Pituitary dwarfism	

As in dominantly inherited disease the action of the responsible gene is not an all-or-none phenomenon, and the heterozygote carrier, although physically normal, may well manifest some biochemical evidence of the condition, for example thalassaemia and sickle cell anaemia. As they are very common conditions they provide an opportunity for population screening and disease prevention. In sickle cell disease it is possible to demonstrate an alteration in the haemoglobin molecule resulting from gene mutation. Sickle haemoglobin has a different amino acid composition from normal haemoglobin. The difference is the result of an alteration in only one of the 146 amino acids making up the haemoglobin molecule. In sickle haemoglobin, valine is substituted for glutamic acid in the beta-chain, a change from the RNA triplet GAA to GUA. Individuals carrying the trait and who are heterozygous have both normal and sickle cell genes. Those who are homozygous suffer from the disease and have the sickle gene at both loci. This was one of the earliest demonstrations of the association between mutation in a gene locus and an alteration in chemical structure. In the thalassaemias there is defective synthesis of one or more of the globin chains and therefore a decrease in the production of adult haemoglobin. The resultant clinical syndrome depends on which of the polypeptide chains is abnormal but all are recessively inherited. Beta-thalassaemia major occurs world-wide and is one of the most common genetic disorders. Alpha-thalassaemia results from gene deletion and this has implications

Relationships

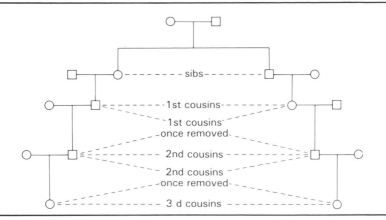

for prenatal diagnosis by techniques such as gene probing.

Each individual carries a few abnormal genes and the possibility of marrying someone carrying the same abnormal genes is considerably increased by marrying a relative, particularly a first cousin. This is because first cousins share an eighth of their total genetic complement, their genome, with each other. With more distant relationships fewer genes are shared. In general there is not a high rate

Galactosaemia (incidence 1:40 000) — a recessive disorder

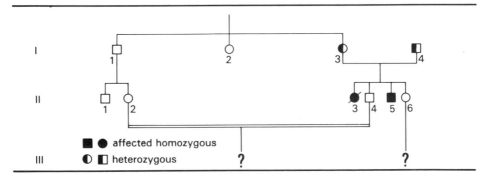

Note:
— Any child born to I_3 or I_4 has $\frac{1}{4}$ chance of being affected.
— Non-affected childen born to I_3 and I_4 have $\frac{2}{3}$ chance of inheriting the gene, i.e. of being heterozygous.
— All offspring of affected homozygotes will inherit the responsible gene.
— The risk of diseases in children born to affected honozygotes depends on the genotype of the spouse.
— If marriage is non-consanguinous then the risk of the spouse carrying the same gene depends on the frequency of that gene in the population and the carrier frequency is approximately twice the square root of the disease incidence, i.e. $2 \times 1/40\ 000 = 1/100$.
— Therefore, the risk of an affected child being born to unaffected female II_6 is $1/100 \times \frac{1}{4} \times \frac{2}{3} = 1/600$.
— If II_4, also with a $\frac{2}{3}$ risk of carrying the gene, marries a first cousin then the risk of an affected child depends on the risk of II_2 carrying the gene. Since the risk of I_1 being heterozygous is approximately $\frac{1}{2}$ (ignoring a new mutation) then the chance of II_2 having the gene is $\frac{1}{4}$. Therefore, the overall risk to the child is $\frac{1}{4} \times \frac{2}{3} \times \frac{1}{4} = 2/48 = 1/24$.

of first cousin marriages in either Great Britain or Europe but among some of our immigrant population consanguinity is common and first cousin marriages are encouraged. Incestuous relationships, although uncommon, do occur more frequently than realised and result in an increased incidence of both physical abnormalities and mental retardation in the offspring. Establishing the degree of relationship helps in assessing the coefficient of inbreeding or the risk of a harmful gene being homozygous in children of related parents.

Summary of characteristics of recessive inheritance
— the disease characteristically appears only in siblings. The parents and other relatives are usually normal.
— the risk of an affected person is 1 in 4 or 25%.
— consanguinity is more likely in rare recessive disorders. In the more common conditions parents are usually unrelated.
— both sexes are affected.

Sex-linked disease. Disease resulting from the action of a gene on the sex chromosomes is said to be sex-linked and the majority are recessively inherited. X-linked diseases are not as numerous as those due to other modes of inheritance, but the 100 or more conditions so far described contain some serious handicapping conditions. They occur with a frequency of approximately 0.5–1.5 per 1000 births.

Some sex-linked disorders

Agammaglobulinaemia (Burton and Swiss types)	Gonadal dysgenesis (female type)	Microphthalmia Mucopolysaccharidosis
Albinism, ocular	Haemophilia A	(Hunter Type II)
Aldrich syndrome	Haemophilia B (Christmas	Muscular dystrophy —
Diabetes insipidus	Disease)	Duchenne
Ectodermal dysplasia	Hydrocephalus (Aqueductal	Muscular dystrophy —
Ehlers-Danlos syndrome (Type V)	stenosis)	Becker
Fabrys disease	Hypophosphataemic rickets	Spastic paraplegia
Glucose-6-phosphate	Ichthyosis	syndrome
dehydrogenase deficiency (variants)	Incontinentia pigmenti	Retinitis pigmentosa
Glycogen storage disease (Type VIII)	Menkes syndrome	Testicular feminisation Wildervancks syndrome

In X-linked disease the abnormal gene is on one of the X chromosomes and the male with the abnormal gene manifests the disease. The female with the normal allele on her other X chromosome is a carrier. Any male born to a carrier has a 50/50 chance of inheriting the gene and manifesting the disease; any daughter has a 50/50 chance of being a carrier. Because it is the X chromosome which carries the abnormal gene, an affected male can never transfer the disease to his sons but all his daughters will be carriers.

Duchenne muscular dystrophy is one of the most common genetic disorders in childhood (approximately 1 in 2500–3000 male births) and the gene is fully penetrant, that is affected males have severe disease. Their reproductive fitness is zero and there is, therefore, complete selection against the gene. It is important to establish the carrier status of any female in a family in which this disease is

Duchenne muscular dystrophy

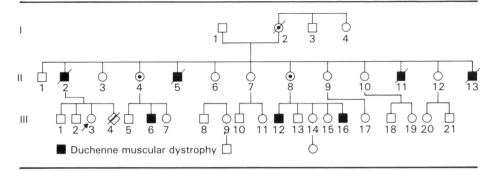

I_2, II_4 and II_8 are obligatory carriers. The risk of III_3 being a carrier depends on the risk of II_3 being a carrier. On pedigree information this can be assessed from the figure. However, in this condition creatinine kinase estimations may be helpful and should be combined with pedigree information to calculate the final risk. The variation in creatinine kinase values in the normal population makes calculations more difficult than in situations without biochemical abnormality.

appearing. This may be apparent from the pedigree and if the mother has an affected brother and subsequently gives birth to an affected child then she is an obligatory carrier. However, where there is a single affected male child only, and no other family history, then this disease could have arisen as a result of a mutation in his mother's gametes, that is on one of her X chromosomes. This is thought to be the situation in about a third of all cases and this, plus the difficulties associated with accurate carrier prediction, produces problems in genetic counselling.

Summary of characteristics of X-linked recessive inheritance
— the trait is normally passed from a carrier female to her male offspring.
— sons have a 50/50 chance of inheriting the gene and therefore of developing the disease; daughters a 50/50 chance of being carriers like mother.
— an affected male cannot pass the disease to his sons but all his daughters will be carriers. (This only applies to X-linked disease where an affected male survives into adulthood and is capable of reproduction.)
— daughters of affected males can pass the disease to their sons.
— in some X-linked disease females may show some clinical evidence of the condition.

This latter point is explained by the inactivation of the X chromosome soon after the formation of the zygote. This hypothesis was proposed by Dr Mary Lyon and explains the wide clinical variability in the 'carrier' female.

X linked dominant disease. Conditions inherited in X-linked dominant fashion are rare. Hypophosphataemic vitamin D resistant rickets and incontinentia pigmenti are seen on occasions and may be a cause of childhood handicap. The transmission of both these abnormalities is similar to that of autosomal dominant conditions from an affected female. If the dominant gene located on an X chromosome is responsible for serious disease, the female with two X chromosomes and hence a normal allele may manifest the condition. The male, without the normal allele of the offending gene, may have a much more serious form of the disease. This may result in fetal or early neonatal death of affected males so that this type of genetic disease is more common in females. The other criteria for this form of inheritance are that each child, irrespective of sex, born to an affected female has a half risk of having the disease, and affected males who survive transmit the trait to all their daughters but to none of their sons.

Summary of characteristics of X-linked dominant disease
— disease is commoner in females and is usually more severe or lethal in males.
— both sons and daughters have a 50/50 chance of inheriting the gene from an affected female and, therefore, of developing the disease.
— an affected male will transmit the disease to all his daughters but to none of his sons.

Chromosomal abnormalities
Overall the incidence of chromosomal abnormalities at birth is approximately 0.5%, but when maternal age and the results of amniocentesis are considered then the incidence at conception may as high as 5% at age 45 years. Disorders of the sex chromosomes and balanced structural anomalies are responsible for more than 50% of the total. Moreover these figures represent only a fraction of the overall burden of chromosomal abnormalities, the majority of which result in early fetal death. Fifty per cent of all spontaneous abortions and 5% of stillbirths are associated with chromosomal disorders. The first and still one of the most common clinical syndromes associated with a demonstrable chromosomal anomaly is Down's syndrome, in which there is normally an extra chromosome of the G group, i.e. trisomy 21. For reasons which are not understood, having an additional chromosome has serious effects on development. The phenotypic abnormalities noted in Down's syndrome are associated with trisomy of the long arm of the chromosome and more particularly with the distal part of the long arm. This contains the locus for the enzyme superoxide dismutase and this suggested the possibility that an increase in this enzyme, a dosage effect of the trisomy, might be responsible for the various abnormalities. However, the similarity of the physical abnormalities with those in other trisomies makes this unlikely. It is more probable that many of the features of the trisomies are a consequence of disruption of normal genetic and hence metabolic balance. Theoretically, it is possible to have trisomy of any of the autosomes but number 21 appears to be particularly vulnerable and there is no satisfactory explanation for this phenomenon. There is no single feature which can be said to be characteristic of a specific chromosomal abnormality and many of them have abnormal physical features in common, e.g. trisomy 21, 18 and 13. Nevertheless, specific clusters of physical abnormalities may combine to produce a characteristic clinical picture such as is seen in Down's syndrome and some of the other classical chromosomal syndromes. Following the demonstration of trisomy 21 in children with Down's syndrome, there have been many other clinical syndromes identified with trisomy of other groups. As with other genetic disease there may be a variation in the clinical severity of these conditions. However, mental retardation is common to most of

Approximate incidence of chromosomal disorders in the newborn

Trisomy 21	1 in 650
Trisomy 18	1 in 3500
Trisomy 13	1 in 7000
Partial deletion short arm 5	1 in 50 000
XXY (Klinefelter's syndrome)	1 in 500 males
XO (Turner's syndrome)	1 in 2500 females
XYY	1 in 650 males
XXX	1 in 2000 females

them and in some can be shown to be due to impaired brain cell growth. There is an increasing number of chromosomal syndromes described; details of the clinical and karyotypic features associated with these are available in standard textbooks of clinical genetics or cytogenetics.

Alterations of chromosome number (Aneuploidy). Down's syndrome has an incidence of 1 in 750 births but the incidence at conception is higher and some fetuses with this abnormality must, therefore, be rejected early in pregnancy (Oakley, 1978). This natural selective termination is of considerable interest but the mechanism underlying it is unknown. The incidence of the syndrome increases with maternal age and an increasing risk of chromosomal non-disjunction. However, the factors responsible for maternal or paternal non-disjunction are unknown although a teratogenic effect on aging maternal ova has been suggested. Occasionally a woman who has had a baby with one type of trisomy, e.g. trisomy 21, may subsequently have an infant with a different trisomy, e.g. trisomy 18, suggesting faulty genetic control of disjunction as seen in some animals. Despite the clear association with maternal age, the majority of babies with Down's syndrome are born to mothers of normal reproductive age and approximately 92% of all children with this syndrome have trisomy 21. In the remainder, some other chromosomal anomalies may be present but the end result, i.e. additional chromosomal material, is the same and the babies have the usual features of Down's syndrome.

Trisomies of portions of chromosomes, either the short or long arm, also occur and may produce recognisable clinical syndromes (Yunis, 1977). Trisomy of the short arm of chromosome number 9 although very uncommon, produces the usual combination of mental retardation and various physical anomalies. As with the full trisomic syndromes it is theoretically possible to have partial trisomy of any of the autosomes, either of the short arm or of the long arm.

Abnormalities of sex chromosomes. As a result of more frequent cytological examination of abortuses and aborted material, the XO constitution has been shown to be a common finding. However, there is a substantial loss of fetuses with this anomaly so that at birth the incidence is 1 in 2000 (approx.). The diagnosis can be confirmed by chromosomal analysis but it may also be suspected by examination of the buccal mucosal cells for the presence of a Barr body. In Turner's syndrome with only one X chromosome the patients are chromatin negative like the male. In trisomy X, as would be expected with an extra X chromosome, there are two Barr bodies to be seen in the buccal cells. The XO and other abnormalities of the sex chromosomes, e.g. Klinefelter's syndrome XXY or triple X female, result from chromosomal non-disjunction. However, some children with all the features of Turner's syndrome may be found to have two X chromosomes instead of just one. One of the X chromosomes is larger than its fellow and this occurs as a result of abnormal division of the chromosome during cell division. The X chromosome divides transversely instead of longitudinally at the centromere. This results in a long and short chromosome instead of two identical halves. The short arm is lost and the long arm, called an isochromosome, survives. There has been sufficient genetic material lost in this process to produce the features of Turner's syndrome.

In Klinefelter's syndrome there are at least two X chromosomes in addition to the Y. This is a common sex chromosome abnormality with a frequency of about 1–2 per 1000 live born males. Some males with this condition go unrecognized, other are picked up at infertility clinics or because of gynaecomastia.

Structural changes in chromosomes. Common types of structural changes are deletions in which there is loss of part of a chromosome and, therefore, loss of some genetic information. The missing portion may be at the end of a chromosome or breaks occur at both ends of the chromosome, and the broken ends then unite to form a ring structure. Such a ring chromosome is generally unstable and during meiosis may not be transmitted intact, resulting in congenital abnormalities. A more common situation is when chromosome breakage occurs and the broken fragment of one chromosome attaches itself to another chromosome. This is referred to as a translocation and it may or may not produce clinical abnormalities. Provided there has been no significant loss of genetic material then the rearrangement of chromosomes in this way may not have any ill effects. However, such translocations may interfere with normal meiosis and the formation of gametes, so that the resultant new individual may have either too much chromosomal material or too little. In either case clinical abnormalities, including mental retardation, may result. Such a structural rearrangement is important in some cases of Down's syndrome and the karyotype in the figure is of a child with a translocation. The karyotype of the carrier mother is also shown.

It is important when a translocation is found in a family that all siblings and the relatives of the carrier parent are examined. By this means it may be possible to detect those with a balanced translocation and therefore at risk of having an abnormal child. They should be offered genetic counselling and amniocentesis during pregnancy. Translocations involving the chromosome number 21 and chromosomes in group 13–15 seem to be more common than translocations of the G group with other autosomes. Balanced translocations of other chromosomes are found in about 10% of women who have frequent miscarriages and in a number of men and women who are infertile. Unbalanced translocations, irrespective of the particular chromosomes, are frequently associated with severe physical and mental abnormalities. It is also recognised that in 50% of pregnancies which terminate in the first trimester, there is a demonstrable chromosomal anomaly in the fetus.

Deletions. Loss of a portion of the short arm of chromosome number 5 and number 4 results in recognised but rare clinical syndromes characterised by mental retardation and physical anomalies.

Translocation; on the top the affected individual, on the bottom the parent

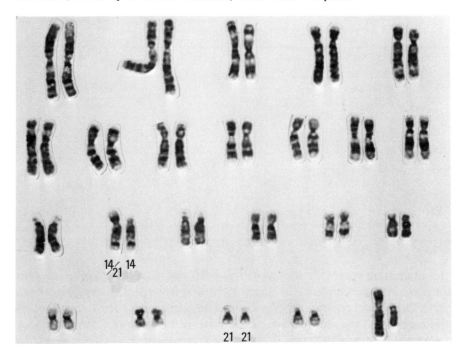

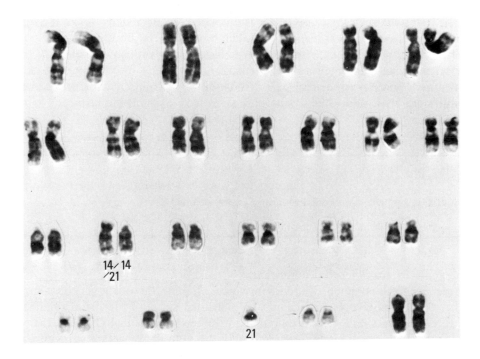

In X-linked recessive mental retardation some 'carrier' daughters are also retarded. Obligatory carrier II1 does not show fragile X. This makes calculations of the risk to normal females difficult. III2 has normal chromosomes and a normal daughter and son. It is unlikely that she is a carrier but she is aged 45 but absolute assurance cannot be given.

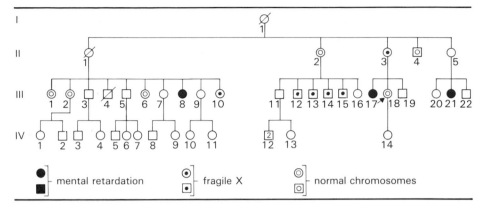

An interesting recent development has been the demonstration of an abnormality of the X chromosome in males and some females with intellectual retardation (Tariverdian & Weck, 1982). The abnormality is localised to the distal part of the long arm of the chromosome and is referred to as a fragile site. It produces the appearance of a constriction in the chromosomes and can be most easily demonstrated if the cells being examined have been cultured in a medium deficient in folic acid. Many males with this abnormality have an associated enlargement of the testes although the cause of this is unknown. Prenatal diagnosis of the fragile X chromosome is possible either in fetal blood or fetal fibroblasts.

It is important to examine the karyotype of any baby with an unexplained cluster of congenital abnormalities and particularly any infant who has an odd facial appearance and developmental delay. Individuals or children with such abnormalities are often said to be dysmorphic or to have dysmorphic features.

Indications for chromosomal analysis

Suspected chromosomal anomaly, e.g. in familial translocation
Unexplained mental retardation
Mental retardation/multiple congenital abnormalities
Ambiguous genitalia/hypo-gonadism/primary amenorrhoea
Recurrent miscarriage, infertility
Unexplained stillbirths and neonatal deaths

Polygenic or multifactorial inheritance

There are many common disorders in which although there is a genetic component, the inheritance pattern cannot be explained simply in terms of dominant or recessive traits and there are no demonstrable chromosomal changes. Instead it appears that the heritable component is the cumulative action of a number of genes and it is this factor, a multiple gene or polygenic effect, which is responsible for the familial tendency or predisposition to these abnormalities. Individuals possessing such a genetic make-up and subject to the appropriate environmental stimulus or teratogen will develop evidence of the disease. Since this results from a combination of genetic and environmental factors it is referred to as multifactorial. In these conditions the severity of the disease may show considerable variation but exactly how the two major components interact is far from clear. Although this concept of multifactorial disease is a useful one, further advances in knowledge of gene action may provide an alternative explanation. It has been estimated that multifactorial diseases have a prevalence of approximately 22–24 per 1000 births.

Neural tube defects are amongst the most common of the serious congenital abnormalities and many features of this disorder can be explained on a multifactorial basis, with evidence of combined genetic and environmental factors. For example, in Belfast the incidence is 7 in 1000, in South Wales even higher, whereas in East Anglia and South East England it is only about 2 in 1000. This increased tendency of those of Celtic stock to have affected children suggests a genetic contribution. It is also well recognised that neural tube abnormalities have a definite seasonal incidence, being commoner in winter months. Lower social classes are more often affected and the disease is more likely to affect the first and fourth children in a family. These various elements may be related to one or more environmental factor. Recently it has been reported that the incidence of neural tube defects is reduced in mothers at risk if they take additional vitamins for the month before, and during the first 2 months, of pregnancy (Smithells et al, 1983). This needs further investigation and if confirmed the particular vitamin needs to be identified. Although some mothers of infants with neural tube defects have dietary histories suggesting an inadequate intake of some essential vitamins, many do not and clinical evidence of malnutrition is not common. Folic acid is the most likely suspect but the role of this substance in the development of the neural tube has not been established, and why some mothers fail to use this substance appropriately or have a deficiency is not known.

Multifactorial disorders. Risks are approximate and the reader is advised to check individual conditions. After two affected children the risk of a third affected child becomes high, 1:10 or greater. The risk of recurrence in some conditions with a marked difference in sex incidence varies with sex of the index patient; where this is the least common sex then the recurrence risk is higher. The risk to an affected parent having an affected child is approximately the same as the risk to normal parents after one affected child

	Incidence	Sex ratio	Normal parents risk of 2nd affected child
Neural tube defects (anencephaly; spina bifida; some cases hydrocephalus)	1:200	1:2	1:25
Cleft lip/palate	1:650	3:2	1:25
Talipes equinovarus	1:1000	2:1	1:30
Hirschsprung's disease	1:5000	4:1	1:50 (male index) 1:12 (female index)
Pyloric stenosis	1:350	5:1	1:50 (male index) 1:10 (female index)
Diabetes (some types)	1:500		1:30
Congenital heart disease (some types)	1:200		1:25 VSD 1:30 PDA 1:50 Transposition
Schizophrenia	1:100	1:7	

It is important to remember that many conditions listed in this group may occur as part of a syndrome with an entirely different mode of inheritance. For example, if congenital heart disease occurs without associated abnormalities, then it may be of multifactorial origin. However, it may be found in about 25% of children with Down's syndrome and is often present in other chromosomal abnormalities such as Turner's syndrome. On occasions it may also be associated with dominantly inherited disease, e.g. Marfan's or Noonan's syndrome, or with recessive conditions such as the Ellis-Van-Creveld syndrome. Any of the conditions listed in the multifactorial group which are part of a syndrome with a single gene pattern of inheritance, has a recurrence risk appropriate to that of the syndrome. Meckel's syndrome is a good example of this principle. In this condition the patient has an encephalocele associated with abnormalities of the kidneys and polydactyly. Encephalocele may occur as part of the spectrum of the neural tube anomalies and the recurrence risk is low. However, as part of Meckel's syndrome it has a high recurrence risk as this syndrome is recessively inherited.

GENETIC COUNSELLING

Genetic counselling is a relatively new type of medical service offered to individuals and families suffering from, or at risk of, hereditary disease (Emery & Rimoin, 1983). A comprehensive service should provide an opportunity for the prevention and in some cases treatment of many serious genetic disorders and in most situations should be seen as an extension of good clinical practice. The counsellor's main task is to establish or confirm the diagnosis, assess the genetic implications of this and advise about the risk of the disorder to offspring or siblings. In addition, it is important to discuss ways in which the disease may be prevented or its effects, social as well as medical, minimised. The diagnostic process is similar to that in other medical conditions and the counsellor needs wide clinical experience and the support of various clinical and laboratory services, including cytogenetics and biochemistry. Appropriate genetic counselling is dependent on the accuracy of the clinical and genetic diagnosis, and if this is incorrect much of what is subsequently said may be misleading or even harmful.

Functions of a comprehensive clinical genetic service

Genetic counselling
Clinical diagnosis
Laboratory diagnosis
Prenatal diagnosis
Genetic screening
Research and education
Support and treatment

Referrals

Patients are normally referred from family doctors and hospital consultants as well as community paediatricians and physicians. Genetic counselling is also more frequently requested for special groups, such as the handicapped school leaver, including young people with severe visual or hearing impairment.

Referrals to Nottingham clinical genetic service 1973–1981

Single Gene	
Dominant	250
Recessive	172
X-linked	132
	554

Multifactorial	
Neural tube defects	240
Congenital heart disease	76
Cleft lip/palate	62
Other	70
	448

Chromosomal	
Autosomal — Down's	160
— Other	95
Sex chromosome	60
	215

Miscellaneous	
Mental retardation-/multiple congenital abnormalities	150
Mental retardation	30
Limb abnormalities	50
Intestinal	40
Stillbirths/Miscarriages	40
Other (consanguinity, suspected chromosomal, etc)	30
	340

Total	1557

The timing of some referrals is important. In families in which there has been the birth of a child with severe congenital abnormalities, the parents have a predictable emotional reaction with varying degrees of depression, self-recrimination, anger and even rejection of the infant. The duration of this reaction varies considerably and some aspects of it may persist for months or even years. In general, it is at least 3 months before the parents are sufficiently emotionally stable to accept, understand and benefit from the information given, and the timing of referrals should take account of this likely emotional response. Most parents appear to benefit from more than one interview, particularly for serious conditions associated with a high recurrence risk and re-attendance affords the opportunity for further discussion and assessment. In many cases home visiting by a genetic nurse may be very helpful and informal discussion 'over a cup of tea' may be more beneficial than formal attendance at the counselling clinic.

A family tree showing consanguinity and the rare recessively inherited condition — neuraxonal dystrophy

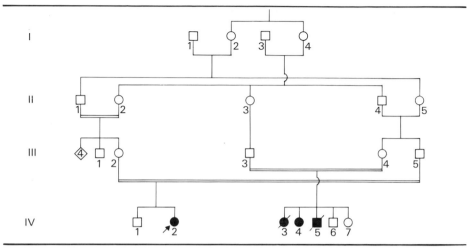

Diagnosis

In every case it is essential to have a firm diagnosis and this, in addition to standard examination and investigations, will also require adequate pedigree information. Community medical and nursing staff should be familiar with the standard symbols. A three generation pedigree provides a clear and easily constructed record of relevant information. In some instances, where the diagnosis may be in doubt, clear demonstration of the hereditary nature of the disease may be helpful. In this respect it is important to remember that some disease may be transmitted in varying ways. This phenomenon is referred to as genetic heterogeneity and implies that the end result of gene action may have similar clinical manifestations irrespective of the position of the gene locus, whether on the autosome or X chromosomes. A good example is hereditary deafness which may be inherited in dominant, recessive or X-linked fashion, with recessive disease being the most common. In some cases, despite detailed clinical, cytogenetic and biochemical investigations a firm diagnosis cannot be made. This often applies to infants and children with unexplained mental retardation and associated dysmorphic features. Such children are commonly referred to clinical genetic services and there has been a marked increase in the literature on syndrome recognition over the years (Smith, 1982). Since many of them are recessively inherited, their identification has important consequences for further offspring.

Risk and burden

When the diagnosis has been made and the mode of inheritance established, the recurrence or occurrence risk can be estimated. The risk of a serious congenital abnormality in any pregnancy is approximately 1 in 40 (equivalent to an incidence of serious defects of 25 per 1000) and it is against this background that other risks are assessed. In general risks greater than 1 in 10 are considered by most people to be high, the situation in most unifactorial single gene disorders; those between 1 in 10 and 1 in 20 as moderate, usually applied to multifactorial conditions; and risks less than 1 in 20 are low. Accurate risk estimation is important and in many cases this may be simple, particularly in autosomal dominant and recessive disease. However, in late or variable onset dominant inheritance, or where the gene shows lack of penetrance, these calculations become more difficult.

In known recessively inherited diseases, where the diagnosis is clear and the family pedigree information adequate, recurrence risks for other siblings are usually straightforward. However, parents may be concerned about the likelihood of the normal siblings having an affected child. This is usually low but can be more accurately estimated using the Hardy–Weinberg formula, and when the incidence of the disease is known, this formula can be used to estimate the gene frequency and hence the carrier frequency. In most recessive disorders this can be approximated to twice the square root of the disease frequency. Further details of the use of this principle are available in standard genetic texts. In families in which there is only one child with an uncommon syndrome, one cannot always be sure of the mode of inheritance. In such situations an accurate risk cannot be quoted but the various possibilities need to be considered. The condition may be the result of non-genetic factors, such as exposure to teratogens during pregnancy, and a careful obstetric history is, therefore, very important. The fetal alcohol syndrome consisting of varying degrees of mental retardation and facial dysmorphism can only be confirmed if mother's alcohol intake is established. Another possibility is that the condition may be recessively inherited and this is more likely if the parents are consanguineous or there have been reports of similar abnormalities in more than one child in other families. Finally the condition may be due to a combination of genetic and environmental factors, i.e. multifactorial or a new dominant mutation.

In sex-linked disease, risks of the carrier state in the female siblings of an affected male may be estimated using either pedigree details alone or combined with biochemical or other information. This is particularly applicable to diseases such as Duchenne muscular dystrophy in which the level of serum creatinine kinase may be of help in calculating carrier risk. In most recessive X-linked diseases, new mutations may occur and this may complicate the calculations. It is important to have an understanding of the basic facts of probability in estimating risks in most genetic problems and Bayes theorem is particularly applicable in the X-linked recessive disorders.

In chromosomal abnormalities the most likely problem is that of a young woman who has had a child with Down's syndrome due to regular trisomy 21. Her risk of another affected infant is increased over that of the normal population but this increase is slight and, provided mother is under the age of 35, her chances are probably not greater than 1%. However, the risk rises fairly dramatically with maternal age and at the age of 45 may be as high as 1 in 40 for a first affected child. Other trisomies recur rarely and recurrence risks are probably even lower than for Down's syndrome.

The chromosomal translocations provide a different problem. If the translocation has arisen de novo, that is, it is not present in either parent, then the recurrence risk is low, less than the recurrence risk of Down's syndrome due to trisomy 21. However, where one parent has a balanced form of translocation, the risk of an unbalanced form of the translocation may be quite high; 1 in 10 where mother carries the translocation and probably about 1 in 15 if father carries the abnormality. These risks are obviously contrary to what one would expect on a theoretical basis but there are various possible reasons for this. There may be abnormal zygotes which are lost early in pregnancy or, in the cases of the male, the abnormal sperm may not be as effective at fertilisation. Most chromosomal abnormalities have a low recurrence risk but each individual problem needs to be thoroughly investigated and discussed with someone experienced in this field.

In addition to risk, an assessment of the burden of the disease is an important step in helping the parents to make a decision about the future. Obviously genetic diseases producing only minimal or treatable consequences, even though having a high recurrence risk, may be viewed in a different light from conditions such as mental retardation which may have a lower recurrence risk but are very burdensome. It is also important to remember that many parents see burden and risk differently at different times. The parents' emotional state is an important factor in how they assess these various aspects.

Options

When the diagnosis has been established, the inheritance pattern identified and factors such as risk and burden assessed, the next step is to discuss the various options available to the individual or couple concerned. There are some disorders of multifactorial origin, such as congenital heart disease and neural tube defects, which are amenable to surgery, and some biochemical disorders, such as phenylketonuria which may respond to early elimination of phenylalanine from the diet. However, there are still only a limited number of genetic disorders which can be treated although this situation may well alter in the future. Where there is no effective treatment then, at present, the only way to prevent the occurrence or recurrence of the problem in further children is for the couple to alter their reproductive lives.

In some cases the recurrence risk or burden of the condition may be so low that the individuals may feel reassured and may decide not to limit their family. Where the risk is higher and the disease serious, such as in the single gene disorders, then reproductive restriction may be an optional course of action. This means that a genetic counselling service must have close links with family planning clinics or ensure that the family doctor advises the couple about reliable family planning techniques. Reproductive alternatives to normal childbearing include techniques such as artificial insemination by donor (AID), which is applicable in situations where father suffers from, or is at risk of, a serious dominantly inherited genetic disorder. A good example is tuberose sclerosis. If the mother is fertilised by donor sperm then she has only the normal population risk of having a child with this disease. However, a child to her affected husband has a 50/50 or 1/2 chance of inheriting the gene and manifesting the disease. It is important to remember if the gene responsible for a disease is common in the population that AID may still be hazardous, for example cystic fibrosis. When a couple are identified as heterozygotes following the birth of a child with this condition, AID still carries some risk. In our community the gene for cystic fibrosis is carried by 1 in 25 or so of the population. The donor sperm, therefore, may carry this gene and the chances of another affected child would be 1 in 100. In rare recessive

Genetic counselling

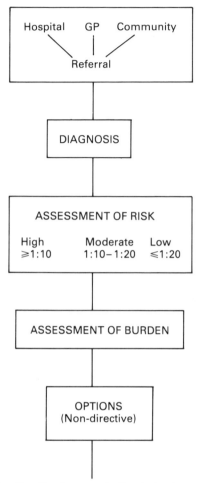

1. No alteration in reproductive behaviour
2. Restricted family size — family planning
3. Alternatives — AID, adoption (remarriage)
4. Prenatal diagnosis and selective reproduction

diseases AID would be justified and is increasingly used in families where there is male infertility for whatever cause.

Adoption, although an option to be considered, is difficult as there are now too few normal babies available for all the couples who would wish to adopt. Remarriage is normally not discussed, or only very rarely when introduced by the individuals concerned. It is, however, important to note that marriages frequently break down in our community and that a change of spouse may alter the risk of a further affected infant dramatically.

Prenatal diagnosis has become increasingly available for a variety of conditions. Although primary prevention is always to be preferred, this technique is increasingly requested by couples at high risk of a serious disorder. In many it provides welcome reassurance that the condition in question is not present and in others with an affected fetus the opportunity of termination of pregnancy.

In all types of counselling, whether for genetic disorders or other problems, it is important that the individuals understand the information given and this may present difficulties and will certainly demand time. It is unrealistic to expect some people to grasp even simple concepts of probability and in some cases even simple biological facts. However, since the information given may have very serious consequences it is important that attempts are made to try and ensure some basic understanding of the situation. The aim, although not always realised, is to ensure that all individuals are in a position to make informed and balanced judgements about their future.

Individuals or families with a genetic problem need the opportunity to identify their difficulties and to discuss ways in which these can be most effectively managed. Initially this very often involves some measure of self-examination and a clearer understanding of their emotional response. At this stage the counsellor's role is usually a very passive one, encouraging discussion and showing a willingness to listen. In genetic disease the need for a firm diagnosis has been emphasised but counselling in other situations also requires a clear identification of the problem. In any serious handicapping condition, for example congenital blindness or deafness, it is clearly important to establish the aetiology. This provides the factual base for the remainder of the counselling session. However, the parents' emotional response to the child's problem, complicated by feelings of guilt, anger or loss of self-esteem, will be important factors in their acceptance and understanding of the information offered. Such reactions may significantly interfere with their ability to cope with the problem and they may need time to come to terms with their feelings. At some stage the counsellor will need to ensure that the parents are made aware of those agencies which can offer help and there are now a number of societies willing to offer support to families with specific genetic

Prenatal diagnosis. Amniocentesis is usually at 16 weeks, chorionic biopsy earlier. Risk of spontaneous abortion following amniocentesis, 1:75–100; fetoscopy approximately 1:30; chorionic biopsy unknown: probably low

Indications	Investigation and material to be examined	Technique
Neural tube abnormalities	Alpha-fetoprotein Acetylcholinesterase	Amniocentesis (fluid)
Chromosomal disorders	Fetal karyotype:	Amniocentesis (cells)
Biochemical disorders	Enzyme deficiency:	Amniocentesis (cells)
Sex-linked disorders	Fetal karyotype:	Chorionic biopsy (cells)
Blood disorders		
Thalassaemia		Fetoscopy and fetal blood
Sickle cell disease	Fetal blood	sampling
Gene identification	Fetal DNA:	Chorionic biopsy (cells)
Skin disorder	Fetal skin	Fetoscopy and skin biopsy
Biochemical disorder	Fetal liver	Fetoscopy and liver biopsy
Bone and limb anomaly		Ultrasonography and/or fetoscopy
Kidney disease		Ultrasonography
Syndrome identification, e.g. those associated with facial clefting		Fetoscopy

problems. Most of these, e.g. those involved with cystic fibrosis, haemophilia or muscular dystrophy, provide a forum for parents to discuss problems with others who have had similar experiences. They also provide easily understood but comprehensive written information about the disease. Parents will also want to be reassured that their child is obtaining optimum treatment and help so that the medical as well as the social and familial consequences of the condition are minimised. Referral to the appropriate specialist is essential and in every case, communication with other professionals involved is essential to avoid families being offered well-meaning but conflicting information.

In certain situations, for example prenatal diagnosis and termination of pregnancy, families may be faced with decisions of a moral or religious nature and these may be very difficult (Hilton et al, 1975). The counsellor's role is to ensure that the facts are discussed, and individuals should be encouraged to make their own decisions. This non-directive approach is usually the most appropriate one and decisions reached by the counsellees in this way are more likely to be seen as the correct ones in the future. There are various determinants of the individual's response to counselling, including reproductive drive, background, education, and religious and moral attitudes. Awareness of these various factors is clearly essential and since they may differ in some instances from those of the counsellor, it is important that the latter does not attempt to influence a course of action which might not suit. There are now a number of texts detailing counselling techniques. As could be anticipated, the counsellor has to learn to listen and to appreciate that even the most uneducated individual can, given the correct presentation of information and time, make a decision about important issues which he or she can live with in the future. Most of us do not know how we would react in certain situations and it would be quite wrong, therefore, to believe that our job is to advise people what to do.

Ethical issues

Over the years, advances in medical technology have produced problems for which traditional guidelines of management may not be available. The ability to keep very handicapped children alive by artificial ventilation is a good example and the wishes of the parents, the views of the medical staff and of the nursing staff may be at variance. In many situations there is no simple answer which will suit everyone and as has happened so often in the past it is necessary to rely on compassion, common sense and professionalism. Medicine has had to adapt to the changing needs of our society and, as some diseases become rare, others are highlighted and present the profession with different problems requiring new solutions. Clinical genetic services have now entered the medical field and some aspects of the work of such services present ethical difficulties for nurses, doctors and the public.

Genetic counselling can be seen as an extension of clinical medicine attempting to answer the question, 'what are the chances of its happening again?' In such a situation there would seem to be no ethical problem associated with the giving of the information required. However, in high risk conditions it is very important that such information is imparted sympathetically and with due regard to the individual's intelligence and cultural background. In many instances, the risk will be such that a couple may well decide not to have further children. This is a very important decision for them to reach and restricted reproduction as a result of genetic counselling advice may produce emotional upset which should be anticipated.

There are other situations which may be more difficult. For example during a pedigree search a number of individuals may be identified who are at risk of a specific disease or of having affected children. Huntington's chorea and other late onset diseases are good examples but the situation can occur with childhood handicap. The pedigree in the figure is of X-linked recessively inherited blindness. Female siblings of the affected males will all inherit the gene and have a 50/50 risk of having an affected son. If they have not come for advice, should they be told about the risk, bearing in mind that there may be no means of identifying the pre-clinical carrier? It is important to discuss the matter with the general practitioner and perhaps with those relatives who have attended the clinic. In all cases, however, the confidentiality of patient information has to be respected and

X-linked recessively inherited blindness

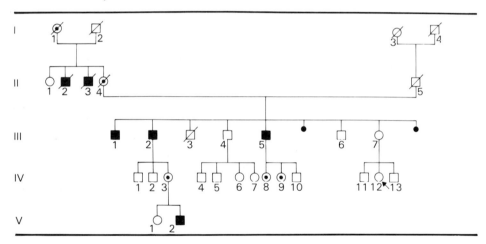

Note:
— I_1 was the obligatory carrier and each daughter had a 50/50 risk of being a carrier (II_4) and each son a 50/50 chance of being affected (II_2 and II_3).
— Any son born to II_4 has a 50/50 risk of inheriting the gene, i.e. of being hemizygous and affected.
— Any daughters born to affected males must be carriers.
— Unaffected males cannot have affected offspring and their daughters cannot be carriers.
— The risk to IV_8 and IV_9 of affected sons is $\frac{1}{2}$ or 50/50; 50/50 risk of carrier daughters.
— Counselling requested by IV_{12} ?Her risk of being a carrier.
The risk of IV_{12} having an affected son is estimated as follows:
— Her risk of being a carrier depends on the risk of her mother (III_7) being a carrier.
— Probability (A) of III_7 being a carrier (a priori) is $\frac{1}{2}$. Probability a that she is a carrier but has two normal sons is $\frac{1}{2} \times \frac{1}{2}$, so probability (A)a is $\frac{1}{4} \times \frac{1}{2} = \frac{1}{8}$.
— Probability (B) that she is not a carrier is $\frac{1}{2}$. Probability b that not being a carrier would have two normal sons is 1. So probability (B)b is $1 \times \frac{1}{2} = \frac{1}{2}$.
— The final risk of III_7 being a carrier is:
$$\frac{\text{Probability (A)a}}{\text{Probability (A)a + Probability (B)b}} = \frac{\frac{1}{8}}{\frac{1}{8} + 4/8} = 1/5$$
Therefore, the risk of IV_{12} being a carrier is $1/5 \times \frac{1}{2} = 1/10$, and the risk of IV_{12} having an affected son is $1/10 \times \frac{1}{2} \times \frac{1}{2} = 1/40$.

this is an important and complicating factor. In some situations it may be difficult to discuss an individual's problem even with a close family member. Experience from counselling clinics of different types suggests that most people expect to be given information even when it may be unwelcome. Few individuals prefer not to be told the facts relating to their particular problem and withholding information may be criticised. Each case has to be carefully assessed and there must be adequate time for discussion with the people concerned. It is important to accept that not everyone 'wants to know'. Having knowledge of their carrier status will upset some people and if they do not want to know then their wishes should be respected.

Large scale screening programmes could obviously multiply this special type of problem many times. It is possible to recognise certain populations at risk for various diseases, for example Tay-Sach's disease in the Ashkenazi Jewish population in America. The carriers of the responsible gene can be identified and the affected fetus diagnosed in utero. There is, therefore, a positive outcome to this screening procedure and it would be seen by many as beneficial to the at-risk population. However, the community involved needs to be properly informed about the condition and the profession must be sensitive to the many social and individual issues which may be involved.

After identification that they are carriers some couples may decide not to have children. This decision should be reached on an informed basis and is a very personal one. However, when prenatal diagnosis is offered this may present moral and ethical issues to doctors, nurses and members of the public. There is a strong anti-abortion lobby in this country and elsewhere, anxious to prevent abortion and to change the law on this procedure. This may be a consequence of strongly held religious beliefs in many instances and it is reasonable that people who have such views should be allowed to express them. Nevertheless, it is difficult for those who criticise this new medical development to understand the issues if they have not had personal involvement. Prenatal testing should not be withheld from those couples who could benefit from it and officially request it. On the other hand this does not morally justify the procedure to those who object to the whole approach.

Genetic counselling staff and obstetricians involved in this work need to be aware of these issues and of the emotional problems involved with termination of pregnancy. It is important that prenatal diagnosis should only be carried out with the consent of both husband and wife. Full discussion is mandatory and sufficient time must be available so that the families concerned may ask questions and voice some of their anxieties. X-linked disease presents a difficult problem and determination of fetal sex with termination of a male pregnancy is an unsatisfactory and clumsy way of dealing with this problem. Intra-uterine diagnosis of the disease is a much more positive approach although not always possible. However, identification of the responsible gene by gene probing techniques is very likely to help in this and other such situations.

Some individuals equate genetic counselling and prenatal diagnosis with the practice of eugenics and because of this find it unacceptable. However, doctors and nurses working in this field would normally see their role as helping individuals and families with a genetic problem in the same way as they offer help for non-genetic disease. For this reason it is important that the individual and family interests are always accepted as more important than the interests of society as a whole. Nevertheless, the natural progression of society will always be towards some form of improvement and most of us would wish to see the elimination of serious handicapping diseases from our community. Although concern has been expressed about the possible increase in deleterious genes as a result of the management of patients with inherited disease, any change is likely to be slow and the effects gradual. In the meantime research continues and may eventually provide a means of primary as opposed to secondary prevention of some of these disorders.

A recent development which has produced widespread interest is genetic engineering and gene manipulation (Antonarskis et al, 1982). This technique has been made possible by the discovery of restriction endonucleases which are enzymes present in various bacterial species and capable of cleaving the large DNA molecule into smaller pieces containing specific genes of interest. There are several hundred such enzymes now known and they are named according to the organism from which they are derived, e.g. Eco RI from E. Coli. All have the ability to recognise and cleave a specific sequence of DNA. The fragments obtained after such cleavage are double stranded and various techniques are available to render them single stranded. They are then exposed to a solution containing a radioactive copy of a specific gene, e.g. that coding for human beta-globin, and fragments that contain the complimentary DNA sequence will bind with this gene. The beta-globin DNA fragments thus obtained can then be examined and their size estimated.

This technique is already being used in the diagnosis of thalassaemia and sickle cell disease from fetal DNA obtained by chorionic biopsy in the first trimester of pregnancy. Sufficient DNA for analysis can be obtained from small amounts of chorionic tissue and this has considerable advantages if termination of pregnancy is necessary. The DNA is fragmented by the appropriate restriction enzyme depending on the specific type of thalassaemia. Until these newer techniques became available the diagnosis of these blood disorders relied on direct examination of fetal blood obtained at fetoscopy. It was the consequences of the abnormal gene which were employed to make the diagnosis. Now restriction enzyme technology makes it possible to examine directly for evidence of the abnormal gene at molecular level and DNA from any tissue can be utilised. As specific gene probes become available for other single gene mutations it should be possible to make a diagnosis of the heterozygous state in individuals with various genetic disorders including late onset conditions such as Huntington's chorea. This would have considerable benefits although, like other developments, is likely to introduce other problems for the individuals concerned. In addition, these techniques are also being applied in the biosynthesis of substances such as insulin, growth hormone and vaccines. They are also invaluable in gene mapping and investigation of gene structure. Inevitably there has been discussion on the possibility of using cloned normal genes or suppressor genes in the treatment of some genetic disorders. This is a formidable task and unlikely to be possible for some time.

There have been few more important developments in medicine than the advances in restriction enzyme technology. Progress has been dramatic over the past few years and the clinical geneticist has the responsibility to ensure that this rapidly advancing knowledge is made available to his colleagues in other specialties for the benefit of the patients with genetic disorders.

REFERENCES

Alberman E 1982 The Epidemiology of Congenital Defects: A Pragmatic Approach. Paediatric Research: A Genetic Approach, p 1. Spastics International Medical Publications

Antonarskis S E, Phillips J A, Kazazian Jr H H 1982 Genetic diseases: diagnosis by restriction endonuclease analysis. Journal of Pediatrics. 100:845

Emery A E H, Rimoin D L 1983 Principles and Practice of Medical Genetics. Churchill Livingstone, Edinburgh

Hilton B, Callahan D, Harris M et al 1975 Ethical Issues in Human Genetics. Genetic Counselling and the Use of Genetic Knowledge. Plenum Press, New York

McKusick V A 1983 Mendelian Inheritance in Man. Catalogs of Autosomal Dominant, Autosomal Recessive and X-Linked Phenotypes, 6th Ed Johns Hopkins University Press, Baltimore

Oakley G P 1978 Natural selection, selection bias and the prevalence of Down's syndrome. New England Journal of Medicine 299:1068

Smithells R W, Nevin N C, Seller M J et al 1983 Further experience of vitamin supplementation for prevention of neural tube defect recurrences. Lancet 1027

Smith D W 1982 Recognizable Patterns of Human Malformation, 3rd ed. Volume VII in Major Problems in Clinical Pediatrics series. W B Saunders Company, Philadelphia

Tariverdian G, Weck B 1982 Nonspecific X-linked mental retardation — a review. Human Genetics 62:95

Yunis J J 1977 New Chromosomal Syndromes. Academic Press, London

8
Nutrition

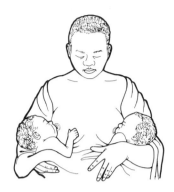

Nutrition describes our knowledge of food requirements and the effects of deficiencies or excesses. It is a much broader concept than 'feeding', which in paediatric practice is sometimes wrongly limited to how a mother feeds her baby often with the implication that the infant is an inactive partner. We, unlike the motor car, survive on all sorts of fuels, we adapt well to changes, and in general we can determine our own intake. However, there are minimum requirements for total energy and individual items, particularly for the growing child, which need to be met. As foods are complex mixtures of the basic constituents — carbohydrate, protein, fat, minerals, vitamins — it is not easy in everyday work to translate any individual child's diet back into these terms. However, there are situations in which it is important to attempt to do so, for example, for a child who through lack of parental knowledge, ability or motivation may not be receiving enough, or for the maintenance of nutrition in a sick child, and for a child with a metabolic disorder on an artificial diet.

MILK

For the first 3 to 4 months of life the infant needs milk only, either human breast milk which is 'tailor made' to fit an infant's nutritional requirements and digestive abilities, or a cow's milk formula which has been adapted to resemble breast milk as closely as possible. The four principal steps in modification of cow's milk are:
— reduction in protein concentration to that in human milk. Relatively indigestible curd protein is decreased and the whey protein mainly lactalbumin and lactoglobulin is increased so that the relative proportion of each of these is similar to that found in human milk. However the lactalbumin differs between cows' and human milk so the amino acid composition of the two milks is still not the same.
— substitution of part or all of the butter fat fraction with vegetable oil mixtures which contain more unsaturated fatty acids, particularly essential linoleic acid which is absorbed well.

— reduction in mineral content, phosphate is reduced to avoid hypocalcaemia and sodium to avoid hypernatraemia which occurs when over-concentrated feeds are given.
— addition of vitamins and iron.

Advantages of human breast milk

Less risk of infection. Human milk contains proteins, IgA, lysozyme and lacto-ferrin, which act against pathogenic organisms and permit the infant's bowel to be colonised by lacto-bacilli which in turn may also inhibit the growth of entero-pathic bacteria responsible for gastro-enteritis. There is a special risk that the bacterial count in powdered milk may become unacceptably high if it is not used when reconstituted particularly where physical conditions and hygiene are poor.

Less risk of metabolic disturbance. The electrolyte content of unmodified cow's milk and of certain of the adapted preparations differs from that in human milk. A high phosphate load inhibits calcium absorption and can precipitate hypo-calcaemic convulsions in the newborn (commonly around the 3rd–5th day of life) and lead to poor dental development later. Renal function of the newborn is unable to cope with the high sodium load of cow's milk thus giving rise to hypernatraemia. The thirst of hypernatraemia results in more feed being given thus adding to the salt load. High sodium feeds combined with dehydration pro-duce a potentially lethal electrolyte disturbance and a risk of permanent handicap in survivors. Neither hypocalcaemia nor hypernatraemia occur with modern for-mulae given in the recommended way.

However, the accurate measurement of powder and water is required, skills which some mothers, particularly those whose educational achievements have been low, do not possess. It is as well to check that parents are able to prepare feeds according to the recommendations.

Low incidence of some important paediatric problems. Cot death is much less common in the children of mothers who are breast feeding, but then, fewer mothers in social classes IV and V breast feed. Eczema is said to be less common in the infants of mothers who breast feed their children though this view is now being challenged. It is presumed to be due to an allergic response to the foreign protein in cows milk; soya based milks also contain a foreign protein and therefore do not avoid this hazard, even if it is present. Obviously, cow's milk allergy is very unlikely to develop in a breast fed baby, though it is not an impossibility. In reactive individuals cow's milk allergy will appear with weaning and the in-troduction of dairy products.

Cost. There are undoubted economic benefits to breast feeding. This particu-larly applies to developing countries. Not only is the cost of the milk formula itself saved, but also that of the bottles and sterilising equipment.

Emotional aspects. It is more difficult to measure the emotional benefit of breast feeding. Bonding is facilitated by breast feeding but feeding by any route can develop into a battle ground or a source of mutual anxiety and uncertainty. For mothers, with the strong feelings of affection and the desire to nurture the infant, come anxieties about their ability to perform that function. There is worry

Why don't mothers breast feed? Breast feeding is strongly related to age, education and social class as shown by the OPCS surveys on infant feeding in 1975 and 1980. The total breast feeding at 6 weeks was 24% and 42% and at 4 months was 13% and 27% in 1975 and 1980 respectively

Incidence of breast feeding in 1975 (%)		The reasons given for choosing bottle feeding first baby (%)		
			1975	1980
Social Class I	77	No privacy/embarrassment	43	18
Social Class V	39	Not tied to baby	38	43
Age less than 20	36	Doesn't like the idea	25	28
Age 25–29 years	74	Experience of others	17	3
Left school at 16	38	You know he has enough	14	18
Left school at 18+	85	Medical reasons	9	2
		Going back to work	6	5

about the adequacy of lactation, and hostility to the baby if he is difficult, unpredictable, 'denies' satisfaction to the mother by feeding and tires her excessively.

The establishment of breast feeding
To help mothers to establish breast feeding they need information and practical help both antenatally and postnatally, combined with confidence, patience and consistency from their advisers. Health professionals can be very critical of mothers who do not wish to breast feed. The neonatal period can be made an unhappy experience for those mothers who only breast feed because of such pressure. It is an unhappy fact that many mothers stop breast feeding soon after leaving hospital. The common reasons given are insufficient milk — 21%, pain in the breast or nipple — 19% and the baby does not suck — 12%.

The establishment of breast feeding requires continuous contact between the mother and baby. 'Rooming in' is not a common practice in the Western World. A recent survey found that only 4% of mothers had their babies with them all the time on the first day and only 32% all the time at day 7. The insistence that all babies are fed at fixed times does not help nor does giving supplementary bottle feeds. The same survey found that only 14% of babies were not given supplementary feeds in the first week. Where mothers were able to put the baby to the breast early, lactation was less likely to be abandoned for the reasons of insufficient milk or failure to suck. In the UK mothers are advised to breast feed for 3–4 months by which time the baby's own defences against infection will have matured, his ability to digest and metabolise and excrete other substances has increased and he is able to learn to chew 'solid food'. However, many mothers will wish to breast feed beyond that time for emotional reasons, for convenience or until the baby can use a cup, thus avoiding the need to make up artificial feeds and sterilise bottles. All these are valid points and the mother who wishes to continue breast feeding should be supported, though solid food in addition to breast milk will be needed. In third world countries where the risk of infection from artificial foods is high, the continuation of breast feeding is encouraged.

Contraindications to breast feeding
There are few situations where breast feeding is absolutely contraindicated. Severe physical illness of the mother or infectious disease necessitating isolation of

mother and infant would fall into this category. Severe mental illness in the mother may be a contraindication to her either breast or bottle feeding her infant. In the child, metabolic diseases such as phenylketonuria or galactosaemia would contraindicate milk feeding by both breast and bottle milk. Some drugs pass into the breast milk and hence to the infant in significant quantities.

Breast feeding technique

Infant feeding is a practical skill requiring teaching. Babies are individual in their feeding habits. Feeding difficulties, positions for feeding, times for feeding and conditions for feeding vary widely from one to another. Feeding an infant is not like putting petrol into a car; to be successful considerably more skill and sensitivity, for example to the baby's responses whilst being fed, are required. Where help is needed it should come from experienced people who have time and patience and who are willing to be available at the time when the baby is being fed and the difficulties arise. Breast feeding counsellors such as those of the National Childbirth Trust, experienced midwives and health visitors, and in many cases relatives and other mothers are the most fruitful sources of help. Preparation for breast feeding should start antenatally; the most important part is an explanation to the mother about the mechanism of lactation. Mothers need to know about the sequence of attachment to the breast, sucking and waiting for the let down reflex to occur. They also need to know that success in lactation is not related to breast

Breast feeding. Let down reflex

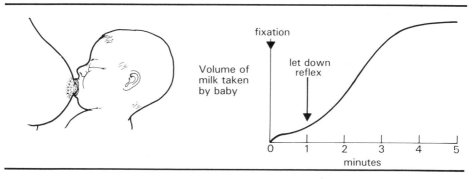

size, and that variations in size are related to the content of surrounding fat and not the content of glandular tissue. Advice is often needed on which brassieres will adequately support the breast during the enlargement which occurs during pregnancy, and which are suitable for infant feeding. Women who have flat nipples may be helped by using a breast shield during pregnancy which encourages the nipples to protrude. Colostrum may seep from the breasts during late pregnancy particularly in first pregnancies, so it helps if new mothers are warned of the possibility. The establishment of successful lactation depends upon adequate stimulation of the breasts by the baby. So the sooner the infant is put to the breast the better after birth. For this, as for other reasons it does not help if mothers and babies are separated and if the baby is offered unnecessary complementary milk feeds.

When feeding, the mother should be comfortably seated and well supported.

Emotional responses to breast feeding!

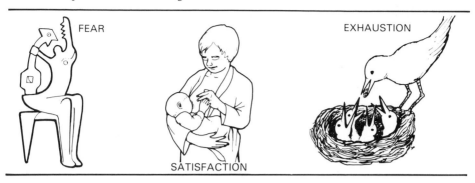

FEAR

EXHAUSTION

SATISFACTION

By allowing the nipple to brush against his cheek the baby will usually find the nipple due to the rooting reflex. He will then fixate on to the breast and the lips will seal firmly around the nipple and areola. As the baby begins to suck the fore-milk will be obtained immediately but the rest of the feed (hind milk) will not be available until the let down reflex occurs. This depends upon sucking initiating the release of oxytocin causing contraction of the myoepithelial cells around the alveoli. The time to initiate this reflex may vary from around 30 seconds to up to 3 minutes. Following the let down reflex the milk will flow, the majority being obtained within the first 5 minutes. However there is considerable variation between the individual breast and the individual baby. At the end of a feed or when changing from one breast to the other, removal of the baby from the breast should be either by the baby voluntarily releasing his grip on the nipple or by gently putting a finger into his mouth to do this. The attachment is strong and the baby cannot simply be 'pulled off'.

More information on the mechanics of breast feeding and sensations of breast feeding and problems which arise is available to mothers from antenatal classes, midwives and health visitors and from many useful books such as 'Breast is Best' and pamphlets from the National Childbirth Trust and the La Leche League.

Ideally breast feeding should be on demand following the argument that babies know when they are hungry and that sucking stimulates milk production. Mothers may need plenty of fluid themselves. If the mother is tired, anxious, or ill, the amount of milk produced will be diminished. Mothers vary just as much as their babies. Some lead very busy and active lives and still successfully breast feed their children whereas others will find themselves tired and in need of additional rest. Some mothers may need to cut down on their household duties if they become tired and lactation is affected. Babies may particularly enjoy their night feed because the mother at rest in bed may produce more milk then than during a busy working day.

Problems in breast feeding

Engorgement. Painful tender breasts in the early days may be due to sudden increase in blood flow into the breasts, but can develop at any time if there is disparity between the amount of milk produced and the amount of milk taken.

Some of the commoner reasons given by mothers for stopping breast feeding at different ages (Infant Feeding, 1980, OPCS)

	Baby's age when breast feeding ceased			
	Under 1 week	2–6 weeks	2–3 months	4–9 months
Insufficient milk	36%	68%	74%	32%
Painful breasts or nipples	24%	15%	10%	1%
Baby would not suck/rejected the breast	30%	8%	4%	17%
Breast feeding took too long	7%	17%	14%	8%
Mother was ill	5%	5%	8%	6%
Baby was ill	2%	2%	5%	1%
Baby could not be fed by others	1%	2%	2%	7%
Returning to work	1%	1%	6%	6%
Had breast fed long enough/as long as intended	—	—	4%	37%

Putting the baby to the breast or expressing excess milk will help to relieve the pain. The breasts need to be well supported and analgesics may ease the pain that might inhibit the let down reflex.

Cracked or sore nipples. Cracked or sore nipples may be prevented by proper fixation of the baby on the nipple and gentle skilful removal of the baby from the nipple. If the condition has developed on one side it may be easier to feed the baby from the other side first. If this is not adequate, milk may need to be expressed whilst the nipple has time to heal. Masse cream or Kamilosan cream may help. Breast abscesses if diagnosed and treated early with antibiotics need not necessitate interruption of feeding from the affected breast. Most can be avoided by general cleanliness and the early and appropriate management of cracked nipples.

Contraception. Oral contraceptives containing oestrogen, particularly in high doses, may interfere with the establishment of lactation. Once lactation is estab-

The left hand column shows drugs that should not be taken by breast feeding mothers (breast feeding should be discontinued if a suitable alternative drug is not available), and the right hand column shows drugs that should be administered with care and the infant observed for possible effects (hazard in brackets) (Drugs and Therapeutics Bulletin, Adverse Drugs Reaction Bulletin, No. 61 December 1976)

Avoid	Take care
Thiouracil, iodides and radio-active iodine cause hypothyroidism in the infant Cytotoxic drugs Metronidazole Indanedione anticoagulants such as Phenindione (Warfarin is a safe alternative) Ergotamine Methysergide	Hypoglycaemic agents (risk of hypoglycaemia) Propranolol (hypoglycaemia and cardiovascular respiratory effects) Diazepam (sedation) Phenobarbitone (sedation) Salicylates in high dose (impaired platelet function) Vitamin D in large doses (hypercalcaemia) Lithium (muscle flaccidity) Anthroquinone laxatives, e.g. Senokot (diarrhoea) Alcohol in large quantities (sedation)

lished some women may continue without difficulty on a low oestrogen contraceptive. However this is often not the case. The progesterone-only pill is generally recommended for mothers to take whilst breast feeding though some have recorded a diminution in milk production on this type of contraceptive as well.

Vitamin supplements for breast fed babies

Supplements of vitamins A, C and D are recommended for breast fed infants from the sixth week onwards. The recommended daily dose is vitamin A 200 μg, vitamin C 20 mg and vitamin D 7 μg. (1 μg = 20 iu). In the UK these are available as drops from Infant Health Clinics under the Welfare Food Scheme at a reduced cost for all children and free of charge to those from low income families. However, vitamin supplements may be unnecessary when the nutritional status of the mother is good. Modified cow's milk already contains vitamin supplements and thus are not needed until the child is weaned. Particularly in Asian children whose diets are low in vitamin D, vitamin supplements should be continued until age 5 years. The danger of overdosage of vitamins particularly vitamin D, should not be forgotten although this is now a very rare problem. Four to 14 times the recommended daily dosage has been associated with hypercalcaemia. Vitamin supplements are also available for antenatal and nursing mothers. These may again be particularly important in Asian families where neonatal rickets occurs due to the mother's vitamin D deficiency. Vitamin drops are preferable to sweet syrups as these may lead to early dental caries. Iron supplements are given to pre-term infants who have not laid down stores of iron in the last trimester of pregnancy.

ARTIFICIAL MILK

There are a number of artificial milks on the market which are intended for infant feeding. Most countries, the European Economic Community and the World Health Organisation have advisory committees which lay down requirements for any product which is the sole source of nutrients for infants. In the UK, the DHSS has recently published the current standards and permitted ranges and given the evidence on which the guidelines are based. The general philosophy is that the artificial feed should resemble human breast milk as far as possible. Most of the products on the European market fall within these guidelines.

When evaluating new or unfamiliar formulae look for the amount and source of the protein, particularly with respect to the relative amounts of curds (casein) and whey (lactalbumin). Is it derived from plants or animals? Has the protein in some way been broken down? Look at the predominant sugar, is it a disaccharide and if so which? Glucose increases the osmolality of the feed. Multidextran is a polymer of maltose which breaks down to glucose, and it requires maltase for its digestion. Sucrose makes the feed taste sweet. Lactose is difficult to avoid altogether. The DHSS guidelines demand that at least some of the carbohydrate is lactose although there is little evidence that either lactose or its component, galactose, are essential nutrients. Look at the fatty acid mixture, particularly how much essential fatty acid, linoleic acid and linolenic are present. Linoleic acid has an 18 carbon chain with two unsaturated bonds and is represented by C18:2. Butter fat contains relatively less unsaturated essential fatty acids than fat from human milk, most vegetable oils contain considerably more. Unsaturated fatty acids are more easily absorbed and metabolised and are less stable than saturated fatty acids, e.g. palmitic acid (C16:0). Babies have been fed on milks with fatty acid compositions up to 45% linoleic acid without obvious ill effects but with no obvious advantage either. The DHSS guidelines recommend that no more than 20% should be linoleic acid. The majority of infant feeds contain fat largely derived from vegetable oils. Some contain fatty acids of medium chain length, C8:0 C10:0. These are relatively water soluble and pass from the bowel via the portal blood to the liver and are metabolised in many respects more like carbohydrate than fat.

Look at the osmolality, and the content of sodium, and the calcium/phosphate ratio. How closely do they match that found in human milk? Some infant feeds contain supplements of vitamins. Vitamin D is controversial, for human breast milk may not contain enough for the rapidly growing infant and supplements are recommended. Therefore some argue that the vitamin D content should exceed that in human milk to a level which avoids supplementation.

Most companies offer two main products — a highly modified formula which closely resembles human milk, with a 40:60 casein:whey ratio; and a less modified formula with a 80:20 casein:whey ratio and higher protein content closer to that in cow's milk. This less expensive feed is entirely satisfactory for the majority of infants. Some mothers report that particularly as they get older their babies find this feed more satisfying, presumably because it makes thicker curds. There is little to choose between the different brands with respect to the constituents and it is rarely justified on the grounds of nutrient content to change a dissatisfied infant from one brand to another.

In some countries it is the practice to feed older infants with 'follow-on' milks, which are thought to help 'build up' the rapidly growing infant and satisfy his increasing appetite. They contain a relatively high protein content and are not suitable for newborn infants. There is also a whole series of special formulae prepared for particular problems — lactose intolerance (lactose free), cow's milk sensitivity (soya protein based feeds), malabsorption (predigested feeds) and inherited disorders of amino acid or carbohydrate metabolism, like phenylketonuria and galactosaemia. Some of these feeds are very expensive.

Constituents of human, artificial and cow's milk

Milks		Human	Highly modified baby milk	Modified baby milk	Cow's milk
Energy	KJ/100 ml	290	275	275	275
	Kcal/100 ml	70	66	66	66
Protein	g/100 ml	1.1	1.5	1.9	3.5
Casein %		40	40	80	82
Whey %		60	60	20	18
Carbohydrate	g/100 ml	7.4	7.3	7.3	4.9
Maltodextrin		—	∓	∓	—
Fat	g/100 ml	4.2	3.6	3.4	3.7
Vegetable oil		—	++	++	—
Minerals					
Calcium	mg/l	35	54	85	117
Sodium	mg/l	15	18	25	50
Iron	mg/l	0.08	0.5	0.5	0.05

Daily milk intake

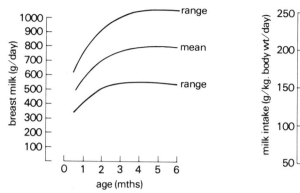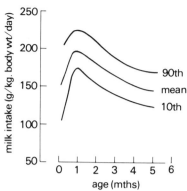

Bottle feeding

Feeding patterns for bottle fed babies should follow the same 'on demand' schedule described for breast fed babies. The first feed will usually be given within 8 hours. A guide to the amount of milk taken is 15 ml/kg/day on day 1, building up to 150 ml/kg/day on day 7. However the normal range is large, 120–200 ml/kg/day on day 7. Babies should not lose more than 10% of their birth weight and all should be gaining weight by day 7 but not necessarily be back to their birth weight.

From the baby's point of view bottle feeding is quite different from breast feeding. They do not have to learn to wait for the let down reflex to occur and the milk arrives by continuous supply with less effort. The supply is also certainly greater. However, babies do seem successfully to resist attempts to overfeed, so like adults they vary in the extent of their gluttony.

Bottle cleaning and sterilisation

Doctors first faced with the task of cleaning and sterilising bottles often feel a little uneasy as sterile gloves are not worn and a 'no touch' technique is not employed. In fact, the process is good general hygiene and comprises cleanliness rather than perfect asepsis. The bottle must first be washed under cold water before the film of milk hardens and then the bottle and teat should be cleaned with detergent and warm water using a bottle brush. The bottle brush should not be used for any other purpose and needs to be regularly washed and boiled. To clean the teat it should be turned inside out and sprinkled with salt and rubbed between the fingers. This loosens the milk stuck to the inside of the teat. It must then be thoroughly washed. Bottles may be sterilised by being placed in boiling water for 10 minutes with the bottle completely submerged or by using a chemical method.

For this a solution of sodium hypochlorite is often used; it must be prepared fresh every 24 hours and the bottle and teat need to be completely submerged. This is easier said than done, for it is surprisingly difficult to exclude air bubbles from some bottles. The bottle must be left in the solution for a minimum of 2 hours. It is preferable to leave it in the solution until it is next used. Parents should avoid the temptation to wash off the few remaining drops of the chemical with fresh water from the tap.

What actually happens in some homes is often far from what is recommended. It is sometimes necessary to go through the procedure step by step with the parents to see exactly what is done. This 'duty' is sometimes performed by the infant's older brothers and sisters and the first step of hand washing is frequently omitted.

Mixing of feeds

In the UK the domestic water supply is generally suitable for making infants' feeds except in time of drought when the ion content may rise. Domestic water that has been repeatedly boiled may contain an excess concentration of sodium. For the same reason water that has been artificially softened is also unsuitable. Lead may also accumulate in drinking water from lead lined tanks and pipes. The water used for making up a milk feed should be boiled previously though not boiled for a prolonged period, and allowed to cool a little. Water near boiling point will destroy water soluble vitamins. The scoops used vary in size from one type of milk to another and should only be used for that particular brand. They should be neither heaped nor packed and each scoop carefully levelled off. The instructions should be followed carefully as in some brands of milk (most) each scoop of milk is added to a fixed volume of water (1 oz) though in some cases the powder needs to be made up to a fixed volume of water. If these differences are not realised, an overstrength feed can easily be made. The bottle once prepared with the teat in place should drip milk at about 1 drop per second. Faster than this and the baby will not be able to keep up with the flow of milk and slower than this the baby will become frustrated by his attempts to receive an adequate amount. Babies of course vary in their needs in this respect. Where there is a refrigerator a whole day's feeds may be made up and the milk fed straight from the fridge. If this facility is not available then each feed must be made up individually as it is needed. It is not necessary to warm feeds and prolonged warming, a common practice for night feeds, encourages bacterial contamination.

Accuracy of measuring milk powder by various groups. They all tend to make concentrated feeds

	Target weight 14 g Mean	Range (g)
10 Primigravidae	16.4	14.7–21.3
20 Multigravidae	17.4	12.4–26
5 Midwives	20.9	18.4–24.1
5 Nurses	17.1	15.6–20.1

MIXED FEEDING

In spite of the recommendation that solids are not required before the age of 3 months, there is considerable evidence that mixed feeding is generally started before this. The 1975 survey of infant feeding practices in England and Wales shows that 3% receive solids in the first 2 weeks, 18% within the first month, 45% within 2 months and 85% by 3 months. These were frequently added to the bottle in the form of cereals.

Mothers can change over from infant milk formulae to 'doorstep milk' from the age of about 6 months. However, there may be advantages in continuing beyond this time particularly in communities where the mixed diet is likely to be poor or where vitamin supplements are unlikely to be given. Parents generally have three options open to them for mixed feeding. The first two are commercially prepared foods available either as powder, which is reconstituted with milk or water, or jars or tins of infant foods. These are convenient and useful foods though somewhat expensive. Quite a number are very sweet and we may be conditioning the child to demand a high intake of sugar with consequent risk of dental caries. The prepared foods may also contain a large number of different food ingredients. Where the parents wish to introduce only one new item of food at a time, where for example there is a family history of atopy or food allergy, these preparations may be unsuitable in view of the large number of substances which they contain. The taste of some prepared infant foods certainly does not appeal to adults and tastes somewhat different from the fresh items.

Many parents prefer to give the child their own food or to prepare meals specially for the child. This is certainly more economical and with the advent in many homes of liquidisers and deep freezers the process is made a lot easier. Food for infants varies only in consistency and salt content from that intended for adults. Although the addition of spices to food for children is generally considered unsuitable there are many instances of children who enjoy such items from their parents' meal plus additions, such as black coffee, without any ill effects.

Solid foods are generally introduced at the end of a milk feed with the baby initially taking perhaps half to one teaspoonful of the new taste initially. Children can usually feed themselves much earlier than parents will allow them to. How-

Recommended intakes of nutrients based on WHO (1974)

	Energy (kcal)	Protein (g)	Ascorbic acid (mg)	Vitamin D (μg)	Calcium (g)	Iron (mg)
Infants						
Under 6 months	117/kg	2.2/kg	35	10.0	0.36	10
6–12 months	108/kg	2.0/kg	35	10.0	0.54	15
Children						
Under 1 year	820	14	20	10.0		5–10
1–3 years	1360	16	20	10.0	0.80	5–10
4–6 years	1830	20	20	10.0	0.80	5–10
7–9 years	2190	25	20	2.5	0.80	5–10
Male adolescents						
10–12 years	2600	30	20	2.5	1.20	5–10
13–15 years	2900	37	30	2.5	1.20	9–18
16–19 years	3070	38	30	2.5	1.20	5–9
Female adolescents						
10–12 years	2350	29	20	2.5	1.20	5–10
13–15 years	2490	31	30	2.5	1.20	12–24
16–19 years	2310	30	30	2.5	1.20	14–28

ever it is a messy process and one which parents hope to avoid for as long as possible. Children will certainly finger feed by about 6 months of age and will be able to use a spoon and a cup by the end of the first year.

CULTURAL VARIATIONS

Doctors and nurses working with different ethnic groups must be aware how diet and custom influence the food available for their children and the beliefs held about it. For example some Sikhs and Hindus believe that the colostrum is harmful and should not be given to the child. Under these conditions the baby may not be breast fed for the first 2 or 3 days, which may be interpreted as another reason for bottle feeding. Proprietary baby foods which we may recommend may not accord with religious dietary rules which is another important consideration when counselling immigrant families. The foods recommended may be unfamiliar to the mother and hence she may not know how to prepare them. Perhaps the best approach is to let the parents teach you about their diet, and then if necessary work out the content and advise the family appropriately.

THE PROBLEM OF TOO LITTLE

Inadequate intake is still the commonest cause of failure to thrive in children investigated for this reason in the UK. In other countries malnutrition coupled with infection remain major health hazards. An inadequate intake may not only reduce overall growth but also brain growth and the prospect for subsequent intellectual development. Improving diet at a later age may give rise to catch up growth but not allow a recovery in brain development.

It is most important therefore that in any child seen a proper assessment of the nutritional status is made. All health workers should be aware of this need and have adequate training in nutritional assessment.

Assessment of diet

Where there is concern about the nutritional status of the child an assessment needs to be made of the adequacy of the individual child's diet. Many processed foods such as breakfast cereals and most types of proprietary brands of infant

Assessment of nutritional status

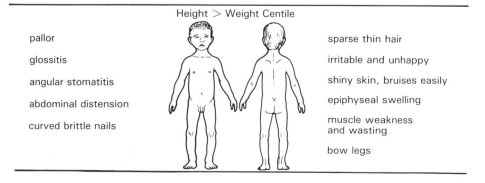

Height > Weight Centile

pallor

glossitis

angular stomatitis

abdominal distension

curved brittle nails

sparse thin hair

irritable and unhappy

shiny skin, bruises easily

epiphyseal swelling

muscle weakness and wasting

bow legs

Nothing for breakfast (from What are Children Eating These Days. Survey supported by National Dairy Council)

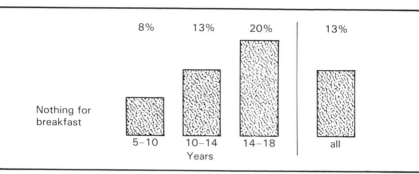

foods are supplemented with vitamins. However where these foods are not used and where the diet contains few sources of meat, fish or animal products, the diet is likely to be deficient in protein, vitamins and minerals. Certain groups of children are particularly at risk of nutritional deficiency. These are immigrant groups, vegetarians, large families or families with low income and families with a low level of care or ability.

Specific deficiency states

Iron deficiency anaemia. Iron deficiency states are fairly common but frequently go unrecognised. Premature babies are particularly at risk as the majority of the infant's iron stores are obtained in the last trimester of pregnancy. The main dietary sources of iron are eggs, meat, and some green vegetables. It is not surprising, therefore, that children on vegetarian diets, particularly Asian immigrants, and those on a largely carbohydrate diet, show a high incidence of iron deficiency anaemia. Handicapped children are also at risk of nutritional deficiency particularly if there are feeding difficulties. Iron deficiency is found surprisingly often in children who have a routine haemoglobin assessment pre-operatively. Where it is specifically sought in deprived populations as many as 60% of the infants may be found to have iron deficiency.

Children most commonly present with irritability or apathy, often combined with an increased susceptibility to infections. They may have clinical evidence of other nutritional deficiencies such as poor growth or rickets. On examination pallor, slight splenic enlargement and a haemic murmur may be found. Haematological examination shows a hypochromic, microcytic anaemia, the serum iron is low and the total iron binding capacity is raised. In immigrant children it is wise to ensure that there is not a coincident haemoglobinopathy. Treatment is with oral iron supplements and these should be continued for at least 3 months. The finding of one child with iron deficiency within a family indicates that siblings should also be investigated.

Rickets is still seen in Britain, particularly in our poor inner city areas and amongst Asian immigrants. It falls into three main groups:
— neonatal rickets due to maternal vitamin D deficiency; infantile rickets

which affects all ethnic groups; and late or adolescent rickets confined to Asian school children. There is some evidence that due to increased awareness of the problem and increased efforts at prevention, the prevalence of rickets is once more falling.

Vitamin D is derived from four sources:

— synthesis in the skin. This is the main source of vitamin D but is deficient in racial groups such as Asian immigrants where the skin is kept covered and where there is little exposure to natural sunlight.

— natural dietary sources of vitamin D, mainly fish, eggs and butter. Milk is a poor source of vitamin D.

— foods fortified with vitamin D such as baby milks and baby foods, cereals and margarine.

— vitamin preparations such as the vitamin A, D, and C drops obtained from child health clinics or cod liver oil.

Chapatti flour used by many Asians is not fortified with vitamin D, and its high phytic acid content inhibits calcium absorption. It is important to look for rickets in high risk groups of children. Likewise the complaint of limb pain in Asian school children should be regarded as due to rickets until proven otherwise. Examination of the blood will show an elevated alkaline phosphatase level. Inorganic phosphorus will be decreased and calcium may be normal or decreased. X-ray of the wrist will show widening, cupping and fraying of the epiphysis.

Welfare foods and vitamins

In the UK the 1940 Welfare Food Act provided free milk for pregnant mothers and all school and preschool children. This is now restricted to children whose families receive supplementary benefit for preschool children and for school children in nursery and infant classes. Children attending junior school are entitled

Good food sources

	Carbohydrate	Protein	Fat	Fe	Ca	Vit C	Vit D	Vit A
Milk Products								
Milk	+	+	+		+			+
Butter	+	+	+		+		+	+
Cheese	+	+	+		+		+	+
Eggs		+	+	+			+	+
Meat		+	+	+				
Liver		+	+	+				+
Chicken		+	+	+				
Fish		+	+					
Vegetables								
Green beans								+
Brussel sprouts				+				+
Carrots								+
Peas				+		+		+
Potatoes	+					+		
Tomatoes						+	+	
Citrus fruits						+		
Whole Meal Bread	+							
Cereals	+							
Spaghetti	+							
Rice	+							
Margarine	+	+					+	+

to free school milk at the recommendation of the school doctor. The decision of the school doctor to recommend free school milk is sometimes a fairly random one. However there is evidence that school children in social classes III, IV and V from families with four or more children, have an increased growth of about 1.5 mm per year, when an additional third of a pint of milk was supplied each day in school. (Cardiff Survey Elwood & Gray.)

PROBLEM OF TOO MUCH — OBESITY

Obesity is a common problem. Our response to it should depend on current knowledge rather than fashion and the diagnosis should be based upon measurements rather than appearance. It is of course accepted that a grossly obese person is obvious without measurement. But bigness and obesity are often confused. Too often the mother of a baby who is long and well built is told that the child is overweight. Weight must always be assessed relative to both height and age. An alternative method of measuring obesity is by reference to skin fold thickness, commonly measured over the triceps and subscapular region. Using the Harpendon skin fold calipers measurements accurate to 0.1 mm can be made.

What happens to fat infants and children?
It used to be held that fat children became fat adults. However over 80% of obese babies will not be overweight in later life. However more fat babies than thin babies will be overweight in adult life and 50% of obese children were obese as babies.

Why do children become fat?
Children tend to resemble their parents in many attributes and obesity is no exception. Overweight 5 year olds have overweight mothers. Early weaning or a higher energy intake in infancy do not, however, appear to be associated with subsequent obesity.

Skin fold thickness

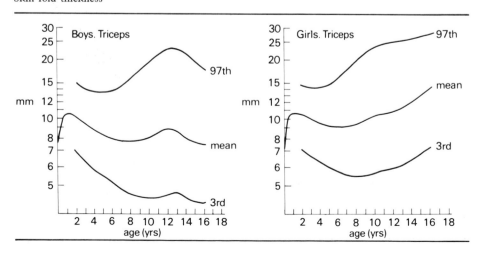

Large and obese!

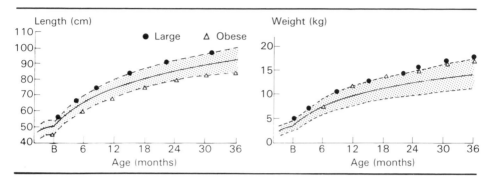

It is common knowledge that many obese people claim that they eat very little, and many thin individuals have what appears to be an excessive food intake. One hypothesis which explains these findings is that thin individuals when overfed, have a system of burning off the excess whereas fat individuals are deficient in this capacity. Although is is pleasanter to explain obesity in terms of bad luck rather than gluttony, the evidence supporting this hypothesis is slight, and what there is, has been questioned.

Consequences of obesity

There are very few fat people who would not like to be thin. Obesity in childhood causes a great deal of unhappiness in terms of self image, comments from other

An obesity index

$$\frac{\text{Actual weight (kg)}}{\text{length (cm)}} = A$$

$$\frac{\text{50th percentile expected weight (kg) for same age}}{\text{50th percentile expected length (mm) for same age}} = B$$

$$\frac{A}{B} \times 100 = \text{index}$$

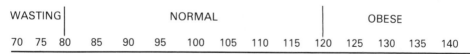

WASTING	NORMAL	OBESE
70 75 80	85 90 95 100 105 110 115	120 125 130 135 140

The incidence of obesity using the obesity index for infants in Dudley, Worcestershire (1972) and for older children and adults from the 1946 cohort are given (Shukla et al, 1972; Stark et al, 1981)

Infants (months)	% obese	Children (years)	% obese male	female	Adults (years)	% obese male	female
0–3	12.5	6	1.7	2.9	20	5.4	6.5
3–6	29.3	7	2.0	3.8	26	12.3	11.2
6–9	10.1	11	6.4	9.6			
9–12	6.8	14	6.5	9.6			

children and lack of success in sports. In adult life obese individuals have a high incidence of ischaemic heart disease, osteoarthritis, post-operative complications, poor obstetric performance and lack of physical fitness. It has also been associated with hypertension, and glucose intolerance. Life expectancy is reduced and insurance companies increase their premiums accordingly.

Prevalence of overweight at later ages according to relative weight at 7 years (males only) (left) and relative weights at earlier ages of overweight 26 year olds (males only) (right)

Relative weight at age 7 years (%)	Percentage of subjects overweight at age				Age	< 100%	101–120%	>120%
	11	14	20	26 years				
< 80	0	0	0	0	6	28	65	6
81–90	0.3	0	0	7	7	29	64	7
91–100	0.7	2	4	7	11	20	53	26
101–110	8	7	4	14	14	17	56	28
111–120	22	24	15	26	20	5	59	35
> 120	70	53	43	43	26	0	0	100

What to do

In contrast to our knowledge of the measurement, incidence, natural history and causes of obesity, our effectiveness in dealing with the problem is poor. Prevention is clearly desirable through education of parents, parents to be, and school children on the elements of nutrition. However there is always a wide gap between knowledge and its implementation. Results are frequently disappointing and children whom we cause to shrink by strict dietary control in hospital, rapidly expand once discharged. Measures to reduce obesity only work in motivated children from motivated families and are only successful where continuing and regular support is provided. The issue of a diet sheet and instruction to go away and come back thin will not be successful. A minimal approach would include the completion of a diet diary by the parents or the child; and an analysis of that diary with the parents and child. It is useful to divide the family diet into green, (good), amber (alright in small quantities), and red (forbidden foods). The child is then allowed to eat as much as he likes from the green column, limited amounts from the amber column and nothing from the red column. The diet is based on the current food that the family has as this causes minimum disruption at home and does not introduce foods which are strange to them (children are very conservative about new foods). The child is instructed either to stay exactly the same weight or to lose weight but at a rate not more than 1 lb per week. He is seen regularly for a period of up to 2 years. The aim is for a horizontal weight chart until it reaches the required height percentile.

REFERENCES AND FURTHER READING

Addy P 1976 Infant feeding: a current view. British Medical Journal 1: 1268–1271
Adverse Drug Reaction Bulletin 1976 Drugs and Breast Milk. No. 61
Davies D 1973 Plasma osmolality and feeding practices of healthy infants in first three months of life. British Medical Journal 2: 340–342

Davies D P, Williams T 1983 Is weighing babies in clinics worthwhile. British Medical Journal 286: 860–866

DHSS 1980 Artificial feeds for the young infant. Report on Health and Social Subjects no. 18. HMSO

DHSS 1980 Present day practice in infant feeding. Report on Health and Social Subject no. 20. HMSO

Drugs which can be given to nursing mothers. Drug and Therapeutics Bulletin Vol 21. No. 2

Editorial 1981 Asian rickets in Britain. Lancet Al: vol no 402

Hull D 1980 Thoughts on obesity. Archives of Disease in Childhood 55: 838–840

Martin J, Mark J 1980 OPCS Report on Infant Feeding

National Dairy Council Study 1981 Taylor Nelson

OPCS 1978 Breast feeding. HMSO

Parkin J M 1982 Free milk for children. Archives of Disease in Childhood 57: 89–91

Peckham et al 1983 Prevalence of obesity in British children born in 1946 and 1958. British Medical Journal 286: 1237–1242

Poskitt E M E, Cole T J 1977 Do fat babies stay fat? British Medical Journal 1: 7–9

Shukla A, Forsyth H A, Anderson C M, Marwal S M 1972 Infantile overnutrition in the first year of life: a field study in Dudley, Worcestershire. British Medical Journal 4: 507–515

Stark O, Atkins E, Wolff O H, Douglas J W B 1981 Longitudinal study of obesity in the National Child Development Study. British Medical Journal 283: 13–17

Wharton B 1982 A quinquennium in infant feeding. Archives of Disease in Childhood 57: 895–897

Wharton B, Berger H 1976 Bottle feeding. British Medical Journal 1: 1326–1331

9
Hazards

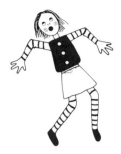

Environmental hazards are responsible for a major fraction of mortality and morbidity in children. In Nottingham, population about 700 000, over 25 000 children each year come to the accident and emergency department of which nearly 70% are because of injuries, cuts, bruises, fractures etc. In the UK accidents are responsible for 50% of the deaths in children aged 1–15 years. Much effort is directed at salvaging the situation once damage has been done. Recently people from many areas have started coming together to try and prevent the problems from arising, surely a more appropriate approach.

ACCIDENTS

Accidents are not only a leading cause of death in children but also of admission to hospital. One in five admissions to hospital of children over 1 year is due to trauma. Boys are more frequently involved than girls. Some children who are perhaps more excitable and overactive, are more accident prone. Accidents occur more often in lower social classes. They are more likely to occur at times of turmoil or stress.

Deaths by accident and violence (%)(from Black Report, 1981)

| Accident or violence | 1–14 | 1–4 | 5–9 | 10–14 |
Number of deaths in years 1968–74	10 887	4371	3712	2794
Road traffic	50.1	34.5	62.2	59.2
Poisoning	2.5	4.1	0.9	2.1
Falls	5.7	6.5	4.2	6.6
Fires	8.3	14.4	5.7	2.3
Drowning	12.9	13.9	14.1	9.6
Inhalation/suffocation	6.8	10.6	2.7	5.6
Electric current	1.4	1.4	1.1	1.7
Suicide	0.3	–	–	1.2
Homicide	3.8	5.7	2.6	2.6

Accidents by social class from occupational mortality figures 1970–72 (reported in Black Report, 1981). N-m = Non-manual; M = manual

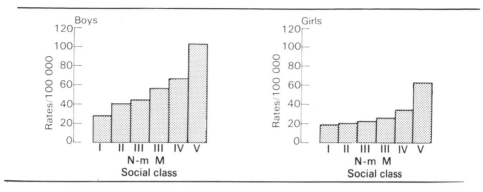

Road traffic accidents

Half the children who die in road traffic accidents are pedestrians. The traffic environment is largely designed from an adult point of view. Youngsters are just not capable of adapting safely to it. For example young children cannot see over cars or over the brow of a hill as easily as an adult can. Immature visual perception and coordination also cause errors of judgement when crossing the road. Adults often do not allow for a child's limited abilities in his behaviour and may be surprised when a 5 year old runs into the road in front of their car. One study found that many drivers who had run into children were male and under 22 years of age, and presumably therefore had little personal experience of children. Some mothers also have unreal expectations of their children. In another study 50% of mothers of 5 year olds and 19% of mothers of 2 year olds thought that their children could safely cross a main road by themselves. Cycling accidents are common amongst older children. Young children do not have the physical maturity to control a cycle in busy traffic.

Vehicle passengers are also at risk. In the UK it is now illegal for a child under 12 years to ride in the front seat of a car and those old enough to ride in the front seat have to wear seat belts. This should reduce serious injuries, but children are still 'legally' allowed to ride unrestrained in the back of the car.

Education of children like the Green Cross Code, teaching materials from

Danger: road accidents (adapted from Play It Safe, Health Education Council)

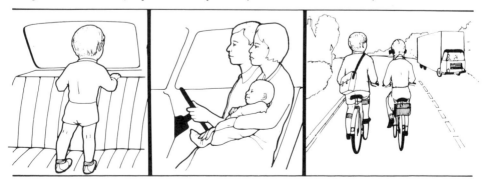

RoSPA, Tufty Club and Cycling proficiency schemes, should contribute towards reducing these problems. There is some evidence that cycle proficiency and teaching road safety are effective if carefully thought out though this has not been extensively studied. Education of parents both to have more realistic expectations of their children and on ways to protect them, and education of the general public on the normal erratic behaviour of children, might also help. Further improvements should follow by (1) altering the environment by providing, for example, more pedestrian precincts and play streets; (2) redesigning cycles and vehicles with safety in mind and (3) legislating for further restraints in vehicles.

Home accidents

Accidents in the home are common in children under 5 years of age, and are particularly common in 2–3 year olds. Boys are more often injured than girls and the incidence is higher in social classes IV and V. Falls, cuts and bruises are the major type of accident seen in accident and emergency departments.

Danger: home accidents (adapted from Play it Safe, HEC)

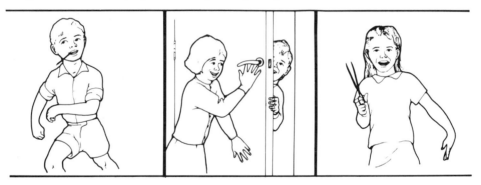

Houses like roadways are designed to cater for adults rather than children, for example, windows poorly secured, low or easily climbed rails on balconies and roof tops, glass panels to floor level, open staircases and lack of play areas. Other hazards are more immediately under the control of the family, such as unguarded fires, stairs and cookers.

Parent education by such methods as television programmes and advertising campaigns is a possible way of increasing awareness, though at present we do not know if they are successful. Individual advice about specific aspects of home safety is possibly the most useful approach and should be a major part of the health visitor's job. In the longer term architects and designers must be more aware of the problems of children living in houses.

Playground accidents

Playgrounds are there to encourage children to have adventures and to take risks. However, poor design and maintenance of playgrounds and equipment can mean that unnecessary risks are taken. In a study of 250 playground accidents the most frequent items of play involved were climbing frames (78), swings (73), slides (44), and roundabouts (33). Swings often caused injury through improper use, falls occurred from climbing frames and slides, and roundabouts caused trapping injuries as young children try to jump off when older children arrive.

The effect of falls can be ameliorated by having earth, grass, or rubber compounds on the ground rather than concrete. Slides placed in a sloping surface prevents falling from the top. Play changes markedly throughout childhood and it is therefore a wise move to separate age groups. Design of equipment should take into account the types of accidents occurring and must anticipate improper use.

IMMERSION AND DROWNING

In the United States, drowning is the third commonest cause of death under 4 years of age and the second commonest over 4 years. With an increase in the number of private swimming pools and aquatic sports in the UK the number here might be expected to increase. Even small quantities of water such as an ornamental pool, a water tank or rainwater in the bottom of a swimming pool can be fatal.

Dangers from immersion result from anoxia, inhalation of water, and hypothermia. Inhalation of water can result in respiratory distress some hours after apparent recovery from the drowning episode. This 'secondary drowning' is possibly due to surfactant loss. Hypothermia can be protective if there is respiratory or cardiac arrest, and normal functional recovery after prolonged arrest has been recorded. However, severe hypothermia can also cause problems with cardiac arrhythmias, which can be induced by handling. Prevention of further cooling is important so remove wet clothes and wrap well. Rewarm the trunk first for rewarming of the limbs will cause vasodilatation and further cooling of the blood.

Pools should be protected by fencing and gates must be kept closed. Awareness that small quantities of water can be dangerous particularly to small children should lead to protection and possible changes in the siting of ornamental pools.

BURNS AND SCALDS

Burns are responsible for 12% of accidental deaths under 5 years and 5% over

Danger: Scalds (adapted from Play it Safe, HEC)

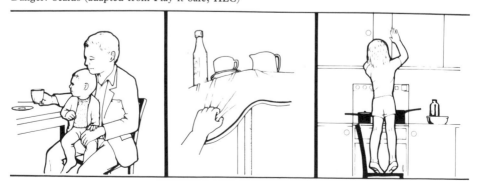

5 years. The chief causes of scalds are spilt hot drinks, kettles and saucepans knocked or pulled over, and immersion in a hot bath. Scalds are common but generally less serious than burns. As even small areas of scalds cause pain and may leave unsightly scars with the risk of contractures, all but very trivial scalds should be treated at hospital.

Burns are less common but more serious. Small burns are likely to be caused by children grabbing hold of electric fire bars, irons, or cooker rings. The more severe burns are associated with conflagration such as clothing catching light or a house fire. In a fire it is often the pulmonary complications from inhaled smoke and fumes that are fatal. Children in house fires have often been left without adult supervision.

Danger: burns (adapted from Play it Safe, HEC)

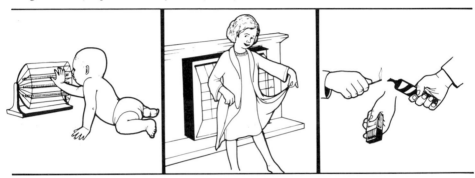

POISONING

In 1972, 25 children died in England and Wales from poisoning and 16 000 were admitted to hospital. Probably 40 000 a year are seen in Accident and Emergency Departments. The major problem is poisoning with drugs, household chemicals, seeds and berries, with drugs causing the majority of the serious problems. Eighty per cent of the children are under 5 years. Salicylates and benzodiazepines are currently the commonest drugs ingested but salicylates and tricyclic antidepressants the most likely to cause death. Salicylates are often being used for the child or a sibling at the time and tricyclics may have been prescribed for an older child for nocturnal enuresis. Other drugs are generally prescribed for an adult, often grandparents who carry their tablets around with them or keep them handy in order to remember to take them. Household chemicals and plant materials are usually not taken in sufficient quantity to cause problems, but corrosives (bleach, lavatory cleaners) can cause oesophageal strictures, and volatile liquids (turpentine, paraffin) can cause a chemical pneumonitis.

Information about potential toxicity of substances can be readily obtained at any time of day or night from poisons information centres. If there is concern that a toxic amount could have been taken, and the child is conscious, vomiting should be induced rapidly (*unless the substance is corrosive or volatile*) in which case it should be diluted with a drink of milk). Syrup of ipecacuanha should be used

Danger: poisoning (adapted from Play it Safe, HEC)

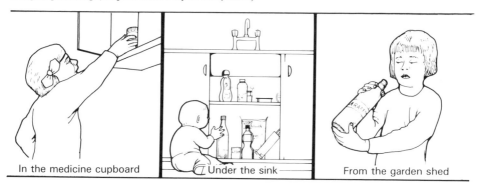

In the medicine cupboard | Under the sink | From the garden shed

with a large quantity of fluid to induce vomiting, *not* saline because of the risk of salt poisoning.

Individual advice by the Health Visitor on places to keep drugs and household chemicals may be the effective approach though general education may help. In the UK child resistant containers have reduced the accidental incidence of ingestion of drugs but people must be aware that these are child resistant not child proof. Clearer labelling of toxic products might be of benefit but parents are usually fully aware of their toxicity. Transfer to unlabelled bottles, particularly bottles previously holding drinks is an obvious invitation to a child to have a drink.

Discharge rates per 10 000 population following admission for injury and poisoning in 1979 (Hospital In-Patient Enquiry, 1979.

	0–4 years	5–14 years
Boys	175.9	138.7
Girls	132.6	79.9

FOREIGN BODIES

Ingested. This is the commonest problem. The majority of objects pass through without difficulty. Certainly once in the stomach, most objects will not penetrate or block the bowel. If they are held up in the oesophagus, they will probably require removal by oesophagoscopy.

Inhaled. Objects that have been inhaled will generally require removal by bronchoscopy. If there is a possibility of inhalation the child should always be seen at hospital. Peanuts notoriously cause problems and their presence is not always recognised. As they fragment they are difficult to remove completely and often give rise to a localised chemical reaction.

Inserted. The presence of a foreign body in the nose, ear or vagina may be recognised only by the resultant discharge or bleeding. If these symptoms occur a foreign body must be considered.

LEAD

There is considerable controversy about the danger of high levels of lead in the blood, and to what extent lead in petrol contributes to this. The level officially considered 'safe' at present is 30 µg/ml or 1.4 mµmol/l. Many reports have related high blood levels to poor scores for intelligence and behaviour but it is hard to prove cause and effect since there are often associated nutritional and social factors. Average blood lead levels in the US have dropped by 37% from 1976 to 1980, a consequence, it is thought, of the use of lead free petrol. More extensive use of lead free petrol in this country has been advocated, for it would at least increase the margin of safety for children.

Lead poisoning presents with the acute symptoms of encephalopathy, or more chronic symptoms of anaemia. It generally occurs in children with pica but has also been reported in Asian children whose eyes have been painted with Surma containing a high lead content. It is illegal to sell Surma containing lead in the UK. Old lead water pipes can still cause problems.

SMOKING

Cigarette smoking starts to affect the child before it is born. Babies of mothers who smoke during pregnancy are significantly lighter and more often born prematurely than those of non-smokers.

During early childhood smoke in the environment, particularly mother smoking, is associated with recurrent respiratory problems in the child. This may be a direct effect of inhaled smoke irritating the airways, or due to infection. Children who themselves start to smoke early have significantly more respiratory symptoms than those who do not and then go on to expose themselves to the risks of chronic bronchitis, vascular disease, and lung cancer.

It is easier to demonstrate the relationship between smoking and ill health than to persuade people to give up smoking or to prevent them from starting. Campaigns in schools to prevent smoking have been unsuccessful on the whole, though attitudes to smoking in school do perhaps have some influence.

Cigarette smoking in secondary school children, London 1979. The columns indicate the percentage of children who had tried or occasionally smoked (occ), who had regularly smoked but had stopped (ex) and who smoked regularly from one per week upwards (from Rawbone & Guz, 1982)

	Boys (%)			Girls (%)		
	Occ	Ex	Reg	Occ	Ex	Reg
11 years	32%	12%	4%	26%	11%	3%
12 years	36%	14%	4%	31%	13%	5%
13 years	39%	17%	9%	33%	15%	12%
14 years	37%	18%	16%	33%	14%	17%
15 years	34%	16%	21%	31%	13%	23%
16 years	35%	13%	22%	33%	13%	19%
17 years	42%	9%	16%	33%	8%	13%
Total	37%	15%	13%	32%	13%	14%

SOLVENT ABUSE

This appears to be an increasing problem amongst children particularly in the 11 to 16 year olds. There are 117 deaths between 1970–1981 attributable to solvent abuse with half from direct toxicity and half incidents occurring during intoxication. The children are generally from deprived areas and have disturbed family backgrounds and other features of delinquency.

The substances used are volatile organic chemicals especially adhesives, but also paint thinners, dyes, hair lacquer, lighter fuels, nail polish remover, aerosols and petrol. Glue is probably the commonest and the least hazardous. The substances are poured onto a rag or into a plastic bag or sprayed directly into the mouth. The effects are similar to alcohol, with euphoria and incoordination possibly going on to stupor, with subsequent depression. Physical dependence is unlikely but psychological dependence may occur. Chronic use may have long term physical effects such as renal damage and neuropathies. The children may go on to abuse alcohol.

Clues to identifying children sniffing regularly are reddening around the mouth and nose, fatigue, loss of coordination, restlessness, and a decline in school performance. As with smoking it is difficult to know how to prevent it. Substances used are so widespread that control of these is not practical, though shopkeepers should be encouraged not to sell such substances to children. Addition of unpleasant substances to glues might discourage some children.

REFERENCES AND FURTHER READING

Black D 1982 Glue Sniffing. Archives of Disease in Childhood 57: 893–894
Drug and Therapeutics Bulletin 1982 Child resistant containers
Jackson R H 1977 Children, the environment and accidents. Pitman Medical, London
Smith M, Delves T, Lansdown R, Clayton B, Graham P 1983 The effects of lead exposure on urban children: the Institute of Child Health/Southampton Study. Developmental Medicine and Child Neurology Supplement No. 47
Yule W, Lansdown R, Millar I B, Urbanowicz M 1981 The relationship between blood lead concentrations, intelligence and attainment in school population: a pilot study. Developmental Medicine and Child Neurology 23: 567–576

10

Infections

Herpes virus: simplex
EB virus

Adenovirus

Picornavirus: poliovirus
rhinovirus

Myxovirus: influenza

Paramyxovirus: parainfluenza

Infectious diseases are still a major cause of sickness. Falling mortality rates in the Western World have taken much of the fear out of epidemics, but it would be a mistake to become complacent. Problems remain. If one assumes that most of those designated on the death certificate as 'respiratory' are due to infections then in the UK infections are still the commonest cause of death in the post-neonatal period. In less fortunate countries infections like pneumonia, gastroenteritis, tuberculosis, whooping cough, measles, malaria, tetanus and diphtheria, remain collectively by far the most important causes of death in all age groups. Some of this is undoubtedly due to a higher incidence but poor nutrition and lack of adequate facilities for treatment, contribute. Again in the UK infective conditions are the commonest reason for children of all ages being seen by family doctors. Children under the age of 9 can be expected to have six to eight upper respiratory tract infections each year, of which three might be anticipated to be accompanied by constitutional symptoms.

Recording infection
In the UK detailed information on the epidemiology of infections is available from a variety of sources. There are, however, many inherent sources of error in these assessments. The information on death certificates may be inaccurate or incomplete. In some the actual cause of death will be uncertain. Statutory notification

Notifiable infectious diseases (1980) UK

Acute encephalitis	Lassa fever	Relapsing fever
Acute meningitis	Leprosy	Scarlet fever
Acute poliomyelitis	Leptospirosis	Smallpox
Anthrax	Malaria	Tetanus
Cholera	Marburg disease	Tuberculosis
Diphtheria	Measles	Typhoid fever
Dysentery	Ophthalmia neonatorum	Typhus fever
Food poisoning	Paratyphoid fever	Viral haemorrhagic fever
Infective jaundice	Plague	Whooping cough
	Rabies	Yellow fever

Mortality due to infectious disease, England and Wales (1977). Worldwide 17 million children died in 1981; less than 1 in 10 of these had been immunised against the six main child killing diseases; 5 million children died through diarrhoea and dehydration (Grant, 1981)

Cause	0–1	1–2	2–3	Age (Years) 3–4	4–5	5–9	10–14
All deaths	7841	489	350	290	254	1008	992
Gastroenteritis	91	12	5	3	2	3	1
Pertussis	5	1	1	—	—	—	—
Chickenpox	4	—	—	—	7	4	—
Herpes Simplex	4	2	1	—	2	1	1
Measles	1	3	2	1	1	9	3
Hepatitis	—	—	—	—	3	7	3
Laryngitis/tracheitis	14	1	1	2	2	—	—
URTI	29	3	2	—	—	2	—
Bronchitis/bronchiolitis	227	21	8	7	1	2	4
Pneumonia	496	53	33	18	9	31	33

of infectious disease, although a legal responsibility of doctors, is also an incomplete exercise. A fee of £1.30 is payable for each notification! Nevertheless the data do provide a basis for local and national monitoring. The Royal College of General Practitioners produces weekly data from a sample of 30 practices which is particularly helpful for following infections like chickenpox, which are not notifiable and would not be recorded in the Public Health Laboratories.

Susceptibility to infection
Children are not all equally susceptible to infection. Although a certain element of infection is 'bad luck', other factors can be identified.

Genetic. Certain children are more prone to infection, for instance, children with Down's syndrome are much more likely to develop upper respiratory tract infections. Mild and severe immune deficiency states run in families.

Environmental. Environmental factors are important with respect to the spread of infection. Good housing, clean water supplies and adequate sanitation contribute enormously to the control of infectious diseases like tuberculosis. Likewise, poor environment is a major factor in the continual high prevalence of infectious disease in inner city areas. New infections introduced into isolated communities where there is little herd immunity may be quite devastating, for example measles in Eskimos.

Morbidity statistics from General Practice Second National Study, 1970–71

Childhood consultation rates/1000 patients, age 0–15 in rank order	
Acute naso-pharyngitis	148.5
Acute pharyngitis	107.5
Acute otitis media	67.6
Acute bronchitis and bronchiolitis	60.3
'Cough'	42.5
Vomiting and diarrhoea	36.7
Eczema	33.8
Injuries	26.8
Impetigo and other skin infections	24.0
Conjunctivitis	23.1

Age. The prevalence and severity of certain infectious diseases relates strongly to age. Thus the prevalence and severity of whooping cough and bronchiolitis is greatest in very young children whilst tuberculosis peaks in the pre-school child and in early adolescence. Mumps tends to be more severe in adults.

Geographical. Many infectious diseases are largely confined to certain climates or areas of the world. However the effects of rapid international travel mean that children can travel far during the incubation stage!

Background nutrition is of paramount importance in the child's susceptibility and reaction to infection. In the malnourished the death rate of children contracting measles or whooping cough can be very high. Children with any form of chronic illness are also more susceptible to infection, particularly where the disorder or its treatment results in immunosuppression or undernutrition. The child's immunisation history is of obvious importance in determining individual susceptibility to infection.

Prevention of infection
Improving the conditions under which people live, by for example, assuring clean water supplies, adequate sanitation, adequate food supplies and storage, has a major impact on the incidence, spread and severity of infectious disease. Improved housing with adequate light, heating, ventilation and abolition of overcrowding has been shown to reduce the incidence and spread of infection. For some infectious diseases isolation of infected persons and efficient contact tracing can be a very effective means of control. However, it is immunisation which has had the most dramatic effect on the extent to which diseases like diphtheria and poliomyelitis have been virtually eradicated from many countries.

Agencies involved

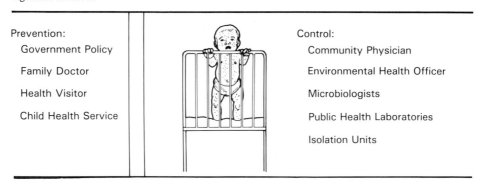

Prevention:	Control:
Government Policy	Community Physician
Family Doctor	Environmental Health Officer
Health Visitor	Microbiologists
Child Health Service	Public Health Laboratories
	Isolation Units

IMMUNISATION

The aim of immunisation is to produce a specific immunological defence against infection without significant risks to the recipient. Historically the first recorded evidence of immunisation was in the 6th century BC in China when dried smallpox crusts were introduced intra-nasally. Modern developments in immunisations start with Jenner who in 1796 demonstrated experimentally the protective effect of cowpox extracts against smallpox.

The theoretical basis of immunisation

During an infection both B and T cell lymphocytes are sensitised. The B cells will then produce specific antibodies against the organism which act to neutralise the toxin (antitoxic antibody), or enhance phagocytosis (opsonic activity). The sensitised T cells multiply on exposure to specific antigens and release chemicals such as lymphokines which attack the organism and invoke a local inflammatory reaction. This specific memory is usually life long. The aim of immunisation is to sensitise the system whilst avoiding the unpleasant features of the natural illness. This may be achieved by using attenuated live vaccines (e.g. oral polio and BCG) or bits of killed organisms, i.e. inactivated vaccines (e.g. pertussis, typhoid). With live vaccines the very low grade infection provides a prolonged stimulus, while with the dead vaccines the stimulus is short lived and has to be repeated.

Reaction to vaccination

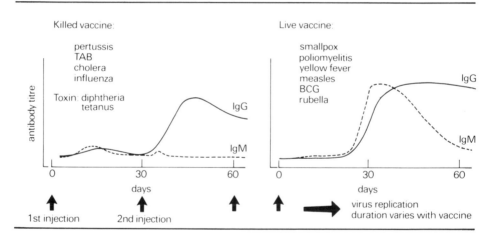

Categories of vaccine

Toxoids	:	Diphtheria, tetanus
Killed bacterial	:	Pertussis, typhoid, cholera
Live bacterial	:	Tuberculosis (BCG)
Killed viral	:	Poliomyelitis (Salk), influenza, rabies
Live viral	:	Smallpox, polio (oral Sabin), yellow fever
		Measles, mumps, rubella

Temporary defence can be given by passive immunisation. Immunoglobulins (antibodies) must be given by injection; they may be given as pooled human gamma globulin which contains a mixture of antibodies against the infections prevalent in the blood donors, or specific gamma globulin prepared from blood taken from patients in the convalescent phase after natural infection or vaccination, or specific antibody prepared from immunised animals such as diphtheria and tetanus antitoxin.

Prospects for a vaccine

These are good if the immunity produced in response to the vaccine is strong; if the incubation period of the natural illness is long enough to enable adequate time for antibodies to be produced in advance of symptoms and if the organism is widespread in the body. Thus the prospects are good for measles which produces a viraemia, but not for viruses which react mainly in the respiratory mucosa. If the infection is localised to one site, access of the antigen to the immune defence system and vice versa may be restricted.

They are poor if the antigenic nature of the infecting organism is variable. If there are many antigenic types, obviously the vaccine must provoke a reaction against those prevalent in the population immunised. If the infecting organism is difficult to culture for, then, on current technology, we do not have the means of producing vaccine in suitable amounts.

Effectiveness and safety

The effectiveness of vaccines within a population can be calculated by the following equation

$$\frac{\text{Attack rate in unvaccinated} - \text{the attack rate in vaccinated}}{\text{the attack rate in unvaccinated}} \times 100.$$

In the laboratory the potency of vaccines may be assessed by inoculation of animals before exposure to the infection, by assay of antibody responses or with live attenuated vaccines counting the numbers of live micro-organisms in a dose. Assessment of safety may be made by injection of large doses of vaccine into laboratory animals and observing for signs of toxicity. Killed vaccines need to be tested for evidence of sterility and all vaccines must be tested for absence of contamination.

Uptake and herd immunity

It is not always necessary to immunise all individuals in order to protect the total population. In some situations, such as tetanus, all individuals need protection because of the ubiquitous nature of the organism. For other infections such as diphtheria where infection is spread directly from one individual to another and where the vaccine is highly effective, a vaccine uptake of just under 80% has proved adequate to eliminate the disease from a country. Vaccinating one group can protect another. Perhaps the only way of avoiding deaths due to whooping cough in infants under 4 months of age is to ensure a high vaccination rate in older children, thus reducing the spread of the infection. Because Bordetella pertussis is carried in the mucosa of the upper respiratory tract eradication is not possible. The issue of vaccine uptake and herd immunity is important in the design of immunisation programmes.

Immunisation programmes

The decision to initiate an immunisation programme, the practical aspects of running such a programme and its final success depend on many factors other than the good intentions of nurses and doctors.

Political. At a national level it is politicians rather than doctors who decide on national campaigns. They are influenced not only by doctors but also by individual pressure groups and publicity. Politicians may also affect people's responses to immunisation programmes, either by support or by casting doubts about effectiveness or emphasising side-effects. Whether they are well or ill-informed, what they say is reported in the press. Moral issues will also influence political discussion. What a discussion there would be if a vaccine against gonococcal infection were to be developed! As it happens this is an unlikely event, for the disease is local and does not itself provoke protection against further infections.

Economic. The budget available for health care is not unlimited, one group of priorities must be weighed against another. In the case of an immunisation programme the cost of prevention must be weighed against the cost of treatment. For instance, in the case of BCG the falling incidence of tuberculosis may, at some time, reach a level where the total immunisation of our teenagers would be an uneconomical proposition. Against the cost of developing a vaccine must be weighed the hours lost from work and consequent fall in productivity caused by the disease. Common respiratory infections must be very expensive in these terms.

Medical. The medical task is to assess the trends in morbidity and mortality from the infection, and assess possible influence of a vaccination programme. Once a programme is established, it is not easy to determine what would be the effects of its withdrawal. Where there are no recorded cases of polio in the country, the presence of a reservoir of infection abroad, combined with the severity of the disorder would seem to warrant continued whole population immunisation. Obviously the benefits of the immunisation must outweigh the risks for the individual as well as the community as a whole. In the case of smallpox the risks of severe complications of vaccination outweighed the risks of contracting smallpox and thus whole population vaccination was discontinued.

Public motivation. Public motivation may range from antipathy and fear when for example there has been adverse publicity, to apathy particularly when the dire consequences of the infection are not within the experience of the community, to panic when an outbreak occurs. All three reactions have been seen with pertussis immunisation over a period of time as short as 10 years. These changes in public attitude stress the need for health education and presentation of precise clear information to public figures and journalists.

Administration of immunisation programmes

I	Register of susceptible individuals
II	Explanation of the benefits of programme — appropriate literature
III	Obtain consent
IV	Appointment system, using computer or manual system
V	Immunisation clinic — appropriate clerical and medical staff
	— arrangements for transport and storage of vaccine in the amounts required
VI	Recording attendance and uptake of vaccine
VII	Arranging payment for those carrying out the service

Recommended immunisation schedule for the UK (1983)

Neonatal	:	BCG Infants of Asian parents or those with a family history of tuberculosis
3 months	:	Diphtheria/tetanus/pertussis and oral polio vaccine
5 months	:	Diphtheria/tetanus/pertussis and oral polio vaccine
10 months	:	Diphtheria/tetanus/pertussis and oral polio vaccine
15 months	:	Measles
5 years	:	Diphtheria/tetanus vaccine and oral polio vaccine
11 years	:	Rubella (girls) and BCG (If Heaf Negative)
15 years	:	Tetanus toxoid and oral polio vaccine

Recommended immunisation schedule in the USA

2 months	:	Diphtheria/tetanus/pertussis and oral polio vaccine
4 months	:	Diphtheria/tetanus/pertussis and oral polio vaccine
6 months	:	Diphtheria/tetanus/pertussis and oral polio vaccine
1 year	:	Measles/rubella or measles/mumps/rubella and tuberculin test
1½ years	:	Diphtheria/tetanus/pertussis and oral polio vaccine
4–6 years	:	Diphtheria/tetanus/pertussis and oral polio vaccine
14–16 years	:	Tetanus

Immunisation schedules

Schedules should not be rigidly interpreted. Primary courses can be commenced at any age after the first 3 months, though clearly the immunisation schedule is designed to protect children against infectious disease as early as possible and at the ages at which they are particularly at risk. Children over the age of 10 should not be given diphtheria vaccine unless they have previously been Schick tested and found to be Schick positive.

The intervals between immunisations must also be interpreted flexibly. In the presence of a pertussis epidemic three doses of pertussis vaccine may be given at monthly intervals to afford rapid immunisation. If the intervals between immunisations in the primary course are longer than those indicated in the immunisation schedule, there is no need to restart the course. This is most important in view of the hazards of reaction when too many doses of tetanus toxoid are given.

For travel abroad no additional immunisations are required for children under 1 year. Smallpox vaccinations should not be a requirement for international travel in view of the eradication of the disease. Yellow fever vaccination is required for those travelling in Central Africa and northern areas of South America. This is obtainable from designated yellow fever vaccination centres. Cholera vaccine is required for parts of East, Central and West Africa, the Middle East and Asia.

Uptake of immunisations (%), England and Wales

Year	Measles	Diphtheria	Pertussis	Tetanus	Polio
1966	—	76	74	76	73
1968	—	79	78	79	77
1970	34	80	79	81	79
1972	52	81	79	81	80
1974	53	80	77	80	79
1976	47	75	39	75	75
1978	48	78	31	79	78
1980	51	80	34	80	80
1981	53	81	41	81	81

Immunisation against typhoid and paratyphoid A and B is recommended for all travel outside Northern Europe, Canada, United States, Australia or New Zealand. In giving these immunisations for children travelling abroad at least 3 weeks should separate the administration of two live vaccines. International certificates are available for yellow fever and cholera immunisation, the former being valid for 10 years, the latter for 6 months. A combined typhoid, paratyphoid A and B, and cholera vaccine is available which can be given in two doses, separated by 4 weeks.

For those travelling to areas of poor sanitation, protection against hepatitis is recommended by means of immunoglobulin; however, there is also a limited supply of live vaccine. Drug prophylaxis against malaria is recommended for Africa, Central and Southern America, South East Asia and parts of the Middle East. Progruanil should begin on the day before travel and should continue for at least 4 weeks after return.

As the requirements for immunisation for travel abroad are subject to variation, up to date advice may be obtained from Ross Institute of Tropical Hygiene, London School of Hygiene and Tropical Medicine (Telephone Number 01-636-8636).

SOME INFECTIONS FOR WHICH IMMUNISATION IS AVAILABLE

Polio

There are three distinct strains of poliovirus — types 1, 2 and 3 — and there is very little antigenic overlap. Clinical diagnosis is confirmed by recovery of virus from faeces (excreted for weeks) or throat swab (present for days) or by serology. Type I has been associated with most of the major epidemics and shows the greatest propensity to cause paralytic forms of the disease. Isolate the patient whilst the virus is present in the stools.

The clinical course of poliomyelitis

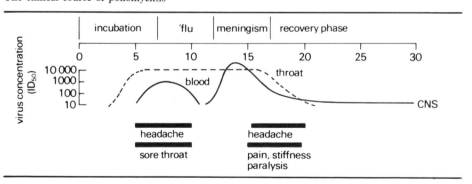

Vaccines. OPV (oral poliovirus vaccine — Sabin) is a mixture of live attenuated strains of virus types 1, 2 and 3, grown in monkey kidney or human fetal diploid cell cultures. This vaccine is given orally on three separate occasions during which both local gut immunity and systemic immunity are established. IPV (inactive poliovirus vaccine — Salk) is an inactivated vaccine given by injection. It is effective but does not give any protection against replication of poliovirus in the gastrointestinal tract and hence there is no transmission to non-immunised individuals.

Effectiveness. Introduction of the two forms of vaccine has led to the virtual elimination of polio in the UK. The duration of immunity is less with IPV than OPV though IPV may be more effective in tropical countries. Antibody in breast milk may diminish its effectiveness. With OPV the attenuated virus is excreted in the stool and may spread to other members of the family, and vaccinate them as well. It is recommended, however, if they are unvaccinated that the parents are offered the vaccine at the same time. UK and USA rely on the cheaper OPV. In other countries, e.g. Holland and Sweden, IPV is used. Recently in Holland 80 cases of polio occurred in a group opposed to immunisation on religious grounds but no cases occurred in the general population.

Contraindications. Polio vaccine is contraindicated in pregnancy and in those with immune deficiencies.

Reaction. Vaccine associated polio resulting from reversion to a more virulent strain in the gut occurs in recipients of OPV at a rate of one case per 4–5 million doses and one case per 2–3 million doses in unvaccinated contacts.

Measles

The maculopapular rash of measles appears first behind the ears and on the face, spreading downwards to form a confluent blotchy appearance. Encephalitis affects 1:1000 children who have measles; 15% of these will die and 25% suffer cerebral damage. In developing countries in the presence of malnutrition, the severity and mortality of measles is much higher than in the UK. Diarrhoea, a sore throat and desquamation of the rash with pyoderma are common. Uncomplicated measles requires only rest, fluids and an antipyretic. Prophylactic antibiotics are not indicated. Where secondary infection does occur this is likely to be a mixed bacterial infection and a broad spectrum antibiotic is required. The patient is infections from a few days before to 7 days after the onset of the rash. Vaccine can be safely given to those incubating the illness or with a doubtful history of the natural illness.

Measles

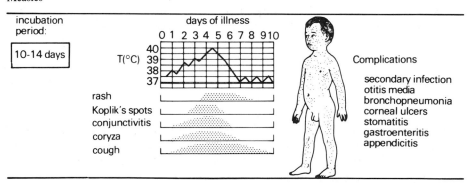

The vaccine is a freeze dried aqueous suspension of live attenuated measles virus grown on fibroblast tissue culture derived from chick embryos.

Measles quarterly notifications, England and Wales

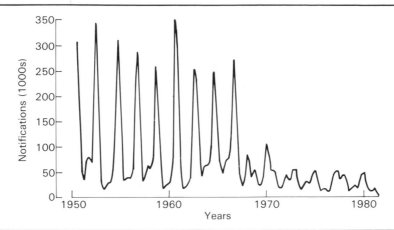

Effectiveness. If the vaccine is given after 15 months of age, protection is greater than 95% and long lasting. If immunised at 9 months, 60% have no antibody rise and at 13 months 10–15% have no antibody rise. Vaccine may be less effective in developing countries because of difficulty in keeping it cool in storage.

Measles vaccine is particularly indicated for children in nurseries or residential care and in those with any chronic debilitating illness. However, the aim is to achieve a high vaccination rate and so suppress measles altogether. They appear to have achieved this in the USA.

Contraindications. Live vaccines should not be given to children with any immune deficiency. Allergy to eggs is not a strong contraindication in view of the purity of modern vaccines. The vaccine contains small amounts of various antibiotics, (polymyxin, neomycin, kanamycin, penicillin, streptomycin) and should not be given to those known to have severe allergic reactions to these. If there is a history of febrile convulsions 0.5 ml of a 2.0 g% solution of human normal immunoglobulin in a separate syringe will reduce the incidence of febrile reactions from 15% to 3% without affecting the immune response.

If there is a history of epilepsy (a strong family history) some would delay immunisation until the age of 2–3 years and others cover the immunisation with a 2 week course of anticonvulsants. However, the benefit of avoiding the naturally acquired measles far outweighs the risk of vaccine.

Reactions. Around 15% develop a fever, rarely a mild rash appears. There is a slight increase in the risk of a convulsion in the second week after the injection (1:10 000). In the National Childhood Encephalopathy Study where encephalitis followed measles vaccination of a previously normal child, 12 out of 14 made an uneventful recovery and two had mild defects. Whether this association can be related to the vaccine is uncertain. However, it does indicate that the risks are very few. The rate of convulsions and encephalitis from naturally acquired measles is far greater than the rates for the vaccine.

Passive immunisation. Suppression of measles can be achieved by giving human normal gammaglobulin and may be indicated at certain times in exposed children with chronic heart, lung or malignant disease. The recommended doses are under 1 year 250 mg, age 1–2 years 500 mg, age 3 years and over 750 mg.

Rubella

Diagnosis of congenital rubella rests on a combination of the clinical features and isolation of the virus from the stool. This may be obtained for up to 1 year after birth. The diagnosis may be supported by serological evidence. High specific IgM titres indicate a recent infection, the complement fixation test remains positive for 2 years, and the haemagglutination inhibition test, HAI, remains positive indefinitely.

Clinical manifestations of congenital rubella in the UK National Congenital Rubella Surveillance, 1971–75

Growth retardation, still births and spontaneous abortion are also common in congenital rubella

36%	Multiple defects	59%	Sensori-neural hearing loss
44.1%	Single defects	25%	Congenital heart disease
7.4%	Neonatal manifestations only	25%	Eye defects, e.g. microphthalmia, cataracts, pigmentary retinopathy
12.5%	Laboratory evidence only	25%	CNS defects, e.g. microcephaly, mental retardation
100%			

The vaccine is a freeze dried suspension of live attenuated virus grown in tissue culture cells of human or rabbit origin. It is given subcutaneously on one occasion only.

Effectiveness. After the initial rise antibody levels slowly decrease over the subsequent years so that reinfection may occur. However, this seems to be asymptomatic and is not associated with viraemia so that the objective of immunisation, fetal protection, is achieved.

Indications. In the UK rubella is offered to girls aged 10 to 14 with the aim of protecting their offspring from congenital infection. It is also offered to sero-negative women post-partum and to sero-negative women attending family planning clinics. In some countries it is offered to boys as well with the aim of reducing the prevalence of the infection in the community as well of course as giving individual protection to the girls.

Contraindications. Rubella vaccine is contraindicated in pregnancy. Women who have been vaccinated should not become pregnant in the next 12 weeks. Rubella vaccine should not be given to those with immune deficiency, thrombocytopenia and those sensitive to polymyxin and neomycin. It has been suggested that children with rheumatoid arthritis should not be immunised because of the possible association of rubella with this disease.

Reactions. Mild fever, rash and lymphadenopathy are sometimes seen. Arthralgia and arthritis are rare complications.

Vaccine uptake. In the UK, the uptake rate has risen from 71% to 83%, since an active campaign has been carried on. However there is wide regional variation with some regions as low as 61%. A higher vaccine uptake rate of 90–95% is re-

Rubella quarterly notifications from Royal College of General Practitioners National Study and the number of infants with congenital rubella by date of birth from the National Congenital Rubella surveillance programme

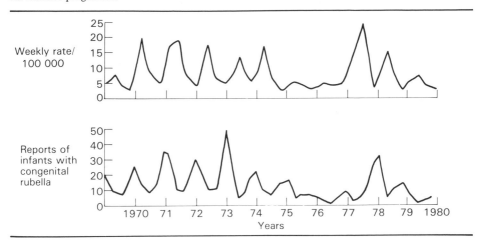

quired in order to reduce the incidence of congenital rubella. Seventy-five per cent of girls aged 11 to 14 are immune anyway due to natural infection so that a low rate of uptake would not materially change the epidemiology.

Whooping cough.
Pertussis is caused by the bacterium, *Bordetella pertussis*, though milder infection may occur from *Bordetella parapertussis* or *Bordetella bronchiseptica*. The incubation period is 7 – 14 days, the catarrhal phase 7 – 14 days, the paroxysmal phase 4 – 6 weeks and recovery usually takes a further 2–6 weeks. Complications include bronchopneumonia, convulsions and rarely bronchiectasis.

Erythromycin given in the catarrhal phase may attenuate the infection and it may be helpful if given as prophylaxis amongst infant contacts. Otherwise treatment depends on good nursing care, which may include oxygen, suction and tube feeding, plus the treatment of complications where they occur.

Prognosis is worst under 1 year of age. There was a case fatality rate of 0.9–2.6/1000 notifications in the 1977–79 epidemic, and large numbers required hospital admission. The infant is infectious from 7 days after exposure to 21 days after the onset of the paroxysmal cough.

Vaccine. Killed organisms of several serotypes of *Bordetella pertussis*.

Effectiveness. Protection rates of 85–90% are achieved, and if the illness does affect an immunised child the illness takes a milder form.

Indications. Pertussis vaccine is particularly indicated in children with chronic respiratory or cardiac problems. Early immunisation is advised because of the severity in infancy. Although not previously recommended over 3 years of age, this may be necessary to protect younger siblings or to increase herd immunity where it is very low. The upper age limit has now been extended to 6 years.

Reactions. Mild reactions are common, these may consist of local pain and

Immunisation history before onset of acute neurological illness in previously normal children in the United Kingdom, for every case there are two controls. The estimated attributable risk of serious neurological disorders occurring within 7 days after immunisation with DTP vaccine in previously normal children irrespective of outcome is one in 110 000 injections (95 per cent confidence limits, 1: 44 000–1:360 000) (From 'Epidemiologic Reviews', Vol 4, 1982 'Whooping Cough and Whooping Cough Vaccine: The Risks and Benefits Debate', by D L Miller, R Alderslade and E M Ross

Vaccine	Interval from immunisation to reference date*		
	0–3 days No. %	4–7 days No. %	8–14 days No. %
Diphtheria-tetanus-pertussis (DPT) vaccine			
Cases	19 2.4	13 1.7	9 1.2
Controls	12 0.8	13 0.8	23 1.5
Relative risk	4.2	2.1	
	(P< 0.001)	(P< 0.1)	NS
Diphtheria-tetanus (DT) vaccine			
Cases	5 0.8	10 1.3	9 1.2
Controls	7 0.4	9 0.6	24 1.6
Relative risk	1.7	1.8	
	(P> 0.2)	(P> 0.2)	NS

* Reference date for case was date of onset of acute neurological illness; reference date for control was date when control reached the same age as index child on day of onset.

swelling or a transient irritability, pyrexia and fretfulness, or very occasionally screaming episodes. They are not contraindications to giving further vaccine. The incidence of serious neurological consequences following pertussis vaccination was investigated by the National Childhood Encephalopathy Study (Miller et al, 1981). Reviewing 1000 cases of encephalitis and encephalitis-like illnesses between the ages of 2 months and 3 years reported from 1976 to 1979, only 35 occurred in children who had been immunised with pertussis vaccine in the previous 7 days. This gave a relative risk of 2.4 compared to control children. Thirty-two of the 35 had no previous neurological abnormality. A year later two had died, nine had developmental retardation and 21 were normal. The attributable risk for serious neurological disorder in previously normal children within 1 week of pertussis immunisation was found to be one in 110 000 injections and the risk of persistent abnormalities 1 year later one in 310 000 injections.

Contraindications. The contra-indications recommended by the UK Joint Committee on Vaccination and Immunisation fall into two categories: those relating to certain groups of children in whom vaccination is absolutely contraindicated; and those relating to groups of children in whom whooping cough vaccination is not absolutely contraindicated but who require special consideration as to its advisability, bearing in mind the need to balance the possible increased risk of vaccination, against the increased hazard to the child from an attack of whooping cough. In such cases it may be considered wise to seek the advice of a suitable specialist such as a paediatrician or paediatric neurologist.

Vaccination should not be carried out in children who have:
— a history of any severe local or general reaction (including a neurological reaction) to a preceding dose;

— a history of cerebral irritation or damage in the neonatal period, or who have suffered from fits or convulsions.

There are certain groups of children in whom whooping cough vaccination is not absolutely contraindicated but who require special consideration as to its advisability. These groups are:

— children whose parents or siblings have a history of idiopathic epilepsy;
— children with developmental delay thought to be due to a neurological defect;
— children with neurological disease.

For these groups the risk of vaccination may be higher than in normal children but the effects of whooping cough may be more severe, so that the benefits of vaccination would also be greater. The balance of risk and benefit should be assessed with special care in each individual case.

A personal or family history of allergy has in the past been regarded as a contraindication to vaccination but this is now no longer regarded as a contraindication. Allergy is but one of many myths that have arisen.

It is advisable to postpone vaccination if the child is suffering from any acute febrile illness, particularly respiratory, until fully recovered. (Minor infections without fever or systemic upset are not regarded as a contraindication).

Whooping cough quarterly notifications, England and Wales

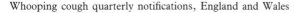

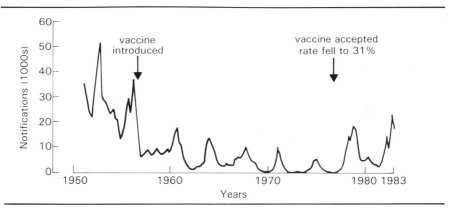

Tuberculosis

Although tuberculosis is declining in incidence it remains an important disorder in the United Kingdom. 613 deaths from this cause were notified in 1979. In developing countries the incidence of tuberculosis is far greater. Transmission is by droplet spread from an individual with open TB. This may be an elderly relative or in the case of school children, an adult with undetected tuberculosis working in the school. Many infections are sub-clinical. The incidence of tuberculosis in the UK is about 30 times higher for respiratory disease and 80 times higher for non-respiratory disease in immigrants from the Indian subcontinent compared to the native population.

Presentation of tuberculosis

Asymptomatic primary infection	Primary infection and its complications	Secondary infection
Routine tuberculin testing	Hypersensitivity phenomenon	Miliary tuberculosis
Routine X-ray Contacts of known cases of tuberculosis	Vague ill health Respiratory symptoms due to primary focus or lymph node obstruction Primary tonsillar infection with cervical lymphadenitis Mesenteric lymphadenitis	Tuberbulous meningitis Bone or joint involvement

Clinical presentations. Unlike chickenpox or measles, the diagnosis of tuberculosis cannot be made simply and quickly on clinical grounds alone. The diagnosis requires a high level of clinical suspicion.

1. Detection in asymptomatic subjects. Tuberculosis may be identified by tuberculin testing of contacts of known cases of tuberculosis or by routine tuberculin testing prior to BCG vaccination. It may also be identified in subjects having routine chest X-rays for any reason. The use of X-ray as a mass screening measure has been abandoned. If a contact has a negative Heaf test it should be repeated after a further 6 weeks for the test remains negative in the incubation period.

2. Presentation of sensitivity reactions. Where primary infection has been recent, children may present with a febrile illness, erythema nodosum or phlyctenular conjunctivitis.

3. Vague ill health. Children may present with primary tuberculosis with very ill-defined symptoms indeed. There may be complaints of lethargy, tiredness and poor growth. Liver or splenic enlargement may be felt.

4. Pulmonary tuberculosis with complications. This may present as (a) pleural effusion, the onset often being acute with breathlessness, pyrexia, pain and occasional cough; (b) caseation and cavitation; the child has a cough, is constitutionally ill, and has a pyrexia. If the cavity connects with the main bronchi, the bacilli may be found in the sputum or in gastric washings; (c) bronchial obstruction due to mesenteric lymph node enlargement. This may cause either collapse or hyperinflation if the obstruction is incomplete.

5. Miliary tuberculosis. This may be acute or slow in onset. The features are

Notification of tuberculosis (numbers) in England and Wales (1979)

	Under 1	1	2–4	5–9	10–14	15–19
Respiratory tuberculosis	19	41	124	242	280	338
Meninges and CNS	2	1	5	3	4	3
Other	5	8	39	67	104	144
Total	26	50	168	312	388	485

again non-specific with fever, weight loss and lethargy. The liver and spleen may be enlarged and choroidal tubercles may be seen as yellow dots along the retinal vessels.

6. Tuberculous meningitis. This is another feature of haematogenous spread and presents with a lymphocytic meningitis, low CSF sugar and bacilli visible on microscopy of the fluid.

7. Bone or joint involvement. This may present as synovitis or osteitis which may affect the spine, hip, knee, ankle, elbow, wrist, hands or feet.

8. Primary tonsillar infection with cervical lymphadenopathy. This is usually caused by the bovine type of tuberculosis.

9. Abdominal tuberculosis. This is a very rare presentation in the UK and is also caused by bovine infection. It presents with abdominal pain and the finding of a doughy abdominal mass. If the mesenteric lymph nodes rupture tuberculous peritonitis will occur. It is of gradual onset with abdominal distention, fever, vomiting and weight loss.

Diagnosis. The diagnosis is not always easy. The various forms of tuberculin testing to be described below probably provide the easiest approach. Radiology is sensitive but non-specific, sputum microscopy is specific but very insensitive, and culture is slow.

Mantoux test. The Mantoux test is not generally used for routine screening because of the difficulty of intradermal injections in small children. An intradermal injection of 10 units of PPD (purified protein derivative) in 0.1 ml is made on the flexor surface of the left forearm. If active tuberculosis is suspected a lower starting dose of 1 unit should be used. The date, time, position of injection and strength of solution are recorded and the site inspected 72 hours later. An area of induration of 5 mm or more is regarded as a positive reaction.

Multiple Pressure Techniques. This uses either the Heaf gun or the Tine test using disposable plastic units. The Heaf gun is set to penetrate the skin at 2 mm, except for children under 2 years when it is set at 1 mm.
The gun is sterilised by dipping into spirit and then flaming. The gun must be allowed to cool before use. Purified protein derivative equivalent to 100 000 units per ml is applied to the skin over the flexor surface of the left forearm. Sites containing superficial veins should be avoided. The dropper used to apply the solution should not be allowed to touch the skin. The Heaf gun is applied over the drop of solution and the handle depressed, which causes the needles to pierce the skin. The result is read at 72 hours.
Using the Tine test, the plastic cover is removed and the four prongs pressed into the skin for a few seconds on the flexor surface of the left arm. This is also read at 72 hours. The Tine test is weaker than the Heaf or Mantoux test, so that severe reactions to it are less common. However this may also be a disadvantage in that it may produce some false negatives. Grade I and grade II reactions may be due to avian tuberculosis or previous BCG. All children with Grade III or IV reactions require X-ray and further follow-up. False negative results may be ob-

Tuberculin test

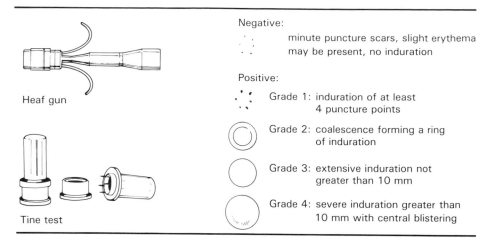

Heaf gun

Tine test

Negative:

minute puncture scars, slight erythema may be present, no induration

Positive:

Grade 1: induration of at least 4 puncture points

Grade 2: coalescence forming a ring of induration

Grade 3: extensive induration not greater than 10 mm

Grade 4: severe induration greater than 10 mm with central blistering

tained from using materials that have deteriorated or if the material is injected too deeply. Negative results may also be obtained if the test is read too soon or too late or if the test was performed near an inflamed area of skin so that rapid removal of tuberculin occurred. If the skin is still wet after cleaning before tuberculin is applied, it may be diluted. False positive results may be obtained by a burn from the Heaf gun which simulates a positive response. Local infection or rupture of small blood vessels may also simulate a positive response.

BCG. (Bacillus Calmette-Guerin) is a freeze dried live attenuated bovine strain of mycobacterium tuberculosis. It is derived from the original bacillus grown by Calmette and Guerin in 1921. The vaccine is given by intradermal injection of 0.1 ml into the skin just above the insertion of the deltoid muscle. It is given to tuberculin negative children following Heaf or Tine testing at the age of 11. It is also given to newborn babies of immigrant families in a dose of 0.05 ml. An alternative technique of administration is by multiple puncture vaccination but this is not suitable for newborn babies. Immunisation results in a small papule appearing 7–10 days later which enlarges over a few weeks and often ulcerates.

BCG is an intradermal injection. Subcutaneous injections cause abscesses and ugly scars

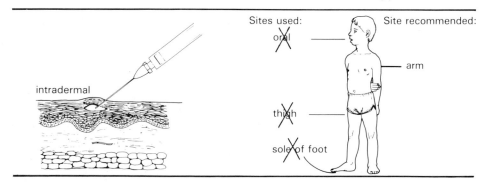

intradermal

Sites used:
oral

thigh

sole of foot

Site recommended:

arm

Peeling occurs in 6–8 weeks with a residual scar forming. Mantoux conversion usually occurs within 3–4 weeks of vaccination though this is slower in babies. It should occur in 100% of subjects vaccinated with potent vaccine.

Abnormal reactions to BCG are often the result of faulty injection technique. Ulcers that are slow to heal are best treated with gauze dressings or with tetracycline ointment should secondary infection occur. An abscess may develop at the site of BCG. These are usually sterile and heal rapidly once they are drained. Lymphadenopathy is common and generally requires no attention.

Effectiveness. Immunity seems long lasting with an 80% protective effect after 15 years. TB can occur after BCG immunisation but it effectively prevents the development of miliary tuberculosis or tuberculous meningitis.

The decision to immunise against tuberculosis at birth depends upon the incidence of the disease. The World Health Organisation recommended that where 5% of children aged 10–14 years have been infected, BCG should be given at birth. Where the rate is more than 2% but less than 5% it should be given on school entry and in places with less than 2% of children affected at 10–14 years, BCG should be given at 12–13 years. As the incidence of tuberculosis is falling a point may well be reached where routine BCG immunisation may be an uneconomical proposal and regular tuberculin testing offered as an alternative. Where tuberculosis does occur in people who have already received BCG the diagnosis may be delayed.

Chemoprophylaxis. Chemoprophylaxis may be given under several circumstances. If the mother of a newborn baby is infected with active pulmonary tuberculosis the baby may be given Isoniazid by mouth and Isoniazid resistant BCG. Secondary chemoprophylaxis is given to those with asymptomatic disease. This will include children with strong tuberculin reactions on routine testing, children who are contacts of patients with tuberculosis whose tuberculin test converts from negative to positive, and any tuberculin reactor under the age of 5. Chemoprophylaxis is generally given for nine months with either Isoniazid alone or combined with Ethambutol or Rifampicin.

Tetanus

Tetanus is caused by a gram positive anaerobic spore bearing organism called *Clostridium tetani*, found universally in soil. The disease is caused by the neurotoxin produced by the organism. After an incubation period of 5–14 days there are progressive intermittent muscle spasms, often triggered by stimuli such as noise or touch.

Tetanus is now rare in this country. It is very easily prevented but the clinical disease still carries a high mortality.

Vaccine. This is a formol inactivated toxoid given in conjunction with an adjuvant by intramuscular or subcutaneous injection often combined with diphtheria and pertussis vaccines. After a primary course of three immunisations and the booster at school entry, immunisation is only required every 10 years. If a wound occurs outside that 10-year period a single booster dose only is required. Too frequent reinforcing doses, as may occur in children who have frequent accidents, are unnecessary and can provoke quite severe hypersensitivity reactions. Human tetanus immunoglobulin may be given to unimmunised persons suffering major wounds with a high degree of contamination.

Diphtheria

Diphtheria is caused by one of three strains of *Corynebacterium diphtheria*. The infection may be caught from infected individuals or healthy carriers. The incubation period is 2 to 7 days after which the toxin causes destruction of the superficial epithelium of the respiratory tract producing obstruction. The toxin can also produce a myocarditis and lower motor neurone symptoms.

The Vaccine is a formol inactivated toxoid adsorbed to a mineral carrier. Diphtheria vaccine should not be given to children over the age of 10 without preliminary Schick testing as hypersensitivity reactions are likely to occur in those already immune.

The Schick test is an intradermal injection of a sterile diluted filtrate from a culture of the diphtheria bacillus injected into the anterior surface of the left forearm. 0.2 ml of a control fluid is injected into the corresponding right forearm. In those who are immune no reaction will occur to the injection of the Schick fluid. The results should be read at 24–48 hours. For a positive reaction the left arm should show a flush 10–50 mm in diameter. Similar reactions in both arms which fade rapidly are non-specific and not due to the toxoid. A reaction on both arms, but greater on the side where the toxin has been given should be regarded as positive. Only Schick positive people should be given diphtheria vaccine.

Mumps

Mumps is most common between the ages of 5 and 15 years. There is a high incidence of subclinical infection and the disease has a low infectivity. The incubation period is 14–21 days. There may be a prodromal disease with fever, headache and malaise lasting 1–2 days before parotid gland enlargement occurs. This can be unilateral and settles within 7–10 days. Orchitis affects 20% of post-pubertal males but sterility following this is rare. Aseptic meningitis is quite common. Treatment is conservative, consisting of analgesia and a fluid diet if mastication is painful.

Mumps may be transferred from 7 days before the onset of symptoms until the swelling has subsided. However, the period of maximum infectivity ends after the first few days of parotid swelling. It is not necessary to exclude contacts because of the low infectivity of the disease.

Vaccine. This is a live attenuated virus grown on chick embryo tissue cultures. It is given subcutaneously on one occasion at any age after 15 months. Contraindications are the same as other live viruses and egg allergy. In view of the rarity of serious complications to mumps widespread vaccination has not been adopted in the UK.

Hepatitis

Hepatitis A is the commonest cause of jaundice in older children and has an incubation period of 15–50 days, commonly 28 days. Passive immunisation may be considered for family and close contacts. The period of communicability to hepatitis A is from 1 to 2 weeks before to 1 week after the onset. Human hepatitis B immunoglobulin is also available and reduces the incidence and severity of disease after parenteral exposure to hepatitis B virus.

Vaccines. A Hepatitis B vaccine has recently become available. It is in short supply and use is restricted to those at special risk such as laboratory workers or dialysis patients.

Other vaccines available

Influenza vaccine is available and can provide 60–70% protection. It is particularly recommended for special risk groups, such as children with chronic respiratory disease. A meningococcal vaccine is also available and its use may be justified in areas with a high incidence of the disease. However the vaccine does not include Group B meningococci which are the commonest cause of meningococcal meningitis in this country.

A pneumococcal vaccine has been developed and is being evaluated. It may be of particular value in those children with sickle cell disease, in those who have no spleen and in certain forms of immune suppression. The pneumococcus is also commonly involved in otitis media and such a vaccine could have a significant effect on the incidence of otitis media.

Rabies remains a threat and a specific rabies vaccine is available. It is a killed vaccine obtained from embryonated duck eggs infected with the virus. Two to 3 primary doses at monthly intervals are required followed by a booster 6 months later. Antiserum is required for unimmunised individuals who are presumed to have been bitten by a rabid animal.

Smallpox immunisation is no longer required due to its global eradication. Some countries (Chad, Cambodia and Madagascar) still require valid international certificates for entry.

INFECTIOUS DISEASE FOR WHICH PASSIVE IMMUNISATION ONLY IS AVAILABLE

Chickenpox

Chickenpox is a highly infectious disease caused by the same virus as that which causes herpes zoster in adults. It is contracted by droplet spread either from other children with chickenpox or from adults with herpes zoster. The lesions appear as crops, being most dense on the trunk. Complications include secondary infection and encephalitis. In the latter case complete recovery can be expected in 80% of cases. A haemorrhagic form does occur as do fetal and neonatal infections but all are very rare. Treatment is conservative and consists of analgesics in the prodromal phase and antihistamines and topical applications such as calamine lotion for the local skin lesions. If infection in the mouth is extensive, oral toilet is most important.

The affected child is infectious from one day before the rash appears until the crusts are all dry.

Chickenpox

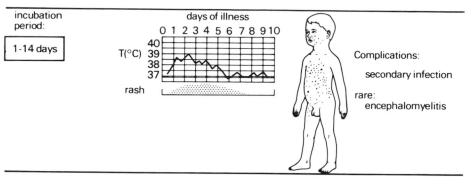

incubation period:	days of illness	Complications:

1-14 days

T(°C)

rash

Complications:

secondary infection

rare:

encephalomyelitis

Prevention. Children with immune deficiency who are known to have been in contact with chickenpox or herpes zoster should be given human Anti Varicella immunoglobulin. This is effective if given within 3 days of exposure.

INFECTIONS FOR WHICH IMMUNISATION IS NOT AVAILABLE

Gastroenteritis

Gastroenteritis remains an important clinical problem. It is still the fifth commonest cause of death in children under 1 year in the United Kingdom and on a global basis accounts for the death of 5 million children per year. In its milder forms it is still one of the commonest clinical problems presenting to paediatricians working in the community.

In any child presenting with gastroenteritis consider the clinical condition and its management; the cause, whether it is infective or whether other conditions such as cystic fibrosis or coeliac disease should be considered; if infective, the source of infection; and general public health measures designed to protect other children.

In outbreaks in schools, nurseries etc. food poisoning should be considered

	Sources	Clinical	Incubation
Salmonella	Common in raw meat and may contaminate cooked or processed meat if not stored properly	Mainly diarrhoea	12–48 hours
Clostridium welchii	Cooked meat. Resistant to heating. Multiplies in anaerobic conditions	Abdominal pain Diarrhoea	12–48 hours
Staphylococcus	Meat Sweets Food handler is a carrier	Vomiting	30 mins–6 hours.
Baccillus Cereus	Fried rice kept warm	Vomiting	1–6 hours
Campylobacter	Poultry	Diarrhoea Abdominal pain Prolonged prostration	12–48 hours

Clinical assessment of dehydration

Sign	5% dehydration	10% dehydration
Skin	Loss of turgor	Mottled, poor capillary return
Fontanelle	Depressed	Deeply depressed
Eyes	Sunken	Deeply sunken
Peripheral pulses	Normal	Tachycardia, poor volume
Mental state	Lethargic	Prostration, coma

The duration of history, the presence of the symptom in other children and any history of recent travel abroad or contact with recent arrivals from abroad, must be obtained particularly when dealing with immigrant populations. If the child is happy, alert and feeding normally and has less than 5% dehydration, then the child should be managed at home.

Children with more than 5% dehydration or where conservative management at home fails, should be admitted to hospital. The treatment of mild gastroenteritis is with clear fluids. Standard glucose electrolyte solutions are available in sachet form and are very easy to use in the home.

The duration of treatment must be indicated and the parents given precise instructions on what to do if improvement does not occur or if there is further deterioration. For the mildly affected child, milk may be given in a more dilute form for 1 day, gradually increasing the strength back to full strength over the next 2 days. In the more severely affected child the glucose electrolyte solution should initially be given for 24 hours, small feeds are then offered every 1–2 hours. Some families may not be able to cope even with this simple routine; in which case the child will need to be admitted to hospital. It has been known for the parents to continue the 'advised' half-strength feeds for long periods and one child was seen recently with quite severe malnutrition because the duration of treatment was not stated and half strength feeds were continued for several months.

Public health measures include isolation of affected children, a search for contaminated food or carriers, ensuring that children are free of infection before they return to school, and investigation of other members of the family. It is important to enquire into the occupation of the parents and others who live in the household. If father is a chef in the hospital, tread carefully. Enquire about basic hygiene and reinforce the need for hand washing and care when handling food.

Respiratory tract infections
These are undoubtedly the commonest conditions encountered by doctors. They probably constitute half of all episodes of illness in pre-school children and a third in older children. Primary school children can be expected to have six to eight upper respiratory tract infections a year. Most are of viral origin. Naturally parents get very concerned particularly if their child misses a lot of school. This usually leads to therapeutic demands which we cannot meet. It always helps to explain about the nature and frequency of the illnesses. It does more good and less harm than unnecessary antibiotics and ineffective linctuses. A minority of respiratory infections are severe and life threatening. In the initial stages they may appear mild and insignificant, only to progress to severe croup or bronchiolitis.

It is often the second rather than the first consultation that matters most. Parents of young children with respiratory tract symptoms must be warned of this remote possibility and positively instructed not to delay a second consultation if the child rapidly progresses to more severe illness.

Colds cause feeding and sleeping difficulties particularly in young babies. They may progress to otitis media or lower respiratory tract infections and may be the prodromal symptoms of other disorders. Young babies can be given nasal drops such as xylometazoline (Otrivine nasal drops) twice daily. Parents however must be shown how to use them properly with the child recumbent and the head lying back. Children over 1 year can be given oral decongestants. Paracetamol or aspirin will relieve discomfort or pyrexia.

Acute otitis media should be considered in any child with an acute illness. A broad range of clinical manifestations may accompany otitis media, from a mild constitutional upset to a high pyrexia, screaming and vomiting. The cause is usually a virus or pneumococcus or *haemophilus influenzae*. Treatment consists of amoxycillin for pre-school children and penicillin V for older children. Analgesics are frequently forgotten in young children who cannot complain directly about pain. Eight weeks later the ears should be inspected to ensure that chronic changes have not occurred and the child's hearing must be tested.

Tonsillitis and pharyngitis usually are viral, but clinical appearances are frequently deceptive. Bacterial causes include *Haemophilus influenzae* and *Beta haemolytic streptococcus* infection. If the latter is diagnosed penicillin V for 10 days is indicated because of the risk of rheumatic fever or glomerulo-nephritis. In young children the symptoms of tonsillitis may be non-specific, such as fever, malaise and vomiting. The throat should always be inspected. Children with recurrent tonsillitis often show a marked flush on the medial border of the anterior faucial pillars. Such children may be considered for tonsillectomy particularly if they miss a lot of school, if they have associated hearing problems or quinsy. The size of the tonsils is usually not relevant as their visible appearance depends upon the degree to which the tonsil is buried in the tonsillar pit. Very rarely the tonsils may be large enough to cause obstruction to the airway and sleep apnoea. The size of the tonsils in children decreases from about the age of 8.

Croup consists of barking cough, hoarse voice and stridor. It is caused by the para-influenza virus, influenza virus or respiratory syncytial virus. The symptoms are frequently worse at night. The treatment for children with mild symptoms is humidified air which in the home is best delivered in the bathroom or kitchen.

Careful clinical assessment is required to observe changes in the child's clinical condition and the need for admission to hospital. An increase in respiratory rate, tachycardia, sweating and increase in intercostal recession with cyanosis, are all reasons for prompt admission to hospital.

Acute epiglottitis. This needs to be distinguished from the viral causes of stridor. It is caused by *Haemophilus influenzae* bacterium and the onset is far more rapid and severe. Attempts to examine the throat in the home are absolutely contraindicated and the child should be referred immediately to hospital.

Bronchitis. Bronchitis in childhood is usually viral in origin. The cough may be productive and children tend to swallow the sputum. Examination reveals widespread rhonchi. Children with asthma are far too frequently diagnosed as having recurrent bronchitis. Where there is obvious wheezing, asthma is a far more likely diagnosis and bronchodilators should be given. For bronchitis antibiotics are not needed unless there is secondary infection. The child will benefit from a light diet, frequent fluids and a cough suppressant can be useful in the night.

Bronchiolitis affects children between the age of 2 and 6 months. It is caused mainly by the respiratory syncytial virus. It commences as a coryzal illness with increasing difficulty in breathing and raised respiratory rate. The child has difficulty feeding and examination shows a hyper-inflated chest with poor air entry and widespread crepitations and rhonchi. In mild cases the child can be nursed at home but increasing tachypnoea is an indication for urgent admission to hospital. Antibiotics are not required.

Pneumonia. In childhood this may be viral or bacterial in origin. Physical examination may correlate poorly with the pattern of consolidation shown on chest X-ray. The child may be severely ill and cyanosed with poor air entry and crepitations. The presence of cyanosis, tachypnoea or severe constitutional symptoms warrant admission to hospital. The most common bacterial cause is pneumococcus or haemophilus. Treatment is with amoxycillin.

Scarlet fever is caused by a group A *Haemolytic Streptococcus*. In its classical form it starts with a follicular tonsillitis. The rash consists of a punctate erythematous eruption which blanches on pressure. The cheeks are usually flushed and there is circumoral pallor. Initially the tongue is covered with white fur which progresses to the classical beefy-strawberry tongue. As the rash fades the skin desquamates particularly on the extremities. Treatment is with penicillin. Following 24 hours of treatment the disease ceases to be infective.

Scarlet fever

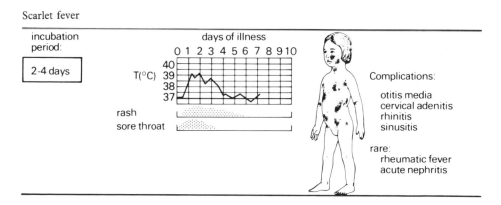

Glandular fever is found most often in older children and in adolescents and is caused by the Ebstein Barr virus. The incubation period is 4–14 days. Tonsillitis, with plaques of white thick exudate, petechiae on the palate, and generalised lymphadenopathy with splenomegaly may be found. A fine macular rash can occur particularly if ampicillin has been given. Complications include hepatitis, pneumonitis, carditis, meningitis and encephalitis. The diagnosis is confirmed by positive Paul Bunnell test and the finding of atypical mononuclear cells.

There is no specific treatment for the condition. Convalescence may be prolonged and may cause particular problems for children at critical times in their education.

Roseola Infantum is characterised by a high fever often reaching 40°C. As the temperature falls, a rash consisting of discrete small macules appears on the trunk. The child improves clinically as the rash appears. Recovery is always uneventful though the high temperature may be associated with febrile convulsions.

Infestations

Head lice are commonly identified by routine examination of school children. They do not respect social boundaries. The reactions of parents and school teachers may be totally out of proportion to the severity of the problem. The louse has a bad name. Simple treatment with Malathion 0.5% solution (Prioderm), which is also used against greenfly, is most effective.

The hair should be shampooed and combed after 12 hours. The solution is irritant and must be kept out of the child's eyes; it is also highly inflammable — no smoking please. Dead nits will be seen in the hair for several days after treatment and merely need to be combed out. Malathion is often alternated with carbaryl to prevent resistance. A female louse can lay up to 300 eggs in a lifetime. They are found exclusively on humans and live on sucked blood. The lifespan of the adult is about 1 month and the eggs take 5–11 days to hatch.

It is not usually necessary to exclude children from school because of lice and they may return to school as soon as treatment has been carried out. With tact and a well organised service parents are usually happy to cooperate which ensures that children are treated promptly. The heavy handed approach, excluding children from school and issuing cleansing orders is not really required.

Scabies. Classically, scabies affects the interdigital spaces, the flexor surfaces of the wrists, elbows, axillae, back, inguinal and genital regions. The red elevated

Scabies and lice

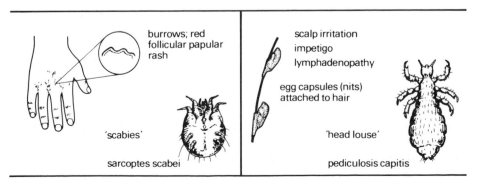

burrows; red follicular papular rash

'scabies'

sarcoptes scabei

scalp irritation
impetigo
lymphadenopathy

egg capsules (nits) attached to hair

'head louse'

pediculosis capitis

tracks are visible and they cause intense irritation. Secondary infection is very common after scratching and in these circumstances the diagnosis may be very difficult and is frequently missed.

Two important principles must be observed: treat all members of the household whether there is clinical evidence of infection or not; and the entire skin surface below the neck should be treated. Gamma benzene hexachloride 1% cream applied once after a bath is usually sufficient. For children under two years it is also necessary to treat the face. Crotamiton cream has the added advantage of being an anti-pruritic. Although the treatment outlined will kill all the acari, itching will continue for several days and patients must be told of this in advance.

The poor acarus has as many friends as the head lice. Children need only be excluded from school until the treatment has been effected.

Fleas. Children with fleas present because of recurrent bites. Not only the child but also their cats and dogs should be inspected to find the culprit. The flea is a small brown wingless creature 2–2.5 mm long with a laterally compressed body. Treatment is with Monosulfiram lotion for the children and DDT for the animals.

Intestinal infestation (Worms and others) There is a very wide range of intestinal parasites. In the Western World they are relatively rare. If they are suspected most can be easily identified in the laboratory by sending freshly passed stools for examination for ova, cysts and parasites.

Threadworms are the most common and present as pruritis ani. Secondary infection may occur because of the scratching. The 'threads' may be seen in the stool or by examination of ova collected from the perineum with adhesive tape swabs. Piperazine for 7 days is the drug of choice and it is wise to treat the entire family. Merbendazole given as a single dose is also effective. Attention to basic hygiene in order to break the cycle of oral/anal infection is most important.

Giardia lamblia, a flagellate protozoon is the other commonly found intestinal parasite in this country. Malabsorption may result from infection and treatment is with metronidazole (Flagyl).

Skin disease

Warts and verrucae. Although these complaints are given very few lines in many textbooks, they are a major drain on the time of the school nurse. Elaborate precautions are taken to prevent children with verrucae from swimming while those with warts on their hands and faces seem to be allowed to enter the swimming bath with impunity. Warts in young children on the hands and face often disappear spontaneously and if they are not causing difficulties, can be left alone. If treatment is required freezing them with liquid nitrogen or carbon dioxide is rapid and effective. The treatment may need to be repeated. If this treatment is not available, verrucae may be soaked daily in 3% formalin after abrasion with pumice. The area should be soaked for 10–15 minutes and treatment continued for 6 weeks. Alternatively 25% salicylic acid can be applied. An adhesive plaster stuck over the verruca with a hole to expose the affected part can be applied with another piece placed on top of the ointment to maintain contact. Podophyllin and glutaraldehyde are also useful preparations to be used in a similar way. However conscientious the treatment many verrucae seem to resist and the wisdom of large scale and frenzied attack on the poor wart virus is to be questioned. Most warts if left alone will disappear in 12—24 months.

Impetigo may be caused by either streptococcal or staphylococcal infection. The lesions start as a vesicle but rapidly develop the typical golden brown crusts. Mis-diagnosis and the application of steroid creams can produce extremely rapid spread of the infection. This error can easily be made and impetigo can easily complicate atopic eczema which is already being treated with topical steroids. Scabies or pediculosis may also be the initiating factor in impetigo. Recurrent impetigo may indicate that the patient is carrying staphylococci. They are usually nasal carriers and the application of chlorhexidine and neomycin cream may relieve this problem. The addition of an antiseptic to the bath water may also prevent recurrence. For severe impetigo, a systemic antibiotic such as erythromycin is given; for limited areas a local application of fucidin or neomycin cream may be used.

Impetigo is highly infectious and children should not attend school until the lesions are healed. Bacteriological confirmation of the diagnosis should be sought wherever possible.

Ringworm infection is commonly seen affecting either the scalp (tinea capitis), the body (tinea corporis) or the foot (tinea pedis). The scalp lesions often present with concern about hair loss, and a circumscribed patch may be seen with scaling of the skin and breaking of the hairs. On the body the ring like lesions are easily recognised. The diagnosis of fungal infections is not always easy on clinical grounds alone. Scrapings for microscopic examination are usually taken. Topical treatment with Whitfield's ointment is effective though newer preparations such as econazole or clotrimazole are probably preferable. It is essential that treatment should continue for at least 10 days after apparent cure. Tinea rubrum does not respond well to local agents and griseofulvin should be used here. This is also indicated for scalp infection, nail infection and animal ringworm. Children with ringworm of the body can normally attend school during treatment though those with ringworm of the scalp should normally be excluded until treatment is successful. Children with infection of the feet (athlete's foot) need not have any restrictions placed on them.

Fungal infections

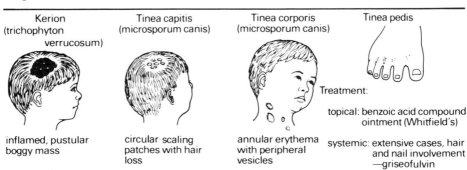

Kerion (trichophyton verrucosum)	Tinea capitis (microsporum canis)	Tinea corporis (microsporum canis)	Tinea pedis
inflamed, pustular boggy mass	circular scaling patches with hair loss	annular erythema with peripheral vesicles	Treatment: topical: benzoic acid compound ointment (Whitfield's) systemic: extensive cases, hair and nail involvement —griseofulvin

FURTHER REFERENCES AND READING.

Adjaye N, Azad A, Foster M, Marshall W C, Dunn W 1983 Measles serology in children with a history of measles in early life. British Medical Journal 286:1478

Campbell A G M 1983 Measles immunisation: why have we failed? Archives of Disease in Childhood 58: 3–5

Christie A B 1974 Infectious Diseases: Epidemiology and Clinical Practice. J & A Churchill London

DHSS 1977 Control of Communicable Disease in Schools.

Dick G 1978 Immunisation. Update Publications

Griffith A 1980 Problems in the use of vaccines. Journal of the Royal College of Physicians of London 14: 184–190

Grant J P 1981 The State of the World's Children, 1981–82. UNICEF, New York

Hull D 1981 Interpretation of the contraindications to whooping cough vaccination. British Medical Journal 283: 1231–1233

Joint Committee on Safety of Medicine and the Joint Committee on Vaccination and Immunisation, Whooping Cough. HMSO (National Childhood Encephalopathy Study)

Joint Committee on Vaccination and Immunisation 1982 Immunisation against infectious disease. DHSS

Miller et al 1981 British Medical Journal 282: 1595–1599

Noah N D 1980 Vaccination Today. British Journal of Hospital Medicine 24: 533–538

Peckham C, Marshall W C, Dudgeon J D 1977 Rubella vaccination of schoolgirls: factors affecting vaccine uptake. British Medical Journal 1: 760–761

Price J F 1982 BCG vaccination. Archives of Disease in Childhood 57: 485–486

Sheppard S, Smithells R W, Peckham C, Dudgeon J A, Marshall W C 1977 National Congenital Rubella Surveillance 1971–75. Health Trends 9: 38–41

Smithells R W, Sheppard S, Marshall W C, Miller S 1982 National Congenital Rubella Surveillance Programme 1971–81. British Medical Journal 285:1363

11
Problems
0–5 years

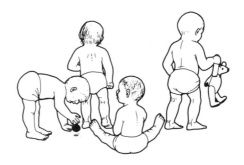

This chapter is concerned with some of the more common paediatric problems encountered in the community. Others are discussed in the chapters on infection and nutrition. Just because they are common, it does not follow that they are trivial, clinically uninteresting or that their management presents no challenge. It requires much time, experience, knowledge and enthusiasm to deal with them correctly. Economically, they consume a large amount of professional time and resource.

When a parent seeks medical advice about some aspect of her child's wellbeing, it is important not only to look at the presenting problem but also beyond it to see what it means in terms of a family's daily life. The doctor may consider the 'problem' of little importance or as a variation of normal development. Comments which are intended to be reassuring like 'he'll grow out of it', 'don't worry it's normal', are not particularly helpful. They take no account of the stresses imposed upon the family or of the secondary effects that the parents' fatigue or frus-

Problems encountered in the first 18 months of life (from Ounsted & Simons, 1978)

Type of problem	No. of children having one or more attacks					
	No. of episodes					Total children
	1	2	3	4	5+	
Upper respiratory (e.g. bad colds; sore throats)	26	24	9	4	7	70
Otitis media	18	—	1	2	1	22
Lower respiratory (e.g. chesty coughs; bronchitis)	11	3	1	1	1	17
Gastro-intestinal (e.g. vomiting and/or diarrhoea)	33	5	—	—	—	38
Exanthemata	27	1	—	—	—	28
Skin (e.g. severe nappy rash, eczema, impetigo)	21	1	—	—	—	22
Trauma	7	1	—	—	—	8
Other	31	4	—	2	—	37

tration might have upon the child. A little time should be spent explaining the wide range of normal behaviour and perhaps also exploring the parents' expectations of their child and his progress.

ADJUSTMENTS IN BECOMING A PARENT

Many of the problems encountered in the first year of life are expressions, at least in part, of the parents' inability to adapt their life-style consequent upon the birth of their child. The mother's own demands now become secondary to the demands of the child. Everyday tasks such as shopping, cooking and housework become more complicated. If the mother previously went out to work she may feel lonely or isolated at home. Fathers also need to adjust. Some may view the baby as a rival, others may resent the restrictions the child imposes on their social life. Some mothers feel that husbands have retained their freedom, whereas they have lost theirs. The prevalence of depression in working class mothers with pre-school children has been found to be as high as 42%. Much lower rates (5%) were found for middle class women and for mothers of older children.

The questions 'Have you looked after any babies before he was born?' and 'Is it what you thought it was going to be like?' may reveal that the expectations of many parents are unrealistic. They underestimate the amount of work and night disturbance and consequent fatigue that a young baby can bring. Many have had no previous experience of the care of young children other than for short periods of time. Some may not have attended ante-natal classes and have little appreciation of the skills required for child care. It is no wonder that such parents feel worried and insecure when faced with the responsibility of looking after a totally dependent baby. The answer to the question 'In spite of all this are you enjoying having the baby?' is usually 'yes'.

How the mother copes with her new baby depends very much on her personality, her ability to learn and adapt, and to seek and accept help from family, friends and professionals. It is obvious, but also needs to be stated, that the wellbeing of the parents is vital for the care of the child.

Bonding

In recent years much, perhaps too much, has been written about bonding. By bonding is meant the powerful, specific attachment between parents and child which enables care, protection, sacrifice and empathy to take place. Its origins are in the parents' own child rearing experience, it is facilitated by early contact between the mother and child and is more likely after a planned pregnancy. The baby is able to fixate on the mother soon after birth and can identify her by scent by the age of 6 days. There appears to be a sensitive period for attachment between mother and child. Bonding is inhibited by separation of mother and child, malformation of the child or an infant who is unresponsive.

FEEDING PROBLEMS

In any feeding problem the contribution of the child, the mother and the technique of feeding all need to be considered.

Drawings used to illustrate to parents the variations in feeding patterns

MR REGULAR	MR SMALL AND OFTEN	MR GUZZLE	MR TOPSY TURVY

A full history of the difficulties, observation of feeding technique, examination of the baby, recordings of growth as well as assessment of the mother's emotional state and the family situation as a whole are required. It is quite difficult to do harm to a child through incorrect feeding practice, however many mothers are led to believe so, and the anxiety that this causes can itself lead to difficulties in feeding. When mothers say '*He* doesn't know what *he* wants' she may well mean '*I* don't know what *he* wants' or '*He* is not doing what *I* expected'.

A baby who is difficult at feeding time creates tenseness in his mother, she may become angry and impatient which only aggravates the situation further. This interaction between the mother and baby needs to be explored. In most instances it is possible to reassure the parents that their baby is growing normally and not coming to any harm. However, advice given in the consulting room may not be adequate to resolve the issue. A visit to the home is often far more successful. This is primarily the role of the Health Visitor but the doctor should not always be excluded. Feeding difficulties can create a great feeling of despair and failure in mothers. The significance to her must never be underestimated and she must be given every opportunity of discussing her feelings.

Regurgitation. Many babies bring back a little of their feeds. Most inexperienced parents do not expect this to occur and interpret it as a sign of abnormality in their child. Telling them that their child is growing and developing normally and 'that there is nothing to worry about', may be reassuring but they still have to contend with constant damp patches on their shoulders, extra washing, the smell of half digested milk and the reluctance of others to handle their baby. Some may accept our reassurance happily, others may not and be unable to cope. The child may end up being admitted to hospital with a 'feeding problem'.

Rumination occurs when the child wilfully regurgitates feeds and seems to enjoy this process. The baby may be observed straining until the milk is brought back into his mouth. The problem may be eased by sitting the baby up after feeds and by thickening the feeds with gum (Nestagel) or the cheaper and more traditional arrowroot.

Recurrent vomiting. The frequent discovery of thick, slimy, half digested milk on the sheet next to the child is very suggestive of oesophageal reflux, with or without a hiatus hernia. Thickening the feeds, sitting the baby up after feeds and the use of alkalis and surface agents are often helpful. Very rarely metoclopramide administration may be justified. Care is needed because of the ease with which overdosage can occur causing symptoms like oculo-gyric crisis.

Projectile vomiting occurs in pyloric stenosis, and may be severe enough to cause dehydration. Visible peristalsis may be seen and test feeding reveals a palpable pyloric tumour. It is more common in male first born infants and tends to run in families.

Vomiting in the child who is ill and who is not feeding may be due to a wide variety of causes. Investigation of the child is required, and infection is the commonest cause found.

Crying with feeding

Crying associated with feeding may be a conditioned response to a tense and unhappy situation. It might be that the infant cannot cope with milk delivered too rapidly or too slowly. The child's screams may be due to impatience or the discomfort of swallowing air. The presence of local lesions in the mouth needs to be excluded.

The explanations of 'wind' or 'colic' are unhelpful, if they lead to tension in the mother-baby relationship being overlooked. Serious conditions such as intussusception with vivid attacks of screaming may go unrecognised if the diagnosis of wind or colic is allowed to overshadow other possibilities. In some cases antispasmodics such as merbentyl are of benefit.

Babies vary as much as adults in the time taken to feed. Feeding may be prolonged but still normal, however respiratory or cardiac problems giving rise to breathlessness or fatigue need to be excluded.

Nasal obstruction also causes prolonged difficult feeding and is helped by decongestant nose drops given before feeds. Mothers need to be shown how to use these drops properly or they will be totally ineffective.

Immature babies or babies with neurological damage who have difficulty coordinating sucking and swallowing, can have great difficulty with feeding.

Stools

The appearance and smell of the stool and the frequency of bowel action can all cause anxiety if they differ from the parents' (or their advisors') expectations. They fear their child is not having enough or not eating the right food. Some breast fed babies pass infrequent stools every 2 or 3 days whilst others pass several stools a day. Those who pass infrequent stools can fill their napkins with devastating effects, and the need for a total change of clothes and a bath! The passage of green stools is often very worrying to parents though this is frequently a normal finding in breast fed children. The stools of a bottle fed baby are firmer and more smelly. Small dark dry stools may be due to inadequate feeding. The presence of fresh blood in the stool alarms most parents. It is usually due to an anal fissure caused by the passage of a large bulky stool, but sometimes there is no obvious cause. The use of local preparations such as 1% amethocaine or Anusol, with plenty of oral fluids usually allows a fissure or local inflammation to resolve.

In true diarrhoea the stool may be so liquid that it is mistaken by the parents for urine. The presence of black stools, very offensive stools or stools containing fat, mucus or large amounts of blood must be investigated.

The parents' description of the baby's stool may be exaggerated or inaccurate. It is therefore necessary but never a pleasant task personally to observe the stools that the parents described as abnormal.

Failure to thrive

Failure to thrive describes babies who fail to gain weight in the expected way. In a wide sense it may also include an associated developmental delay, misery or apathy. All need to be investigated, even in the absence of other abnormalities. Initiation of investigations should not occur after a single measurement unless the child is grossly underweight. He may be a small normal child growing below but parallel to the 3rd centile and whose parents are also small. Weighing without reference to a centile chart is worthless. Centiles for length and head circumference also need to be recorded and plotted. Weighing of babies must be properly performed. Scales must be calibrated and checked and the baby must be unclothed. Undressing the baby for weighing provides an opportunity for checking the overall appearance and nutrition of the child as well as identifying any signs of a non-accidental injury.

Factors in the giver. This is by far the commonest cause of failure to thrive seen in clinical practice. The phrase, failure to rear, is more precise. A wide range of factors may be involved and a detailed history of the entire family with particular enquiries about their infant feeding practices is required. In many cases it is found that an insufficient amount of food is being offered for the child's needs. In others the feed is too dilute. One mother was unaware that she had to increase the child's feed with growth and another when she was advised to give half-strength feeds because of vomiting and diarrhoea, continued to do so for 2 months after the child was better. In other families the diet may be nutritionally inadequate, consisting of bought sandwiches, chips from the shop and a variety of cheap crisps, soft drinks and sweets. Lack of money or, more commonly, poor budgeting may lead to the babies not being given enough. Those families who spend their limited income on cigarettes, alcohol and gambling also have a zero credit rating with the local stores.

Maternal depression may be another underlying factor, the mother may be so depressed or withdrawn that she is unable to respond to the child's needs. Other types of mental illness and any type of chronic illness in the mother will also reduce her capacity to meet the child's needs. Mothers suffering severe anaemia secondary to menorrhagia, thyrotoxicosis, tuberculosis, epilepsy, multiple sclerosis and arthritis fall into this category. The demands placed upon a mother with a large family particularly if she has no support, must not be underestimated.

Some parents, particularly those who themselves have come from very deprived backgrounds seem unable to perceive the child's needs. Their own needs may be so great and unsatisfied that they are unable or unwilling to put their child first. This lack of perception of the children's needs leads to other areas of neglect and non-accidental injury. The child may respond by becoming apathetic and non-demanding due to the lack of stimulation and social interaction. More specifically, parental indifference or irritability may condition the child to act negatively when fed.

Factors in the child. Within the child, immaturity or disorders of the central nervous system frequently give rise to difficulties in the mechanics of feeding. There may be difficulties coordinating sucking and breathing, and delay in the development of the ability to manage solid food. Any chronic disease, particularly respiratory or cardiac disease which gives rise to breathlessness or fatigue, can lead to failure to thrive. The child should be examined and investigated for signs of infection, particularly urinary tract infection. In spite of adequate intake the child may fail to thrive because of abnormal losses. Disorders such as cystic fibrosis, coeliac disease, bowel infection and infestation need to be excluded. Abnormal utilisation of food and inborn errors of metabolism are rare causes which need in-patient investigation. Surgical causes include oesophageal reflux and hiatus hernia; problems such as rumination rarely give rise to inadequate growth.

Management. Unless the problem is gross, initial examination with serial measurements of length, weight and head circumference, together with observation of the child's general condition, development and social history enable us to distinguish the child who is constitutionally small from one who is failing to thrive. Where the cause is underfeeding due to deprivation the infant usually gains weight on admission to hospital. Management involves not only improvements in the child's nutrition but also a broad educational and supportive programme aimed at improving parenting skills and helping the parents cope with their physical, mental and emotional problems. This second task is far more demanding than the first. Organisations such as family centres which can provide close support and education over a period of months, or intensive home visiting schemes by health or social work professionals or volunteers in programmes such as Homestart are helpful.

Failure to thrive?

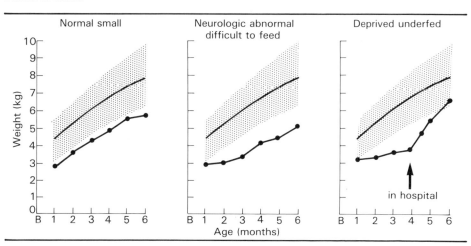

Toddler's diarrhoea

Toddler's diarrhoea is the name used to describe chronic diarrhoea commonly starting between the ages of 6 and 24 months and ceasing spontaneously before the age of 4. Characteristically the stools contain undigested food materials such as peas and carrots. The cause is probably a decreased transit time. The children are otherwise well and growth is normal. All that is required is reassurance to the parents. In persistent troublesome situations a course of aspirin which inhibits prostaglandins is worth trying.

Food forcing

Many children do not eat what their parents think they should eat. They deny their parents the satisfaction of providing them with good food. Food is central to many cultures and refusal to eat may be viewed almost as a personal rejection by parents. It may be a continuation of infantile feeding problems where anxiety by parents at feeding has conditioned the child to act adversely. Food forcing only leads to increased food rejection. In other instances the parents may only supply the food which the child will happily eat in order to avoid the conflict. This encourages the development of food fads and it is certainly not uncommon to see children brought up by desperate parents who claim that they are living on a diet of chips and fizzy drinks only.

One simple approach is to reassure the parents that the child is growing and developing normally (if that is the case) and then recommend they provide for the child the same meal as for the rest of the family and make no comment whether it is eaten or not. Quantities given should be small initially. Foods like biscuits or sweets between meals are withheld. This strategy is usually effective though the level of anxiety experienced by many parents makes it extremely difficult for them to carry out and they require a large amount of support during the programme. Occasionally admission to hospital is required to sort out just what is going on. Children do vary widely in the amount of food which they require and this variation in normal intake must also be explained.

Postnatal growth curves — all normal (from Davies & Williams, 1983)

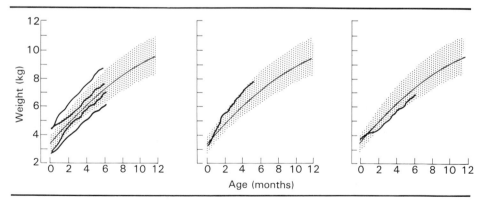

SLEEP DISORDERS

These are not disorders in the usual sense of the word in that failure to sleep through the night is sufficiently common to be recognised as part of a spectrum of normal sleep behaviour. However, it can be very disturbing for parents and often leads them to seek medical advice. By 3 months of age approximately 30%

of babies wake at night, this drops to 20% at 2, 14% at 3 and 10% at $4\frac{1}{2}$ years of age. However parents' expectations are that children should sleep through the night and that failure to do so is abnormal. There is also a wide variation in the amount of time spent asleep, normal 2 to 3 year old children may sleep from 8 to 17 hours. Without active management the problem is self-limiting and is rarely seen after the age of 5.

Anyone who has done a midnight ward round on a children's ward will know that children do not sleep solidly through the night but go through a sleep cycle with periods of wakefulness. Adults have similar patterns though their reaction is to turn over and go back to sleep after the period of wakefulness whereas the child may call out.

Sleep problems require individual analysis. Enquire about the child's daily routine and the parents' reactions when the child awakes. Anxiety in the child, fear of separation, particularly after episodes of hospital admission for the child, or the mother going away to have the new baby, may underlie wakefulness. Physical illness or discomfort from nappy rash, eczema or upper respiratory tract infection need to be excluded.

It is important to find out what really happens when the child wakes up, how soon the parents go to him, whether they respond with anger or comfort or whether they excessively reward waking by play and bringing the child downstairs. There are no rigid rules as to how a child should behave at night and what does occur depends on cultural patterns and what is considered tolerable or intolerable to the parents. Some parents will grasp the simple solution of bringing the child into their own bed while for others such a solution would be totally unacceptable. Inviting the parents to keep a record of the child's sleeping patterns may help them as well as you to get the problem into a better perspective. Although sleep problems can usually be managed from a clinic setting, it may be necessary to visit the home in the evening to record what really happens, rather than what the parents say happens or to support them in carrying out any particular programme.

Only an anaesthetist can effectively make a child sleep when he is not tired. The aim of management and investigation is to decrease the night disturbance for the parents. Admission to hospital is not necessary other than when parents are desperate for some form of relief which cannot be provided in any other way.

Sleeping problems in the month prior to interview (from Ounsted & Simons, 1978) age 18 months

	No. of children	%		No. of children	%
Getting off to sleep			*Waking during night*		
Always very difficult	11	7.0	Wakes more than once a night	17	10.8
Screams for 10 minutes	5	3.2	Wakes most nights	22	13.9
Cries few minutes	18	11.4	Wakes about twice a week	23	14.6
Talks, no crying	70	44.3	Rarely wakes	65	41.1
Drops off instantly	54	34.1	Never wakes	31	19.6
Total	158			158	

The following suggestions are offered for management of night time waking. None is a panacea but all may be helpful in a variety of families.

Stopping the struggle. Frequently the situation arises whereby the more the parents try and put the child to sleep the more the child is determined to stay awake. This is an unequal struggle. The instruction 'go to sleep' is usually totally ineffectual. One strategy is to advise parents to stop putting the child to bed but to observe for a few days the time at which he spontaneously falls asleep. Bedtime is therefore initially determined by physiological need rather than social custom. The child will often sleep earlier than he would under the previous conditions. The same sort of management is often useful in feeding difficulties, where food forcing by parents results in the child eating less and not more. Having established the normal physiological pattern of sleep for the child, it is usually possible to move bedtime in the required direction by 15 minutes per day until a more satisfactory result is achieved.

A good supper. Occasionally babies awake because they are hungry. This applies particularly to those infants who are slow to be weaned on to solid food. In this situation increasing the amount of food given at bedtime by the addition of solids may be useful.

A bedtime routine. A fixed bedtime routine is often useful in preparing for sleep. Thus putting the toys away is a concrete sign to the child that part of the day is finished. A bath and a bedtime story complete the ritual. Children cannot be expected to switch suddenly from active energetic play to sleep. A bedtime ritual helps the child to make the adjustment. Children may easily succeed in gradually increasing the length of the ritual to unmanageable proportions. This should be resisted. As with much of the advice given by paediatricians it is far more difficult to implement when the parents are tired at the end of the day.

Rocking. Rocking at a rate of 60 per minute is probably the oldest method of inducing sleep in infants. It is effective and calms both the parent and the child.

Don't over react. Sometimes it is a mistake to go to the child immediately he cries in the night for the child may cry briefly during a period of wakefulness and will go back to sleep spontaneously. Too quick and active a response may reinforce this undesired behaviour. However, leaving the child to cry for long periods goes against most parents' instincts, and prolonged crying may cause more parental discomfort than picking the baby up. Leaving the baby for up to 10 minutes (by the clock) followed by comforting the child, is far more effective than responding rapidly but with anger. In the case of breast fed babies the smell of mother's milk will arouse excitement and hunger in the baby so it might be more appropriate to send father instead; alternatively, if his mother awakes, the baby's cry may condition the let down reflex so feeding is a comfort to both. It is worth demonstrating to the older child that it is night time and that everyone else is asleep.

Comforters. Most children have some sort of comforter at night, be it a dummy, a favourite cuddly toy or a blanket. These are often a suitable stimulus for sleep and are vital equipment. A small light left on so that the child can see his surroundings when he wakes up has often been found to be useful. A waking up bag of assorted toys left in the cot at night, may effectively delay the child calling for his parents.

Star charts. For older children a star chart system with rewards for undisturbed nights can be very effective.

Drugs. Young children are surprisingly resistant to the effects of hypnotic drugs. Sometimes the only effect is an irritable child the next morning. However, trimeprazine tartrate (Vallergan) in a dose of 3 mg/kg given at night can be very effective. If it is, parents should not feel guilty about its use.

Outside factors may have a considerable influence. Complaints by neighbours about crying babies may cause considerable anxiety to the parents. Overcrowding, noise from the general environment or other discomforts may also be implicated.

A calm, sympathetic and systematic approach will be of benefit in most cases. There remain, however, a small number of children who require very little sleep and in whom the aim should be to prevent disturbance of the parents rather than to make the child sleep. Explanation to parents that the child is not coming to harm through not sleeping and that the child takes the amount of sleep that he needs, is most helpful.

Nightmares occur in most children at some time. However, frequent nightmares may reflect underlying anxieties. Encouraging children to talk about their dreams or to draw them, may give us better understanding. Close examination of social, family and school factors may indicate possible sources of anxiety leading to fear at night.

CRYING

The crying baby is a most potent stimulus for parental action. The reaction may range from comforting, to anger and to non-accidental injury. It may be a source of confusion or frustration. One mother commented that if a baby cries in a room of adults, half the adults will criticise the mother if she picks the baby up and the other half will criticise her if she does not.

Mothers are adept at recognising the cause of a child's cry. It may be hunger, boredom, tiredness, pain, the need for companionship or the discomfort of a wet nappy. Responding to the child's distress positively enables the baby who is totally dependent, to develop a sense of trust and confidence in the world about him. Failure to respond or a negative response to crying, increases the child's distress or eventually can lead to a withdrawn, apathetic state where the child whimpers or sobs. Although complaints of crying are most frequently a symptom of a problem in the child, it may also be a symptom of a problem in the family. Anxiety, marital disharmony or any other form of stress may present as 'a crying baby'. The conflict is between the needs of the child to be comforted and the needs of the parents to be relieved of the discomfort of the baby's cry and to carry on their own independent activities. Baby's demands may seem endless and the mother's ability to cope with them limited.

Management. The first stage is to exclude a physical cause. This is particularly likely in babies who do not usually cry excessively. Commonly found causes such as upper respiratory tract infection and otitis media can be excluded by examination. Crying may be a presentation of a more serious disorder such as intussusception or meningitis. To ascribe crying to teething or to 'wind' can be dangerous; it leads to serious problems being overlooked, and is often unhelpful.

Carrying and comforting the baby is the most obvious approach. Very often the use of a baby sling enables the mother to fulfill her daily activities and keep her baby in close physical contact with her. The use of the baby chair so that he can see his mother is another approach. Lying in a carrycot provides very little stimulation for a baby who is awake and alert. The hum of a vacuum cleaner or the rattle of a washing machine often fascinates young babies and distracts their attention.

Screaming accompanied by reddening of the face may be due to colic when dicyclomine (Merbentyl) may help. Taking the baby out in the pram or pushchair is also effective.

Excessive persistent crying which the mother is unable to settle requires admission to hospital not only to investigate the cause but also to relieve the mother. Parents must have this lifeline open and be made aware that this option is readily available even if other health workers are already involved. Some authorities provide a 24 hour crying baby service staffed by Health Visitors to advise when further action is required.

Teething

In the past, teething has been held responsible for a wide range of paediatric problems, such as convulsions, diarrhoea or bronchitis. In 1839 the Registrar General attributed 5016 deaths in England and Wales to teething. However, the claimed associations of teething with illness in the child are not causal. Teething probably does cause pain in some infants indicated by food refusal and thrusting of fingers into the mouth towards the site of the erupting tooth. Analgesics such as paracetamol do seem to be useful. The excess salivation associated with teething may cause coughing or choking if the infant does not keep pace with this excessive production. This may be wrongly interpreted as a sign of respiratory infection. The danger is that too many conditions may be ascribed to teething and that this diagnosis masks the search for other more important conditions.

Teething problems and temper tantrums (from Ounsted & Simons, 1978)

Teething troubles			Temper tantrums at 18 months		
	No.	%	Frequency of tantrums	No.	%
Very severe	4	2.5	More than once a day	10	6.3
Considerable upset	43	27.0	Every day	32	20.1
Minor upset	62	39.0	Two or three times a week	44	27.7
Negligible	36	22.6	Once a week or less	41	25.8
None	14	8.9	Never	32	20.1
				159	
Total	159				

FEBRILE CONVULSIONS

Febrile convulsions affect 30 to 33 children out of every 1000 in the first 5 years of life. There is often a family history of febrile convulsions. They are associated with a rapid rise in temperature leading to a generalised convulsion. The overall risk of recurrence during the next 2 years is 30–40% though the risk is higher overall for children under 18 months than those over 18 months. In children who are previously neurologically and developmentally normal, the long term risks are small. A few do go on to develop temporal lobe epilepsy and other forms of neurological damage as a result of a prolonged convulsion. The experience for the parents of dealing with a febrile convulsion is very alarming. Many believe that their child is dying. Much explanation and counselling is an essential part of management.

Usually, by the time the doctor arrives on the scene the child has ceased convulsing. If the child (or the doctor) is not that fortunate, then intravenous or rectal diazepam may be used. The latter is easier. Once the convulsion has ceased, a search must be made for the source of infection. This is generally an upper respiratory tract infection, though urinary tract infection and the possibility of meningitis cannot be ignored. In infants under 18 months a lumbar puncture is recommended to exclude meningitis (viral or bacterial) and in all children if there is any evidence suggesting meningitis.

When the initial episode is over, the nature of the convulsion and its relationship to the sudden rise in temperature must be explained to the parents. Parents still tend to wrap up children when they get hot and this should be discouraged. Some also tend to panic when the child is convulsing and may rush away from the child leaving him on his own while they summon help. Parents therefore need advice on how to manage a convulsion should it recur. The most important step is to put the child on his side in the recovery position. Forcible attempts to introduce spoons into the mouth to keep the airway 'open' are unnecessary and may cause damage to teeth and soft tissues. Rectal diazepam can be given by the parents. The management of further febrile episodes also needs to be discussed. The parents should be encouraged to undress the child, to cool him using tepid sponging and to give either paracetamol or aspirin to lower the temperature.

With repeated fits long term treatment may be indicated. However compliance

Febrile convulsions, age incidence and recurrence rate

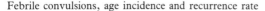

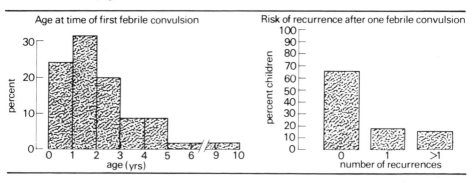

is often poor, so each case needs to be assessed individually. Features which would influence a decision in favour of prophylactic treatment are complex convulsions, prolonged convulsions, children under 1 year of age and those with a strong family history. Children with idiopathic epilepsy may also have febrile convulsions but they, in addition to this, have other convulsions unassociated with pyrexia. Likewise, children with previous neurological abnormality are more likely to need anticonvulsants.

Phenobarbitone, sodium valproate or phenytoin have all been used for prophylaxis. Some would use intermittent prophylaxis by giving rectal diazepam when the child has a pyrexia.

SKIN PROBLEMS

Babies are by nature spotty individuals and parents are by nature concerned by these perceived imperfections in their child. Most are harmless and transient, disappearing without treatment.

Capillary naevi or stork marks. They consist of small dilated capillaries usually on the eyelids, forehead or nape of the neck. They always disappear and parents can be reassured.

Strawberry naevi. These are not usually obvious at birth but appear shortly afterwards. They are raised, bright red lesions which grow over the first months of life. Many disappear by the age of 5 years and all will disappear by the age of 10. They go pale in the centre and gradually resolve. Except when they are at certain critical sites no interference is justified for they disappear without trace. Surgical removal will leave a scar.

Mongolian blue spots are seen in babies of African or Asian origin. They are usually found in the sacral areas but may be widespread on the back and legs. They disappear by the age of 3. They have been misinterpreted as bruises by those without experience, though fortunately such embarrassing incidents are rare.

Milia are tiny yellow-white spots seen over the face and nose of the newborn. They disappear within several days of birth and parents can be reassured.

Erythema Neonatorum is a very common erythema seen in the first weeks of life. As it may be quite widespread the parents may be most disturbed by the appearance. In addition to the general erythema, papules and pustules may develop. The lesions contain eosinophils and the blood picture shows an eosinophilia. The lesions disappear without treatment though the appearance may be unwelcome in baby's first photographs.

Port wine stain. The unilateral port wine stain on the face does not disappear as the other lesions do. In the Sturge Weber syndrome it may be associated with intracranial calcification and convulsions. Treatment is generally cosmetic.

Areas of depigmentation. Coloured skins often develop areas of depigmentation where there has been trauma, infection, ammoniacal dermatitis or other eruptions. Parents are often upset by the blotchy appearance that results after the initial rash has healed. However they can be reassured that it is only temporary.

Ichthyosis. The dry scaly skin of ichthyosis is generally inherited as an autosomal dominant condition and thus one or other parent is usually affected. The application of local oils or emulsifying ointment results in improvement but usually some evidence of the condition remains. It tends to improve as the child gets older. Urea cream is effective but is painful to apply if there are any small abrasions in the skin.

Seborrhoeic dermatitis is a common erythematous greasy yellow lesion found in the napkin area, behind the ears, on the scalp (cradle cap), forehead and eyelids. In its mildest form no treatment at all is required. Lesions behind the ears are easily missed and these should be treated as they can cause considerable pain and discomfort to the child as he is dressed and undressed. The lesions respond rapidly to topical cortico-steroid preparations but as secondary infection is common, the introduction of a combined preparation with an antibiotic or nystatin for monilial infection may be required. Cradle cap in its mildest form can be left untreated. However parents often press for treatment of even minor degrees of the condition. Wash the hair to remove the scale and apply salicyclic acid and sulphur preparations.

Ammoniacal dermatitis. This is basically an ammonia burn caused by breakdown of the urea in urine by bacteria. The rash consists of a widespread erythema in the napkin area with individual ulerated lesions. It does not involve the flexures. Prevention by changing napkins at adequate intervals is important. The use of one-way nappy liners keeps the bottom dry. The simple measure of washing the bottom with clean water when nappies are being changed is probably a more effective measure than applying creams on top of the damaged skin.

Where ammoniacal dermatitis is established leaving the bottom exposed to the air usually leads to rapid improvement. Many proprietary preparations consist merely of creams containing a weak acid to neutralise the alkalinity of the ammonia. Adequate washing and rinsing of napkins is important. The use of fabric softeners is not recommended. Rinsing the napkins in a weak vinegar solution of one tablespoon of vinegar to a gallon of water and letting this dry, is a traditional but effective therapy. The vinegar acts as a weak acid to neutralise ammonia. If simple means are not effective or if circumstances make it impractical to follow this advice, then the use of topical corticosteroids also works. Secondary infection is common particularly with monilia so if the rash fails to clear up add an antibacterial agent or nystatin.

Monilia. Infection causes a bright red erythema in the napkin area spreading from the anus and involving the flexures. Monilia may also be seen in the mouth as white spots on the buccal mucosa or tongue which unlike milk cannot be removed. Nystatin applied to the skin and mouth lesions is treatment of choice. It is important to continue it for sufficiently long to prevent recurrence. Frequently the mouth lesions have not resolved after a 7 day course and a further few days treatment is required. Recurrence of monilia after successful treatment suggests an outside source of infection and it is wise to check the mother for monilial vaginal discharge and treat her if necessary.

MINOR INFECTIONS

Snuffles. When parents bring the infants to Child Health Clinics they commonly complain that the child has, or has just had a 'cold'. Where the child is well, the discharge is clear and where there is no associated feeding difficulty, generally the parents can be reassured and no treatment provided. If nasal discharge is associated with other symptoms, particularly difficulty with feeding, then treatment is required. The use of ephedrine before a feed and last thing at night or xylometazoline nose drops twice daily often relieves the difficulty. However, parents must be shown the correct technique of instilling nasal drops with the head well down. They should be advised to see their doctor again if this difficulty persists. The nasal discharge may be an initial symptom of a more generalised upper respiratory or lower respiratory infection or may be the prodromal symptom of any of the ordinary infectious diseases of childhood, such as measles. Where the discharge is purulent, many infants tend to spread the infection over the rest of their body surface. A nasal swab is often useful in the identification of organisms causing associated skin lesions.

Sticky eyes. Eye infections are another common finding in infancy. Most infections can be treated with chloramphenicol eye drops. As with the use of nasal drops, parents need to be instructed in their use or the drops may never effectively reach their target. They need to be used 4 hourly and the parent encouraged to continue the treatment for an adequate period of time and not to stop after 1–2 days when the eye appears better. Recurrent infections or clear, watery discharge from the eyes may be due to blocked naso-lacrymal ducts. In this situation a mild discharge needs no treatment. If it persists beyond the age of 8 or 9 months then the child should be referred so that the naso-lacrymal ducts can be probed and syringed. Most however resolve spontaneously before this time.

Administration of medicine!

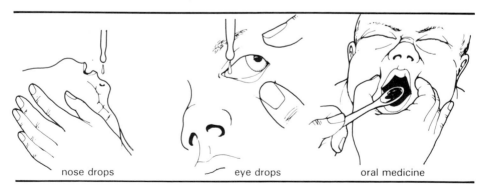

nose drops   eye drops   oral medicine

MINOR SURGICAL PROBLEMS

Tongue-tie

In the past tongue-tie was a fashionable diagnosis treated by cutting the frenulum of the tongue. Normal growth of the tongue ensures that the insertion of the frenulum into the base of the tongue becomes sited further and further back. If the infant cannot protrude the tongue through the lips then the tethering may be sufficiently severe to interfere with either feeding or the development of speech. Both are very rare.

Undescended testes

This ought to be an easy condition to diagnose in the newborn period before the cremasteric reflex has developed and therefore before the testes are retractile. However, many are still not identified until the child is much older when clinical examination can be far more difficult. If both testes are found to be well down in the scrotum at birth, repeated examinations which are extremely unwelcome to schoolboys are not indicated. The incidence of undescended testes at birth in full term normal deliveries is 2.7%. Fifty per cent have descended by 7 months and 75% by 1 year, giving an incidence of 0.7% at 1 year. After this age spontaneous descent does not occur and referral for surgery is required. Eighty per cent of undescended testes are ectopic and have strayed from the normal line of descent. They are most commonly palpable in the superficial inguinal pouch but may be also found in the perineum, femoral triangle or pubic area. Incomplete descent of the testes accounts for the remaining 20% of cases in which descent of the testes may be arrested at any point during the migration from the abdomen, through the inguinal canal into the scrotum. The testis may be intra-abdominal or within the inguinal canal, muscle coverings usually causing it to be impalpable in this position. Retractile testes are easily confused with truly undescended testes in older boys. Examination of the boy in the squatting position enables muscle relaxation and for the testes to be easily seen to come well down into the scrotum. Eighty per cent of undescended testes are unilateral.

Surgery is required for the following reasons:

— *Cosmetic and psychological*. This may well be the most important reason for treating the children before they enter school.
— *Fertility*. In bilateral cases almost all are sterile if the testes are not brought down into the scrotum before puberty. Histological changes are seen in undescended testes at the age of 2 years. Results in terms of fertility are very good after surgery but are much better for cases of ectopic testes than in those where descent is incomplete. Fertility after surgery is not 100% because some testes have not descended because they are abnormal. Sometimes at operation very little testicular tissue can be found. This may warrant investigation for chromosomal or endocrine disease. The undescended testis is also more prone to trauma and torsion.
— *The risk of malignancy*. There is an increased risk of malignancy in the undescended testes. The risk might not be avoided by orchidopexy but does bring the testis into a position where it is easily palpable and observed.

Treatment for the ectopic testis is usually easy and orchidopexy is performed by an inguinal approach. In cases of incomplete descent an abdominal approach is required. Early surgery may be required because of an associated hernia or because of pain suggestive of torsion. Surgery is usually performed between the ages of 3 and 5 years unless associated hernia or pain suggestive of torsion demand earlier action.

Circumcision

Circumcision is one of the most ancient of all surgical procedures, it is still widely practised today though largely for religious reasons. Approximately one-sixth of the male population of the world has been circumcised.

Whilst the child is in nappies the foreskin acts as a protective device for the glans and meatal ulcers are not seen in uncircumcised children. Parents often expect the foreskin to retract at an age when the foreskin is still adherent to the glans. Eighty per cent are still adherent at 6 months and 10% at 2 years. Forcible retraction of the foreskin can cause tearing of the adherent tissues which heal by fibrosis giving rise to phimosis.

The medical indications for circumcision are phimosis or paraphimosis. In true phimosis the foreskin is tight, leading to ballooning of the foreskin during micturition and a poor stream of urine. Paraphimosis results from forcible retraction of the foreskin with the latter being trapped in the retracted position. Simple pressure on an adrenaline soaked gauze may relieve this but a general anaesthetic is often necessary. A dorsal slit may be required to reduce the paraphimosis.

Hypospadias

Minor degrees of hypospadias may be easily missed on examination particularly when the orifice is glandular. In more severe cases there may be associated curvature of the penis and surgical repair is required. Circumcision is contraindicated as the foreskin may be required for the reconstructive procedure.

Hernias

Umbilical hernias are extremely common in the newborn period and nearly all disappear spontaneously by the time the child goes to school and most much earlier. Parents should be reassured of the likelihood of spontaneous disappearance. In the past they have been treated with various forms of strapping and it is still not unusual to see them treated in the 'traditional' manner with an old penny stuck on with sticky tape.

Inguinal hernias are far more likely to strangulate in the infant than in the adult. The child should therefore be referred for urgent surgery. A narrow processus vaginalis which does not permit herniation of bowel, may present as a hydrocoele. If it does not resolve in the first few months of life then referral for surgery is indicated.

ORTHOPAEDIC PROBLEMS

Children are frequently seen because of parents' concern about their legs. Parents may worry that the legs turn in (in-toeing) or that they turn out (out-toeing), that the feet are too flat or the toes crooked. There is a large range of variation in the posture and gait of young children. Virtually all of these eventually correct themselves without any external interference.

Intoeing

This occurs when the child stands or walks with one or both feet deviated medially. There are three major causes for intoeing: metatarsus varus, medial tibial torsion and persistent anteversion of the femoral neck in relation to the shaft.

Metatarsus varus consists of an adduction of the forefoot in relation to the hindfoot. A deep vertical crease is seen medially. The majority correct spontaneously without intervention. If the adduction is rigid and cannot be passively corrected or if there are associated neurological signs, then orthopaedic assessment is indicated. Full spontaneous resolution may take to the eighth birthday to be complete.

Metatarsus varus

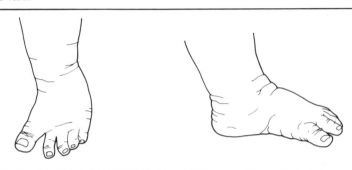

Medial tibial torsion. Outward bowing of the tibia associated with medial tibial torsion (twisting) commonly gives rise to an intoeing gait. If this intoeing is passively corrected and the feet placed in the neutral position, then the patellae point outwards. Medial tibial torsion usually resolves by the age of 3–4 years.

Medial tibial torsion needs to be distinguished from rickets in which the whole skeleton is affected and from Blount's Disease. Instead of the smooth curve of the tibia normally seen there is a sharp medial angulation just below the knee. In this condition osteotomies are often required to prevent progression of the deformity.

Orthopaedic problems

Medial tibial torsion and outward bowing   Knock knee   Femoral retroversion

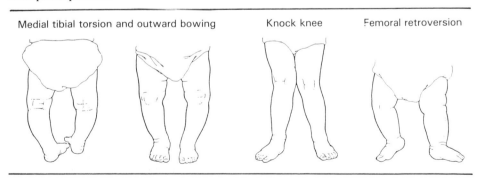

Anteversion of the femoral neck in relation to the shaft. In this condition the femoral neck is anteverted (twisted forwards) and causes the rest of the lower limb to turn inwards. An intoeing gait alters the range of internal and external rotation of the hip. The normal range of internal rotation of the hip is 50–55 degrees. In patients with femoral anteversion internal rotation may exceed 90 degrees and external rotation is reduced. Observation shows that the children stand with the patellae pointing inwards, the so-called squinting patallae, and they run in an awkward manner throwing their legs out to the sides. They sit in a characteristic position which has been labelled the television position with the hips in a high level of internal rotation. Nearly all correct spontaneously by the age of 8. A few remaining cases may be treated by osteotomy after that age though this is probably seldom justified and it does not appear to cause any significant functional disability.

Anteversion of the femoral neck, standing, sitting and clinical demonstration

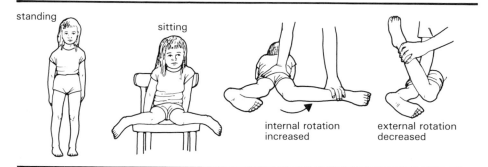

Out-toeing

In this condition the children develop a characteristic Charlie Chaplin type stance with feet rotated outwards. The cause of this is retroversion (outward twisting) of the femoral neck in relationship to the shaft. The effect on rotation is to increase the range of external rotation to 90 degrees or more and there is often no internal rotation at all. The position therefore is the opposite of that found in femoral anteversion. Provided there is no associated neurological abnormality, the condition corrects spontaneously by the age of 2.

Knock-knees (Genu valgum)

Knock-knee is present to some degree in 75% of all children during growth and may be increased where there is joint laxity. Its progress may be plotted by measuring the inter-malleolar distance. Distances of up to 9 or 10 cm can be expected to correct spontaneously without treatment. In the few cases that persist, treatment by osteotomy in late childhood or early adult life is satisfactory. Knock-knee can of course be associated with other orthopaedic conditions such as rickets.

Flat feet (Pes Planus)

In this condition, if it can be regarded as a condition, the medial arch of the foot rests on the ground in the weight bearing position. Reassurance is all that is required; valgus insoles or foot exercises are unnecessary. If shoe wear is excessive then an insole might reduce the cost of shoe repairs until the condition improves spontaneously.

The common and benign type of flat foot must be distinguished from pathologically flat feet. Here the foot may be painful and rigid. When the child stands on tiptoe the medial arch is not restored. In addition there may be evidence of neurological disorders such as cerebral palsy, increased joint laxity such as in Marfan's syndrome or abnormalities of the tarsal bones such as in congenital vertical talus.

Crooked toes.

Children are frequently brought with complaint that their toes are not straight. The toes may be seen to be either over-riding or under-riding one another. In the newborn this does not matter and many seem to improve with weight bearing. The feet may become painful with callous formation when the toes are squeezed into shoes that are too tight. Strapping the toe to its straight next-door neighbour may result in some improvement. Most require no active management other than the wearing of comfortable supportive shoes.

BEHAVIOUR PROBLEMS

Toilet training

Toilet training can be a time when the child's desire to please his parents may be constructively concentrated or a time when the child's own will and negativism reaches its peak. Toilet training needs to be carried out in the right atmosphere, a mixture of calmness, enthusiasm and praise. Under conditions where there is much discord at home, where there is a new baby or where there are other stresses and changes occurring within the family, toilet training is much more likely to be presented as a problem. Some parents have unrealistic expectations of the child's ability to control his bladder and commence toilet training at the age of several months. However, 2 years is a far more realistic age. By then the child has independent mobility to get to the toilet or pot and can be taught to pull his pants down and up and also to wash his hands. Thus toileting can become a totally independent function. It is also a powerful weapon. When all else fails to gain the parents' attention, the agitated cry of 'wee-wee' is guaranteed to secure rapid cooperation from the attending adult. Likewise the anger associated with such manipulations by the child or by failure may result in increasing negativism and resistance.

Although 2 years is the average age for commencing toilet training, there are still many children who are not ready to appreciate what is required of them. The competition amongst parents to have their child dry or the temptation to relieve themselves of the volume of nappy washing may cause demands to be made of the child which he does not understand and which he cannot fulfil. Motivation also varies, some children dislike the discomfort of wet nappies more than others.

Toilet training may be simply introduced by demonstration. Children copy what their parents do, however parents vary in their reluctance to provide this experience for their children. Without it however, what is required of the child will appear to them as somewhat of a mystery; a secret and private act. Putting the child on the pot at regular periods during the day and providing praise for micturating into the pot is usually all that is required. The length of time needed for success may vary considerably and parents must be willing to accept accidents in the early days, to wash extra pairs of trousers and dresses and to mop up the occasional puddle on the floor. Training pants are useful. Toilet training is more easily carried out in the summer in the garden than in winter indoors on the best carpet.

Various aids are available; these range from musical potties which play a tune as soon as the child micturates into it, to wetting dolls which may be used as a model for teaching the child. Azrin and Fox have described a system of toilet training in less than a day. This involves the use of behavioural principles, a wetting doll and encouragement of the child to consume large volumes of fluid to provide more intensive practice of micturition. It requires total concentration on that day for the purpose of toilet training. Not only can it be successful, it can also be fun for both parents and children.

Temper tantrums

Temper tantrums are sufficiently common to be regarded as normal! Only 20% of children of 18 months were reported never to have temper tantrums. It is one form of the negativistic behaviour commonly seen at this age. However the frequency and severity varies widely from one child to another. Temper tantrums are an expression of the child's own will.

On this topic as in many others it is much easier for the doctor to give advice to the parents than for the parents to take it. Regular support on a weekly basis is required.

One recommendation is to ignore the unwanted behaviour. This rests on the observation that the tantrum soon ceases once the child realises he is not being observed. The reverse of this, in which the child receives attention or is given the object that has previously been refused and which initiated the temper tantrum, only serves to reinforce the undesired behaviour. However, in the short term it is often easier for the parents to 'give in' for the sake of peace and quiet than to stick to their decision. It is well to remember our own behaviour as parents. Who, at some time or other, has not given in to tantrums for the sake of personal comfort or to avoid social embarrassment? Where temper tantrums become more persistent, it is useful to record the situation in which they occur and to get the parents to produce a written record of the temper tantrums from day to day. With this written information it is often easy to see that they only occur in particular situations and that with a bit of planning these situations can be avoided. The parents may also be able to observe the early events leading up to a temper tantrum and to divert the child to some other activity before this occurs. Some parents would do this naturally and instinctively and others require instruction. Demonstration, which may also place the paediatrician in a vulnerable position, is a more concrete method of teaching the parent than by verbal advice. Punishment is ineffective as this in itself may represent a form of attention to the child. Extreme uncontrolled anger by the parents provides a model of behaviour similar to the child's own temper tantrum and from which appropriate behaviours cannot be learned. Parallel to telling the child the behaviour is not acceptable, it is probably far more important to reward appropriate behaviour and to teach the child what these appropriate behaviours are. From the child's point of view it may seem that the most frequent word the parent uses is no, and from the parents' point of view a similar statement may be made. It is far more difficult to deal with temper tantrums if the parents are tired or suffering from other types of social or environmental stress.

Breath-holding attacks

In some children, either caused by temper or pain, the child ceases respiration at expiration and becomes cyanosed. In a few children this may progress to unconsciousness or a convulsion. Although alarming to the parents these attacks are benign and cause no permanent harm. Their history is typical. They need to be distinguished from other causes of loss of consciousness or convulsions.

Head banging

Head banging in normal children, as opposed to the mentally handicapped, does not carry with it any evidence of damage or psychological disturbance. It occurs at bedtime and usually stops spontaneously before the age of 5. Head banging may be associated with emotional deprivation.

Rocking

This also has little significance other than in the mentally handicapped. A few children who are deprived and withdrawn, may exhibit excessive rocking as a satisfying means of self stimulation though for the majority of children this symptom has little significance.

Thumb and finger sucking

Sucking is part of normal development. It provides comfort for the child and should not be discouraged. Although the favourite finger or thumb may become pale and soggy from being kept wet, drastic measures to prevent thumb sucking are not indicated. A few children might develop dental problems consequent on thumb sucking but again it hardly seems sufficient justification to design measures to eliminate the habit. In the older child thumb sucking might be related to continued insecurity and any intervention should aim at the cause of the child's insecurity and not at the thumb sucking itself.

Nail biting

Nail biting may result in an unsightly appearance but results in little real harm. Constant nagging of the child to stop it may cause more damage. If the nail biting is associated with anxiety then the underlying problem should be dealt with rather than the presenting symptom. With girls the application of nail varnish might represent a pleasant acceptable way of preventing nail biting.

Masturbation

Masturbation is a normal feature of childhood for both boys and girls. However, traditional views may lead parents to become greatly alarmed. Some may attempt to punish the habit and others may describe it as 'dirty'. They should be reassured that this activity is normal and that if any action is felt to be needed, then they should divert the child into some other activity. The rhythmical rocking of the child and the power of dissociation with the environment, has sometimes caused confusion with epilepsy.

SUDDEN AND UNEXPECTED INFANT DEATHS (SIDS)

About one in every 500 babies dies suddenly and unexpectedly. Not all of these deaths remain unexplained. At necropsy some are found to have had infections like gastroenteritis and meningitis and from the history to have had symptoms which were not recognised for what they were or were not acted upon. In this group of unexpected deaths the most common symptoms reported were unusual drowsiness, irritability and excessive crying, an altered character of cry and missing feeds. Others had had diarrhoea, vomiting, rapid breathing and wheezing. Thus some of those recorded as sudden infant deaths are due to disease which might have been diagnosed and treated.

Aetiology

After exclusion of the group where death was unexpected but not unexplained, there remains a group where there are not previous symptoms and no specific findings at post mortem. It has been suggested that defective control of respiration may be a cause. The 'near miss' cot death in which the child is discovered to be apnoeic and commences respiration after external stimulation may or may not be a precursor of cot death in a susceptible child. Spells of apnoea may be associated with clinically minor upper respiratory tract infection.

Another suggestion is that overheating may be a factor in some unexpected infant deaths. Some were found to be excessively clothed and to have a raised temperature and pathological changes of the kind associated with heat stroke.

Symptoms found in children dying unexpectedly at home compared with controls (Stanton et al, 1978)

Symptoms	Children who died	Controls
Respiratory symptoms		
Snuffles	26	21
Cold	19	5
Cough	31	8
Rapid breathing	6	0
Wheeze	6	1
Noisy breathing	7	1
Gastro-intestinal symptoms		
Loose stools	4	1
Diarrhoea	12	1
One vomit	9	2
Vomiting	14	2
Non-specific symptoms		
Undue drowsiness	36	3
Irritability and excessive crying	37	8
Altered characters of cry	14	0
Missed one feed	3	0
Off feeds	26	5
Fever	13	1
Excessive sweating	10	0
Rash, excluding nappy rash	10	6

Post neonatal infant deaths per month and by Social Class, 1975–79. England and Wales (from Studies in Sudden Infant Death, OPCS No. 45)

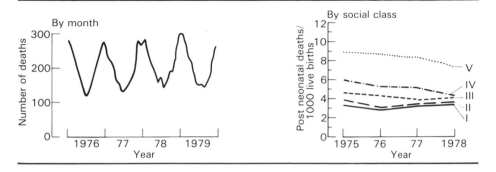

Certain cases of sudden infant death have been attributed retrospectively to infanticide in which a pillow is held over the child's face causing suffocation.

High risk groups

Research into unexpected infant deaths has revealed social and medical factors which are associated with a higher incidence of the problem. Examples of social factors are young mothers, illegitimacy and residence in certain disadvantaged areas. Examples of medical factors are low birth weight, twin pregnancy and bottle feeding. Using a combination of such factors a variety of birth scoring systems has been devised. These identify infants at high risk and trigger increased contact of the family with health visitors. Evidence from Sheffield suggests that this may be effective in reducing post-neonatal death.

Management

When a baby has died unexpectedly at home, the Coroner's Office must investigate, and there will be a post mortem examination. Parents need to be warned that the police will visit, though this is clearly a very sensitive and distressing time for the family. Counselling and explanation about the death of the child is provided by a paediatrician. Parents may feel guilty about the death of their child; mourning and grief may be prolonged. Parents and indeed the whole family must be able to discuss their own feelings in relation to the event.

Prevention

Strategies which might help include:
— informing parents by health education to recognise symptoms of illness and to respond effectively.
— providing access to medical help 24 hours a day. In practice this means a telephone and at the other end, a medical service that is able to listen and respond.
— giving clear advice on follow-up after initial consultations so that parents are able to recognise a worrying condition and know that their doctor *wants* to be called upon.
— avoiding medicines like cough mixtures which give false security to parents

and delay further medical help being sought.

— developing sensitive birth scoring systems so that increased professional help can be given to high risk groups.

— apnoea monitors combined with appropriate counselling and instruction may be of value when a 'near miss' cot death has occurred.

REFERENCES AND FURTHER READING

Apley J, McKeith R, Meadows R 1978 The Child and his Symptoms. Blackwell Scientific Publications, Oxford

Bax M C O 1980 Sleep disturbances in the young child. British Medical Journal 1170–1179

Bleck E 1982 Developmental orthopaedics. 3. Toddlers. Developmental Medicine and Child Neurology 24: 533–555

Carpenter J et al 1983 Prevention of unexpected infant deaths. Lancet 723–727

DHSS 1969 Screening for the detection of congenital dislocation of the hip. HMSO, London

Editorial 1975 Teething Myths. British Medical Journal 604

Fixsen J A 1977 Borderline orthopaedic abnormalities in children. Hospital Update 185–191

Hensingen R, Jones E 1982 Developmental orthopaedics. The lower limb. Developmental Medicine and Child Neurology 24: 95–116

Illingworth R S 1979 The Normal Child. Churchill Livingstone, Edinburgh

O'Callaghan M J, Hull D 1978 Failure to thrive or failure to rear? Archives of Disease in Childhood 53: 788–793

Ounsted M, Simons C 1978 The first born child: toddlers problems. Developmental Medicine and Child Neurology 20: 710–719

Richman W 1981 Sleep problems in young children. Archives of Disease in Childhood 56: 491–493

Stanton et al 1978 Terminal symptoms of children dying suddenly and unexpectedly at home. British Medical Journal 1249–1251

Taylor E, Emery J 1982 Two year study of the causes of post perinatal death classified in terms of preventability. Archives of Disease in Childhood 57: 668–673

Wolkind S 1981 Depression in mothers of young children. Archives of Disease in Childhood 56: 1–3

12
Problems
5–15 years

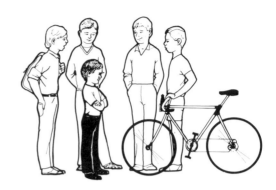

Infectious diseases and physical injuries following accidents are the common reasons for school children visiting family doctors. By contrast it is longstanding rather than acute problems which bring the child to the school medical clinic.

The practice of routine school medical examinations is being progressively abandoned for a more selective approach based on the school nurse's appraisal of the children's health and wellbeing, coupled with teachers' reports and parent's requests. Medical records from the pre-school period and information given by the hospital medical service or social services also contribute towards the identification of which children should be seen by the doctor.

Children should also be encouraged to refer themselves, particularly in the later school years, if they are concerned about some aspect of their health. It should be part of the health education programme to let the children know what services are provided within the school by the school nurse and doctor and the range of problems that are seen. Problems which worry adolescents but might not be reported or put down on parent questionnaires, include worry about exams, being shorter than one's peer groups, and being less advanced in pubertal development.

School Medical Service

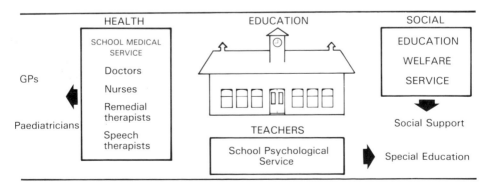

Results of medical examination of 124 nursery and infant school children in Nottingham

Abnormalities detected	48
No. identified by school nurse	40
No. identified by teachers	15
No. identified by parents' questionnaire	10

Conditions of significance that might have been missed if school medical not carried out were, one child with a contracture of right knee and another with enuresis, though both were recorded in past notes of the child health service. One child had asthma which failed detection but he was being treated by his GP; another had in-toeing which did not cause functional impairment.

Success depends on a good working relationship between the medical service and the school staff. The doctor should be readily available and known to them, and viewed by them as an important integral part of the school. The hit and run or perhaps more precisely the hit and miss approach of 'medicals' conducted as a block exercise for one short period during the school year is not seen as valuable by many teachers. Teachers require ongoing advice about individual children throughout the year. Causes for concern may present at any time and some need to be attended to before the next pre-arranged visits. Continuity for both the school doctor and the school nurse from primary school to secondary school is very important for much depends upon relationships that are built up between them, the parents and the children.

Clinical findings in school entrants and leavers — Scotland, 1978 (rate per 100 000 children examined)

	Entrants		Leavers	
	Boys	Girls	Boys	Girls
Total abnormalities	37 301	35 709	38 947	38 323
Disease of tonsils	6 834	6 939	1 453	1 970
Refractive error	5 091	5 391	12 227	13 678
Enuresis	5 592	4 909	490	305
Speech disorder	4 871	2 562	537	214
Obesity	684	1 151	2 193	3 687
Underweight	214	260	339	235
Squint	3 005	2 901	1 035	929
Impairment of hearing	1 654	1 610	1 253	1 206
Asthma	1 265	529	1 954	1 023
Hay fever	252	140	1 012	754
Eczema	1 263	1 229	655	785
Acne	3	6	2 135	3 395
Congenital abnormalities of genital organs	3 952	6	436	—
Congenital heart disease	303	269	149	130
Scoliosis	48	48	177	214
Renal disease	504	151	46	5
Neoplasm	94	193	85	76
Diabetes	38	45	200	157
Blood disorders	88	62	59	125
Behaviour disorder	847	619	429	483
Epilepsy	209	160	298	311
Mental handicap (including borderline)	239	177	1 220	864

NOCTURNAL ENURESIS

Nocturnal enuresis is a common and an important condition. Estimates of its prevalence vary depending upon the population studied. Between 10 and 20% of 5 year olds and 5 to 10% of 10 year olds wet at night. The problem does not always disappear in adult life. Figures for army recruits have indicated that 1.2% wet at least on one night a week. Enuresis is more common in boys, and in social classes IV and V. Daytime wetting (diurnal enuresis) was found in up to 10% of the younger children referred with nocturnal enuresis.

Causes

Enuresis is not a single entity, a number of factors may be involved in any one child, so individual assessment is necessary.

Organic disorders. It is dangerous to assume that all cases of enuresis have a non-organic basis. Urinary tract infections have been found in up to 9% of children presenting with enuresis. Appropriate investigation and treatment of the urinary tract infection will cure the enuresis in many but not all. Although a previously unsuspected urinary tract infection may be found, the discovery of a previously unidentified neurological disorder is an unlikely event, though it needs to be considered. Diabetes mellitus may present as secondary nocturnal enuresis. Two children with diabetes were identified in a 4 year period in a busy school clinic for children with nocturnal enuresis.

Immaturity. Many of the children presenting with nocturnal enuresis simply represent the tail end of the normal distribution, and there is no obvious psychological, social or organic disturbance. It is so common in pre-school children that enuresis may be regarded as the normal state of affairs rather than an exception. (Some parents may disagree and demand dryness at night at an age where it cannot reasonably be expected.) Nocturnal enuresis does not seem to be related, as many parents may claim, to the child sleeping 'too deeply'. Likewise attempts at water deprivation lead only to thirst and not to dryness. However, the converse, allowing an enormous water load at bedtime, is perhaps unwise. The commonly adopted practice of lifting the child at bedtime often results in a dry bed and clearly has the practical advantage of keeping the bed sheets clean and avoiding conflict. However the sleeping child usually does not remember being lifted and in terms of helping him to acquire bladder control it is often ineffective. Sleep is not a uniform state; children go through cycles of lighter and deeper sleep throughout the night. Many children wet the bed during the phases of lighter sleep or during the process of waking up, though the converse is true for others.

Anxiety. Enuresis is often seen in association with life events that are particularly stressful for the child. For instance it may be seen when the child starts school or with the birth of a younger sibling. With some children the pattern of enuresis has been seen to follow the school time-table with periods of dryness occurring during the holidays. With others it may relate to family illness, to discord amongst other members of the family or to frequent moves and instability. However, being away from home may be therapeutic. Many children who wet the bed, are dry on holiday or when staying with friends or other members of the family. However, children who wet the bed often find themselves excluded from school camps and planned holidays because either they or their parents fear they might 'misbehave' at night.

Stressful toilet training, a highly punitive approach, or unreasonable expectations of dryness may lead to persistent nocturnal enuresis. Perhaps not surprisingly sexual assaults have also been reported to precipitate secondary enuresis.

Bladder capacity and frequency of micturition. Children with enuresis do not have structurally smaller bladders than other children. However children who are enuretic seem to pass smaller volumes of urine more frequently than other children. Those children who pass smaller volumes of urine often have urgency as well. They are well known to school teachers. Their mothers when out shopping with them may be seen anxiously trying to find a lavatory. Many get by during the day without diurnal wetting, either by frequency of micturition or by voluntary restriction of fluid input. Improvement in enuresis is associated with an increase in urine volume passed.

Average urine volume passed at each voiding by enuretic and normal children, and average bladder capacity in enuretics with and without urgency compared to controls (from Kolvin et al, 1973)

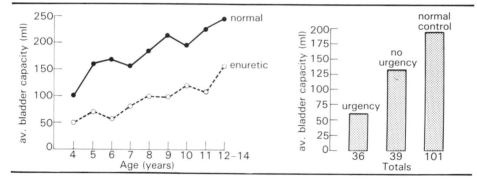

History
First establish whether the enuresis is primary or secondary. Primary enuresis occurs in a child who has always been wet at night and has had no long dry spells. Secondary enuresis occurs after a long period of established bladder control at night. Secondary enuresis is likely to be associated with a precipitating event such as starting school, or a urinary tract infection.

Enquire whether there is a pattern. Is it confined to certain days of the week or related to school holidays? Does it occur at the weekend? It is also useful to record the time at night when the child wets the bed. For instance if a child's bedtime is 7 o'clock, and the wetting occurs between 3 and 4 am, he can be encouraged with the achievement of being able to stay dry for 8 hours of the night; he has more hours dry than wet. Some children wet within a short period of being put to bed and others shortly before getting up in the morning. With improvement the child may wet at progressively later times during the night until he is able to hold on throughout. Some children may wet the bed more than once. This also needs to be recorded. The amount of urine passed needs to be assessed roughly.

Occasionally the child wakes up and passes part of the urine in the bed but is able to get to the toilet to pass the remaining urine. These records provide a proper basis on which to judge any change.

What are the sleeping arrangements in the house? Does he share his bed with a sibling? This is far more common than many people would imagine. Problems with bed linen and inadequately protected mattresses are frequently of major concern to parents. The child's nightwear is also very important. Some parents put even their teenage children into nappies and plastic pants at bedtime. Removal of these is often the only therapeutic measure that is required in order to ensure dryness.

What is the reaction of the parents to enuresis? A critical or punitive approach will undermine the child's confidence in himself. Giving the child credit for any of the nights that he is dry is a more positive approach. Is the child given general responsibility for himself or do the parents encourage dependency?

Enquire about the pattern of micturition during the day, particularly with respect to frequency and urgency. Has the child ever woken up at night to go to the toilet? Are there any practical difficulties in him so doing, for example an outside lavatory, dark and cold and spiders? There is little point recommending a behaviour programme if the child has irregular sleeping habits and no fixed bedtime and bedtime routine.

What does the child do after he has wet the bed? Does he get into his sibling's bed or parents' bed? Does he hide the sheets? Does he change the bed himself, does he wash to remove the smell of urine from his skin? Is he ashamed about the enuresis and frightened that others will find out? Is he restricted in school visits, visiting friends and holidays, etc?

Lastly, is there a family history of enuresis?

As can be seen from the detail required in history taking, enuresis cannot be treated in a hurried manner and much time may be required to elicit the full history from parents and the children. More than one consultation is often required in order to obtain sensitive information such as the 15 year old wearing nappies at night.

Examination

A physical examination is required, largely to reassure the family that no organic abnormality is present. This can also be linked to the explanations given on the anatomy and physiology of micturition. Culture of the urine and urine testing for glucose, are essential. Neurological examination is very seldom rewarding in children with enuresis. Attention to the roots S1 and S2, responsible for bladder control, by testing ankle reflexes, and looking for clawing of the feet and testing for anaesthesia in the saddle area, are sufficient.

Treatment

Each clinician will develop his own approach and preferred therapies. Evaluation of various methods of treatment is difficult, for there is a large placebo effect and it is the doctor's interest and enthusiasm which play the major part. A combination of treatments, such as a star chart and an alarm, are often more effective than simple treatments used on their own.

Explanation. This is, perhaps, the most important aspect of management. It is essential that the child understands what in fact we are asking of him. Children, and indeed many adults, are usually fairly ignorant of the anatomy and physiology of the urinary tract and the means by which normal continence is acquired. The mystery of being wet needs to be explained in terms of the origin of all 'that water' and the means by which its exit from the body is controlled.

One approach is to start with a simple drawing of the abdomen putting on the kidneys, ureters and bladder, and then explaining that the kidneys work all day and all night and that they act rather like very fine tea strainers which clean the blood and that the urine goes down the tubes, called ureters, into the bladder. Children are interested to learn where the bladder and kidneys are positioned. The bladder may be described as a bag made of muscle, which fills up with water coming from the kidneys. Then we reach the nub of the matter. The child may be told that the exit from the bladder is controlled by a sort of little tap, which he can control himself during the day but which in some people falls asleep at night together with the rest of the body, when in fact it should stay working. The next step is discussing with the child ways of getting the system to gain better control. Most children understand that muscles work better after a period of training, so it helps to describe various forms of treatment as a means of training.

The nature of sleep also needs to be discussed with the child. Children know that when people go to sleep not all bodily functions are switched off. Daddy snoring in his sleep is a good illustration. Furthermore, they may appreciate that they can control their own waking and sleeping, perhaps the best example is when they go away on holiday. Did they need an alarm clock to get up very early? Could they, if they tried very hard, manage to wake up on their own 2 hours earlier? Likewise if they did not have to go to school, did they find that they automatically slept in a little bit later that day? Most children accept this and it is not too big a jump to get them to understand that they could wake up at night to go to the toilet if the bladder is full, or remember 'to save it up' until the next morning.

The various types of treatment offered are 'walking sticks'; the system will not work if the child does not cooperate. Their aim is to help the child to help himself. The concept of personal responsibility in control is important in many areas of child health but is particularly so in the treatment of enuresis.

Chart Systems consist of small rewards given for appropriate behaviour. The child is seen at weekly intervals. The issue of a chart and a follow-up appointment for 6 weeks, with an instruction 'come back dry' is pointless. The chart system — say a blue star in the morning every time that he is dry — is explained to the child and is built into a night time routine; that is, it is produced at bedtime when the child is asked by the parent to go to the toilet, and hopefully will act to remind him about the explanations previously given about how the kidneys work and the nature of sleep. If he does wake up on his own at night he may go to the toilet or try and hold on till morning. In the morning with great ceremony, dry nights are rewarded by sticking on a star. Variations of star charts abound. Animal stickers may be used or the stars collected may act as tokens that can be exchanged for more desirable goods later on. Children get easily disillusioned if they do not have rapid success and some cheat. As so many of them desperately desire to be

Enuresis chart

dry, cheating can be dealt with sympathetically rather than by reproach. With children who seem to have a scatter of dry nights around the time that they see the doctor, an approach whereby the child writes each day a letter which he can 'post' to the doctor, is often successful. With other children it may be more desirable to give the reward for getting up and going to the toilet at night. For some there is clearly a very big jump from being wet to being dry, so the child may be rewarded for wetting later at night or by the bed being less wet and trying to finish it off in the toilet. The chart therefore is an approach which needs to be tailored to the child's individual history and to the response.

Influencing the family's attitudes. By the time medical help is sought the family's reaction may be one of despair or anger and hostility which may continue throughout the day. Positive help and encouragment of the child are essential for success and this, together with a system of treatment described above, which gives both the parents and the child something to do, usually works. Clearly there is no place for nappies during the training programme.

The child's commitment must be reinforced. If he is one of those children who does not seem to mind being wet, then there is little motivation for change. As far as it is possible the child should be responsible for carrying out the treatment, with of course, the support of parents. The child can also be asked to be responsible for making his own bed and changing the sheets. This is a measure which in itself can be dramatically successful. The child is relieved that the parents will not be nagging him about his enuresis as the responsibility for the sheets no longer rests with the parents. This system of wider responsibility can be extended outside the immediate area to evolve to other functions such as washing and dressing. Many children dramatically 'grow up', become more confident, take greater pride in themselves, and, happily, also become dry at night. The questions of responsibility and control are often deeply engrained in the structure of any particular family. Parents often want to do things for children because the child's own performance although satisfactory, might not be up to their standards.

However, success gained from activities such as washing and dressing may provide the confidence for success in other areas, such as bladder control.

Interval training. As children with enuresis tend to micturate more frequently and pass smaller volumes of urine, encouraging them to increase their bladder control seems a reasonable approach. It is thought that a few only remain dry during the day by severely restricting their fluid intakes. For this small group of children increasing their fluid intake can result in daytime as well as night time wetting.

In interval training the child micturates according to a fixed timetable and then gradually increases the time interval. Thus the child might begin by drinking half a pint of fluid on the hour and go to the toilet on the hour from 9 a.m. till 3 p.m. Many will find this impossible and it provides the opportunity to illustrate to the parents the sorts of difficulty that the child is having. Once the hour interval is achieved, it can be gradually extended by half hour until $2\frac{1}{2}$ or 3 hour intervals are reached. Up to 50% of children may become dry on interval training routines but for success the intensity of training and the level of adult commitment to the programme must be high. The use of alarm clocks or cooking timers is helpful to remind the child or parent when the time for a drink or micturition is due, and the use of rewards when the required target is met is a helpful reinforcement.

Enuresis alarms. On average, these give about 80% cure in 4 months. In enthusiastic hands higher rates than this may be obtained.

The principle consists of a detector mechanism which becomes activated when wet. This may consist of two foil mats on which voided urine completes an electric circuit or a single sensor as in the smaller Malem alarm. The sensor, of whatever type, is linked to a battery and a loud bell. Using either system the bell goes off when the child wets and the child should get out of bed, turn the alarm off and go to the lavatory.

Alarms are suitable for children over the age of seven. The first stage is instruction in the use of the alarm, combined with demonstration and rehearsal. The instructions are addressed mainly to the child. The rehearsal is completed by triggering the alarm with a little saline!

Initially the parent may need to sleep in the same room to waken him or to avoid confusion or fear when the alarm first goes off. It is obviously important to ensure that the parents are willing to do this before the alarm is issued. The

Enuresis alarm

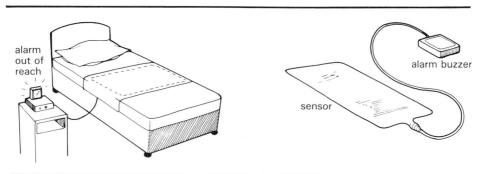

use of the alarm may be more difficult if parents work at night or irregular hours or if the child shares a bedroom or indeed a bed with a sibling.

A record needs to be kept each day of the result, showing whether the child is dry or wet, the time of wetting and the degree to which the bed is wet. If the alarm is triggered, then the bed needs to be remade and the alarm reset before the child returns to bed. Using the standard type alarm the child should not wear pyjama trousers as the first drop of urine is required to trigger the alarm. When using the Malem alarm the child may wear pants to keep the pad in place.

An alarm is generally issued until the child has been dry for at least 3 weeks. Using this routine 80% of children will be dry within 4 months. Ten per cent relapse but a further course of the buzzer is usually successful.

Failures with the buzzer are more often due to failures in implementation of the technique rather than of the method itself. False alarms may occur if the circuit is completed by perspiration or if the mats or their connections are allowed to touch. Initially the child may not awaken to the alarm and it is often necessary to obtain parental help in these early stages. Some children will just switch the alarm off and go back to sleep and it is important to site the box as far away from the bed as possible. Failure of the alarm to sound may be due either to low batteries or to a connection which has come adrift. Failures occur more often in the unmotivated or where conditions required for its use are difficult. The alarm is obviously of no benefit to deaf children. An alternative version using a vibrator as opposed to a buzzer is available.

Use of imipramine. Anti-depressants such as imipramine and amitriptyline have been shown in properly controlled trials to be effective in the treatment of enuresis. They have their maximum effect in the first week of use but a very high number relapse subsequently. Up to 50% cure rate has been claimed using this method which is definitely superior to placebo. However, bearing in mind the high rate of relapse long term success is probably achieved in only up to 20% of children.

Management of nocturnal enuresis

Management:	art or science?
	— unique condition for studying the placebo effect (and the gadget effect of alarms)
	— thorough history
	— exclude organic causes by examination and investigation
	— regular review and support (weekly)
	— personal responsibility of the child
	— appropriate teaching
Treatments:	— charts, suited to individual needs
	— interval training — requires full-time commitment by child
	— suitable for use in school holidays
	— alarms — over 7 years
	— own bed and own bedroom
	— requires (a) motivation as nights are disturbed
	(b) teaching vital
	(c) maintenance of equipment and correct techniques of use vital
	— Imipramine — easy to use
	— high relapse rate
	— needs to be combined with other method
	— dangers of accidental poisoning

In spite of the short-lived response to imipramine it is certainly of value when combined with other methods of treatment, such as star charts and altering family relationships. It does give some rapid success to many children which can be continued providing another method of training is carried out simultaneously. An initial dose of 25 mg is recommended but this is certainly too low for secondary school children who may require up to 75 mg. A trial would be for 4 to 6 weeks and if the child becomes dry I continue for at least 3 more weeks. Parents and children always need to be reminded of the dangers of imipramine if taken as an accidental overdose by a younger child.

SOILING

Soiling is included in this section because it mostly presents as a problem at school age. It is often found in younger children when it may be regarded as an extension of the normal variation. The principles of management in soiling are very similar to those already described for enuresis. Three main groups of children with soiling can be identified.

Children with constipation and overflow. These children are constipated, the rectum is usually dilated with impacted faeces around which liquid stool is allowed to leak. Abdominal examination usually reveals a mass of impacted faeces in the abdomen. Stretching of the rectum due to the faeces causes the muscle to be inefficient and unable to expel its contents. The constipation may have started with a painful perianal lesion such as a fissure which caused the child to hold on to faeces in order to avoid pain. In other children disruption at the time of toilet training may be pinpointed as a cause. Undue pressure by parents or unrealistic expectations of children's bowel control may also result in soiling as a negative response to the parents' demands. Some children may begin soiling when they start school and this may be related to fear of using school lavatories which the child may find to be cold, draughty or lacking in privacy. Some children who require a little help are frightened to ask the school staff. Problems with school lavatories are encountered fairly commonly by school doctors. They are often asked for their views on the adequacy of cleanliness of the lavatories (and the school kitchens)!

Causes of chronic constipation

Behaviour	*Neuromuscular*
	Mental handicap
Nutrition	Cerebral palsy
Low residue diet	Spinal cord lesion
Excess cow's milk	Congenital absence of abdominal wall
	muscles
Anatomical	Generalised hypotonia
Anorectal stenosis	Hypothyroidism
Aganglionosis (Hirschprung's disease)	
	Metabolic
	Diabetes insipidus
	Diabetes mellitus (early stages)
	Hypercalcaemia
	Renal tubular acidosis

Soiling with no constipation. These are children who have not been adequately toilet trained. Some may use the toilet at school but not at home. Others are just inadequate in self-help skills, whereas others are reluctant to give up the attention that they get from their parents through soiling.

Encopresis. This is a different matter in that the stools are passed in inappropriate places. They may be found hidden in drawers or under the settee. The encopresis here is a manifestation of an underlying emotional problem.

Management

Management, as with enuresis, starts with an explanation of the anatomy and physiology of the gut. For the child the gut may be likened to a long tube along which the food is pushed rather like toothpaste. When the tube is stretched it is too weak to squeeze the food onward. Although children with nocturnal enuresis very rarely need in-patient management, children with soiling occasionally require admission to introduce the training routine. The child is encouraged to use the toilet after each meal, a record is kept of the result and a star or other reward given for success. A 'pooh' chart is perhaps a better system of symbols than the somewhat abstract star chart. The child's attitude to faeces is different from the adult's and he may take pride in counting and drawing his produce. If rewards are merely given for clean pants, then some children may tend to hold on to their stools rather than let go. It is therefore more appropriate to give the reward for using the toilet, rather than for not soiling. However in some children both systems of reward may be required.

The concept of personal responsibility is more difficult to introduce. A careful history should indicate the family's attitudes towards self-help for the child. The parents' support should be engaged, criticism or apathy on their part would be a major stumbling block. Within a training programme the child can be rewarded for using the toilet on his own initiative as opposed to being sent there by an adult.

Some children are frightened of using the toilet, so clearly there is a need to distinguish between children who are frightened of going to that particular place and children who are frightened of a bowel action because of the pain that they have associated with defaecation. Such children need help and encouragement (as opposed to criticism or despair) in tackling their fear of the lavatory. They may be brought nearer and nearer to it, encouraged to spend longer periods in the toilet and learn to associate using the lavatory with more pleasurable tasks, such as a music box or reading a story. Therefore, if attention is diverted away from soiling towards appropriate use of the toilet a remarkable number of children

Soiling

Management	Explanation— anatomy
	— physiology
	— treatment
	Training routine
	Personal responsibility
	Laxatives
	Modification of family attitudes
	Psychotherapy

can be helped by a 'communal approach' to the problem. Later on, the company and support may be gradually withdrawn.

Laxatives are needed in most children with underlying constipation. They are mandatory where the rectum is dilated. The rectum needs to be emptied initially; oral laxatives in adequate doses usually work. Enemas should be avoided if at all possible, for the procedure is distressing to children. If an enema is required then this should be done on 'a once only' basis at the introduction to a hospital based programme. In order to help the bowel to return to normal, a combination of a faecal softener such as dioctyl sodium sulphosuccinate and a stimulant laxative such as senokot, is usually used. A dose of 5 ml of the dioctyl syrup tds and 5 ml of the senokot started at night is recommended. The senokot may well need to be increased up to 10 ml. However, parents' expectations of bowel actions may be too high and they may continue to increase the dose of senokot for their own satisfaction rather than the child's needs. Senna, in excessive dose, does cause abdominal pain which clearly is the reverse of what we are trying to do therapeutically. Many other laxatives are also effective. It is most important to become familiar with one or two and the appropriate therapeutic ranges that are required. Anal dilatation under general anaesthesia is used as an initial procedure in some centres.

Encopresis, is less likely to respond to the simple strategies of training, explanation and laxatives. The child may be improved by admission to hospital, away from the stresses and hostilities at home. However, usually some form of psychotherapy involving the child and the family is required so that the symptoms may be understood, and alternative outlets for the child to express his feelings are encouraged.

Although soiling is a much more distressing condition than enuresis, it does not continue into adult life and most children cease before secondary school age.

RECURRENT ABDOMINAL PAIN

Recurrent abdominal pain is a common problem affecting up to 10% of all children. There is often a family history of recurrent abdominal pain — the incidence is six times higher in the mothers of such children than in the rest of the population. Other disorders which are more commonly found in the relatives of children with recurrent abdominal pain are migraine, peptic ulcer, nervous breakdown, appendicectomy and convulsions.

In practice distinguishing between organic and non-organic causes is not usually a difficult task. Extensive investigations should be avoided for they only serve to fix the parents and children on a search for an organic cause. A fruitless series of investigations serves to enforce their lack of confidence in the doctor for he has failed to discover what is wrong.

Clinical assessment

A thorough history is important, for example the site and nature of the pain may not only help to exclude an organic cause but may also identify particular problems at home or at school which might be acting as triggers to the pain. We need to discover what the parents do when the pain occurs, for example, does the child

Features of 200 children with recurrent abdominal pain (from Apley, 1975)

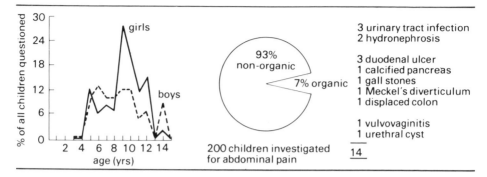

still go to school, is he able to watch TV, what are the child's reactions to the pain? Children with recurrent abdominal pain are often highly strung, fussy, excitable, or anxious and timid. They may have other evidence of emotional disturbance such as sleeping or eating problems, phobias or nocturnal enuresis. The family history is important. In 'painful families' there is a high incidence of such disorders.

A careful and thorough physical examination is essential when the child is first seen. It is reassuring to the parents to know if nothing abnormal is found and that the child's weight and height are satisfactory. Further investigations are usually not required though simple tests such as a full blood count, ESR, urine test and a plain abdominal X-ray may be found to be therapeutically, if not diagnostically, useful.

Management

Again explanation is a most important part of management. Explaining to the child the anatomy of the gut and the mechanism of normal gut motility (like toothpaste being squeezed from a tube) is useful in giving the child a proper understanding of what might be a mystery and what might be frightening to him.

Features pointing to an organic cause of recurrent abdominal pain

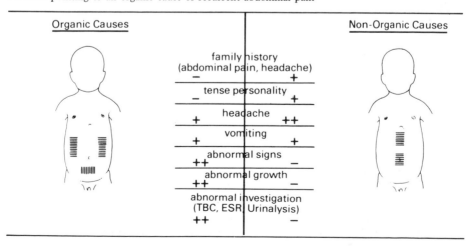

Associated symptoms in recurrent abdominal pain (Apley, 1973)

Vomiting	60%
Nausea	50%
Pallor	50%
Sleepiness afterwards	25%
Fever	5%
Diarrhoea	4%

The vomiting may become severe, leading to dehydration and the need for hospital admission.

During the examination it is useful to explain to the child what you are doing. For instance that the kidneys, liver or spleen are being examined and that they are normal.

It is important that sources of stress should be discussed and relieved wherever possible. Occasionally the child may 'be feeling the pain inside the mother's abdomen' and dealing with the parent may be more successful than dealing with the child.

It is easy for children to meet any new or stressful situation with abdominal pain and hence escape. It is permitted to give them reassurance and comfort but long periods away from school create more stress rather than less, as the child's school work slips farther behind.

Recurrent abdominal pain cannot be dealt with in a single consultation, by definition the condition is chronic. Regular follow-up, repetition of reassurance, explanation, support and discussion of stressful situations are needed. The child has to learn how to deal with challenges. The parents who are so often of similar emotional make-up are not able to provide either good examples or wise control.

The relationship between emotional stress and physical symptoms is often difficult to explain to children and parents. However the concepts of blushing with embarrassment or going pale with fright are examples which most people will understand. It is important that parents appreciate that the child is not putting it on but that it is an involuntary response like pallor or blushing. Both can to some extent be controlled with increased confidence and social skill. Secret fears

Follow-up of 30 treated and 30 untreated cases of abdominal pain 10–14 years after initial presentation (from Apley, 1973)

Abdominal pain in 30 treated children at follow-up		New symptoms — comparison of treated and untreated groups	
No pains	19	*No abdominal pains, no*	
Rapidly ceased	14	*other symptoms*	
Slowly ceased	5	untreated series	9
Mild and infrequent pain	7	treated series	9
Moderate less frequent pain	2	*No abdominal pains but*	
Severe and frequent pain	2	*other symptoms*	
		untreated series	9
		treated series	10
		Abdominal pains continuing	
		with other symptoms	
		untreated series	12
		treated series	11

about organic disease (for example grand-parent's malignancies which were associated with abdominal pain),feelings of guilt or unexpressed feelings of anger must also be explored.

The prognosis is worse in 'painful families', in boys, in those presenting under the age of 6 and in those with a period of over 6 months before presenting for treatment. Girls commonly develop new symptoms instead.

HEADACHE IN CHILDHOOD

Headache is common in childhood, particularly amongst secondary school children. The incidence rises with age, with 85% of boys and 93% of girls of secondary school age reporting recurrent headaches. Estimations of the incidence of migraine in this population are generally around the 3–5% level. However, many children have frequent severe non-migrainous headaches. Recurrent headaches can seriously impede the child's educational progress.

Acute headache with no past history of headache
These are most commonly a presenting feature of a systemic febrile illness. Symptoms of the causative infection such as one of the ordinary infectious diseases of childhood or an upper respiratory tract infection may not initially be shown. Intracranial infection (meningitis and encephalitis) should be suspected in children who have accompanying drowsiness, irritability, photophobia, focal neurological signs or signs of raised intracranial pressure. It is important to exclude a recent history of head injury as a haematoma resulting from a bang may present as headaches.

Recurrent headaches
An organic cause in all cases of chronic headache must be sought by taking a full history and making a thorough examination.

An organic cause is more likely if:
— the child is under 5 years old
— the headache is not relieved by weak analgesics
— they are increasing in severity and frequency, particularly if the pattern is that of recurrent morning headaches, or they awaken the child from sleep
— there are associated symptoms such as vomiting which may indicate raised intracranial pressure
— there is slow physical growth
— there are neurological signs suggesting hydrocephalus or focal lesions, particularly those related to the eye, e.g. squint, changes in the fundi, or impairment of visual fields or acuity
— any slowing of intellectual performance clearly points to some brain pathology.

These features refer mainly to the early identification of brain tumours; happily they are rare (5.2 per 100 000 population age 0–9) but early identification is necessary for optimum treatment to be provided.

Migraine. Migraine is the commonest cause of chronic headache in childhood. Classically the headache is unilateral, associated with vomiting and a visual aura. There is usually a strong family history of migraine.

Particular precipitating factors need to be looked for. They may be related to hunger and hypoglycaemia or to the ingestion of particular foods, particularly cheese and chocolates. Others may be precipitated by fatigue often in association with working for exams, and various forms of stress. Many other factors have been claimed as precipitators of migraine and clearly, their identification and avoidance are useful aspects of treatment.

Treatment early in an attack with simple analgesics such as paracetamol or aspirin, combined with rest, is usually very effective. Parents and children should be warned that allowing the headache to build up results in a much more prolonged and severe incapacity than treating it early on. Continuous prophylactic treatment with drugs such as prochlorperazine, propranolol or combinations of analgesics and anti-emetics is rarely needed in childhood.

Ocular causes of chronic headache in childhood. Eye strain is frequently diagnosed as the cause of headaches. Many children with minimal errors of refraction have been prescribed glasses unnecessarily on the assumption that they will relieve the headaches. However, occasionally bilateral frontal headaches can be caused by hypermetropia, astigmatism or ocular imbalance.

Sinusitis rarely presents in childhood as headache without the underlying cause being identified. The presence of local tenderness and other features of upper respiratory tract infection are usually obvious.

Other 'unexplained' headaches

This broad remainder contains the majority of children with recurrent headaches. Once we have satisfied ourselves that there is no organic cause, we must remember that the parents and child are still dissatisfied because the child continues to have incapacitating headaches. The pain is usually bilateral and is often described as a heaviness or fullness.

Precipitating factors such as anxiety about school work, stresses at home, worries about the relationship with school friends should be explored. This may, and usually does, require several sessions with the child and family with the intention of enabling the child to discuss and deal with his anxieties. Where headaches do occur the reluctance to start analgesics early on should be discouraged and aspirin or paracetamol given at the first hint of a headache rather than waiting to see what develops.

Again an explanation to the child is most important. The commonness of headaches needs to be emphasised; children who do *not* have headaches in the secondary school group are a minority rather than the majority. The child and his family need to be reassured that headaches very rarely mean any underlying disease and that the history and examination excluded these possibilities. An explanation that the pain is caused by muscle tension can be likened to the aching felt in other muscles after excessive use. Explanation that the pain arises from muscles outside the brain rather than structures within it can be most reassuring.

PAINS IN THE LEGS

Almost all pains in the legs may be ascribed by parents to growing pains. In immigrant children or any who may be thought to be deficient in vitamin D, rickets needs to be excluded by clinical examination supplemented if necessary by X-ray and blood alkaline phosphatase estimation.

Other children have evidence of trauma or past injury. Children commonly injure their legs in sports and conditions such as greenstick fractures and soft tissue injuries to the knees or ankles may not be identified if appropriate examination is not done.

Cramp in the legs, which particularly seems to occur either at night or during exercise, can be very painful and distressing. The affected muscle goes into spasm which can be relieved by gentle massage and stretching.

In children who are getting recurrent cramps, calcium or vitamin D deficiency should be excluded. Others are helped by the use of quinine. The most palatable version of this is tonic water.

Joint pains, particularly where there is general systemic illness can be the presentation of Still's Disease or leukaemia. In the early stages of both disorders there may be very little to see on examination.

Osgood Schlatter's Disease (tibial apophysitis) consists of pain and tenderness over the tibial apophysis. The condition is benign and self limiting and responds simply to rest. Other disorders such as Perthes' disease of the hip, osteochondrosis affecting the ankle bones and ligamentous injuries of the knee, should not be forgotten. Malignancies of the bones of the lower limb are fortunately rare but present with pain and swelling of the leg. Likewise the possibility of osteomyelitis, although rare, should not be forgotten.

Apart from cramp, which is common, the so-called growing pains remain the only other large category of pain in the lower limbs. Children do seem to localise the site of pain to the insertion of tendons or the junction between the epiphysis and metaphysis of the bone. These are clearly the areas where the greatest tension is likely to be felt. Exclusion of a physical cause by careful examination, and if necessary investigation, plus reassurance are usually all that is needed. The pain is rarely severe and it is the length of time over which the pain lasts that seems to cause anxiety in parents.

GROWTH PROBLEMS

Short stature

School children are routinely screened in order to detect those with short stature. In order to be meaningful, measurements must be performed accurately by properly trained staff and interpreted with reference to standard centile charts. It must be remembered that centile charts only apply to the population on which they were standardised and the time at which it is done. The heights of children have increased progressively over the last 100 years. Height is also strongly related to social class and to ethnic origin.

On the basis of these measurements, three groups of children need to be identified for further investigation:

— Children who are crossing centile charts in a downward direction
— Children who are below 3 standard deviations from the mean in height
— Children who are below the 3rd centile (1.9 standard deviations from the mean) but whose parents are tall.

The following questions should be asked at the initial consultation.

How tall are the parents? Measurement of the parents is important because of the genetic influence on final height. Both parents' heights may be plotted on the same centile chart as that of the child; 12.5 cm is subtracted from father's height if it is a girl who is under observation or 12.5 cm added to mother's height if it is a boy who is under observation. This measurement represents the average difference between the heights of males and females. On this basis a child who is below the 3rd centile but above 3 standard deviations whose parents' height also falls into the same area does not require further investigation.

Is there any evidence of general illness? Any severe gastro-intestinal, respiratory, renal, cardiac, haematological, hepatic or metabolic disease may result in short stature. Usually such an underlying cause is obvious. However some disorders may not be easily recognised. For example, the child may present in advanced renal failure with short stature as the only abnormality.

Does the child look normal? Many recognised genetic disorders, syndromes and endocrine disease present with typical facial and body appearances. These are well summarised and classified in the book 'Recognisable Patterns of Human Malformation' by Smith. Some disorders such as achondroplasia may result in disproportionate short stature; others such as Cornelia de Lange syndrome with characteristic facies; and others such as thyroid deficiency with associated symptoms such as constipation, dry skin, umbilical hernia and delayed deep tendon reflex relaxation. Turner's syndrome may present in an apparently normal looking individual and would only be identified if buccal smear or chromosomal analysis is requested.

Assessment

Three pieces of information enable many of the children with short stature to be divided into broad groups. These three measurements are growth velocity, bone age and parental height.

In one group the parents are short, growth velocity is normal and bone age is equivalent to the chronological age (bone age is obtained from analysis of an X-ray of the left hand and wrist with comparison with established standards). These children will be short adults and no active intervention is required.

In a second group the height velocity is again normal but the bone age is delayed: however, height plotted for bone age is normal. There is usually a family history of delayed puberty. These children will also have delayed puberty but eventually attain normal adult height. No treatment is required.

In a third smaller group the growth velocity is subnormal with bone age retarded in relation to height age. Such children require further investigation as treatable disorders such as growth hormone deficiency, thyroid deficiency and severe generalised illness may be found. Investigation in addition to the anthropometric measurements mentioned previously include: visual field assessment and

Longitudinal growth assessment

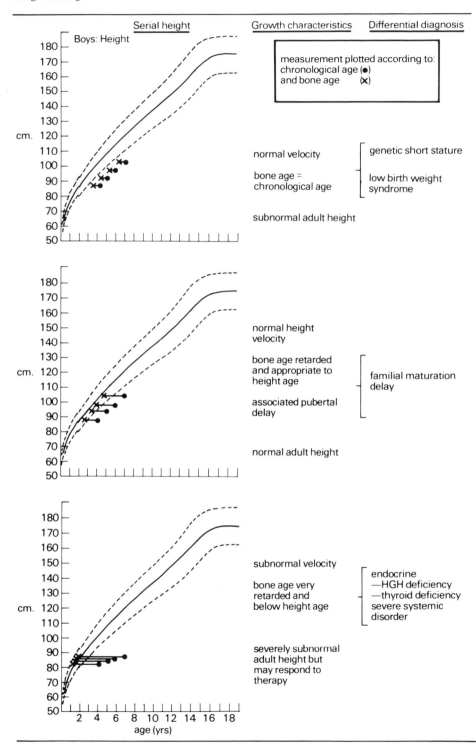

examination of the fundi to investigate the possibility of pituitary tumour; full blood count; urea and electrolytes; calcium, phosphate and alkaline phosphatase measurements, thyroid function tests; exercise tests to measure rises in growth hormone; wrist X-ray; X-ray of pituitary fossa; chromosome analysis; and in some children a jejunal biopsy.

Children with suspected growth hormone deficiency need to be referred to regional growth assessment centres from whom supplies of human growth hormone are available once appropriate criteria have been met for diagnosis.

Psycho-social deprivation

In the United Kingdom inadequate intake of food is not generally a cause of growth retardation. However, there is some evidence that children from large families in social classes IV and V, do in fact increase in height velocity when given supplemental foods like school milk.

Children who have suffered deprivation have impaired growth due to depression in release of growth hormone. This is reversed by improvements in their environment. The cause does not seem to be lack of intake of food as many of these children are quite obsessed with food and they eat excessively. Psycho-social deprivation is discussed further in the chapter on 'Child and Family Psychiatry'.

Tall stature in girls

Socially, excessive height in females is not considered desirable. Although the girls are normal some have argued that curtailment of growth by means of oestrogens is desirable. Treatment must be given before puberty. They must be assessed very carefully before this is undertaken.

PROBLEMS AT PUBERTY

Delayed puberty

Puberty consists of a series of changes involving not just growth and alteration in physical appearance, but emotional and psychological changes. Delayed puberty, or what is seen as delayed puberty by parents and children, can cause a considerable amount of distress. It can be defined simply as no sign whatever of pubertal development by the fourteenth birthday in boys and girls. Three per cent of children have some delay; in 50% of the boys and 15% of the girls it will be constitutional in origin. Of the rest, 30% will have pituitary problems, 10% of boys and 14% of girls will have gonadal failure and in the remaining 10 to 15% delayed puberty is associated with chronic and severe disease such as coeliac disease, renal failure or cystic fibrosis. Delay in puberty is also related to anorexia nervosa and is seen in thin girls who take part in intensive sports activity, such as gymnastics.

Constitutional delay. There is often a family history of delayed puberty and on occasions it is found that the parents themselves have also been investigated. These children have short stature and delayed bone age though the actual height is compatible with the bone age. Growth velocity is normal.

Pituitary disease. Delayed puberty may be associated with a deficiency of gonadotrophin releasing hormone. This may be an isolated deficiency or associated with other hormone deficiencies. The possibility of a space occupying lesion in the pituitary fossa must be excluded so that both endocrinological and neurosurgical investigations may be required.

Gonadal problems. These are far more common in females and about half of these are found to have Turner's Syndrome. Another third have other X chromosome abnormalities. Elevation of gonadotrophins in both boys and girls indicates gonadal failure. In boys where the testes are not palpable they may be found to be unresponsive to gonadotrophins or releasing factors are deficient.

As far as the community paediatrician is concerned the major task is to identify correctly the children with no sign of pubertal development by the fourteenth birthday. Measurement of growth velocity and bone age will help to identify those with constitutional delay and the history and examination will also identify those with other severe medical conditions. Investigation in a few remaining children with pituitary or gonadal problems is a task for a children's endocrinology clinic.

Precocious puberty

This is far more common in girls than in boys and in the former is usually idiopathic. Precocious development may lead to unrealistic expectations of the child in that emotional or intellectual maturity are not advanced. It may also cause considerable embarrassment to the child in being so different in appearance to the rest of the class.

Precocious puberty in girls. This may be a true onset of puberty or only a limited number of aspects of puberty may be advanced. Examples are premature thelarche in which there is premature development of breast tissue and pubarche in which there is premature development of pubic hair. The children are tall with advanced bone age though final adult height may be short because of premature fusion of the epiphyses. Premature puberty in girls is usually idiopathic but may follow inflammatory disorders of the brain such as an encephalitis or hydrocephalus. Precocious sexual development may be related to exogenous sources of oestrogens from ovarian or adrenal tumours. These are frequently calcified and can be seen on plain abdominal X-ray. X-ray examination of the skull may also be required.

Precocious puberty in boys. Precocious puberty in boys is far more likely to be due to an organic cause. Investigations to exclude cerebral tumour, tumour of the testes or adrenals or congenital adrenal hyperplasia should be carried out.

MISCELLANEOUS PROBLEMS

Colour vision defects

Colour vision defects are extremely common in boys. The incidence is around 10% and the defect is inherited as a sex-linked recessive. A much smaller number of girls, perhaps 0.4% also have colour vision defects. Most fall into the category of red–green colour blindness in which there is difficulty distinguishing these colours if equally bright. The underlying cause is a deficiency of one or more pigments in the retinal cone cells. The disability resulting from such a deficiency is trivial and the inability to do the particular tests, such as the Ishihara colour vision test, may be the only problem that such people encounter in their life time. However, it has been argued that on grounds of safety those whose jobs may require colour discrimination under difficult conditions, should be excluded from such occupations. Therefore, pilots, train drivers, police and some areas of the army exclude those with colour vision defects. On less substantial reasons they have been excluded from electrical engineering apprenticeships. Jobs which per se involve accurate colour matching, such as in the fabric industry, would clearly be difficult. Half the boys with colour vision defects have only a partial defect and are able to do many of the items in the Ishihara test.

In the Ishihara test the subject is confronted with printed colour plates consisting of dots of varying colours on a black background. Older children are asked to identify the number displayed by the dots on the plate. Younger children who have not yet learned numbers are asked to trace a wiggly coloured line across the plate. The pattern of responses is recorded and from a record book the degree of colour defectiveness is worked out.

It is argued that on the basis of this test careers guidance can be given to the children to divert them from unsuitable occupations. The prohibited list of occupations is long, probably too long, and the time spent in colour vision testing is not rewarding as there is no treatment for the condition; it produces no ill health and the hazards are only theoretical. Should they be continued?

Acne

Acne is an extremely common complaint in teenage children and in many extends into the early twenties. About 15% of children with acne consult their doctor about the condition. Patients need to be told that for success, treatment must be long term. However in this age group compliance is likely to be poor. At the onset of treatment it must be emphasised that results are not rapid and that treatment usually needs to be continued for at least 6 months and that a large number may expect to relapse without such treatment.

The defect in acne is an increase in sebum caused either by excessive androgen stimulation of the sebaceous glands or excessive sensitivity to androgens. Additional factors are plugging of the sebaceous glands with keratin and secondary infection leading to inflammation. The role of oral contraceptives and their possible androgenic effects also needs to be considered by the paediatrician.

Treatment of mild cases is with benzoyl peroxide used once or twice a day. This is available in 2.5%, 5% and 10% concentrations. Tretinoin acts by separating the obstructing keratin plug and may be used in conjunction with benzoyl peroxide. The benzoyl peroxide is used in the morning and the tretinoin in the evening. Patients must be warned that scaling and erythema may be caused by topical treatment. If they are not warned of this, treatment may be stopped prematurely.

Antibiotics are required to treat severe acne. Treatment is required for at least 6 months and when it is stopped, topical treatment must be continued. The two most suitable preparations are tetracycline 250 mg given 2 to 4 times a day or erythromycin 250 mg. The tetracycline needs to be given at least half an hour before food and should not be taken with milk.

Dental caries

Dental caries is the rule rather than the exception amongst school children. It is however a preventable condition though prevention of course must start long before school age. At age 5, 75% of children have at least one carious tooth and at age 15, 95% of children have at least one permanent tooth affected by caries. The average is of ten decayed, missing or filled teeth in this age group. Amongst the adult population in 1978 29% were edentulous. This is, however, an improvement from 1968 when 37% were edentulous. Dental decay is therefore a major problem to be tackled. The process, once started, is an irreversible destruction of the tooth. Only treatment by removing damaged tissue and replacing it with synthetic material is successful.

Although the means of preventing dental caries are well known the application of this knowledge, both as a nation and individually is poor. Regular and proper tooth brushing should be universal and is not. The sweet consumption of the UK is higher than anywhere else in the world. Pharmaceutical preparations may be just as much to blame as confectionery for most preparations for children are sweetened with syrup.

Fluoridation of water supplies would drastically decrease the amount of dental caries. In spite of this only 10% of the UK receives such fluoridated supplies. Oral fluoride supplements can be given according to the following schedule.

Fluoride in local water (recommended supplements)

Age	Less than 0.3 ppm	0.3–0.7 ppm
0–2 years	0.25 mgF/day	0
2–4 years	0.5 mgF/day	0.25 mgF/day
4–16 years	1.0 mgF/day	0.5 mgF/day
No supplements needed if local water >0.7 ppm		

REFERENCES AND FURTHER READING

Apley J 1959 The Child with Abdominal Pain. Blackwell Scientific Publications, Oxford
Apley J 1973 Which of you by taking thought can add one cubit to his stature? Psychosomatic illness in children: a modern synthesis. British Medical Journal 2: 756–758
Apley J, Hale B 1973 Children with recurrent abdominal pain: How do they grow up? British Medical Journal 3: 7–9
Apley J, Mackeith R C, Meadow S R 1978 The Child and his Symptoms. Blackwell Scientific Publications, Oxford
Brook C G D 1974 Short stature. British Journal of Hospital Medicine 668–674
Kolvin I, Mackeith R C, Meadow S R 1973 Bladder Control and Enuresis Clinics in Developmental Medicine Nos. 48/49. William Heinemann, London
Rayner P H W 1976 Puberty: precocious and delayed. British Medical Journal 1: 1385–1387

13
Long-standing Illness

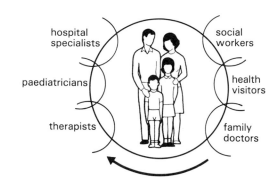

Estimates of the prevalence of chronic disease in childhood vary from 6% to 11%. The medical disorder brings with it other problems, for example, the child may be disappointed because he is not how he would like to be, and that he is not the popular image of a child: lively, free and exploratory. The parents may be disappointed because their child, due to the chronic illness, cannot live up to their expectations. Discipline can cause difficulties. Adolescents particularly rebel against the restraints that some treatment programmes impose. Inability to compete with peers at school and sport, hurts, and sometimes well meant 'kindly protection' does not help. There is uncertainty about the future. This with the fear of the pain and distress of an acute episode, can demoralise the strongest child within the warmest family.

To help combat some of these problems the child with a longstanding illness needs

— *Continuity of care* so that a relationship of trust can develop between the child and his family and their doctors. This requires time.

— *Integration of care*, so that all aspects, medical, developmental, social, educational and emotional are put into perspective. As nearly all will attend ordinary schools it is important that home, hospital and school have the same understanding of the disorder and its management.

— *Accessibility of care* so that what help and treatment is effective is readily available to them at times of acute need.

Principal disorders 10–12 year olds in the Isle of Wight (Rutter et al,)

	Rate per 1000
Asthma	23.2
Eczema	10.4
Epilepsy	6.4
Orthopaedic conditions	3.4
Heart disease	2.4
Diabetes mellitus	1.2

ASTHMA

The diagnosis of asthma should be considered in any child with a recurrent wheeze. It is the most common chronic illness of childhood, with a prevalence of approximately 5% overall. Rates between 1% and 11.3% have been reported in different populations. It is also a common cause of loss of schooling and referral for special education. Even so it often goes undiagnosed or is treated inappropriately or inadequately with the result that the child experiences unnecessary distress, or is subject to inappropriate restriction of activities and very occasionally death occurs which is avoidable. Clinically, the spectrum of asthma is wide, ranging from children with mild intermittent attacks of wheezing who do not miss school and do not require continuous treatment, to those with continuous wheezing and superimposed acute exacerbations which precipitate hospital admission. Boys are affected twice as often as girls. Thirty per cent have eczema compared to 3.7% in the general population, 50% of patients with eczema eventually develop asthma. About half the children with asthma have a family history of asthma, eczema or hay fever. Any programme of care must consider the management of all the members of the family with allergic reactions. Asthma appears to be more common in social classes I and II, but the more severe forms are seen more often in social classes IV and V.

The diagnosis of asthma or its severity may be overlooked in a child presenting predominantly with cough, in a child who is not seen in an acute attack and who between attacks is clinically normal, and in a child with continuous bronchospasm who cuts down his activities to match his exercise tolerance so that he does not experience breathlessness.

Clinical features

Answers to the following questions should be sought before considering management. What is the frequency, severity and length of attacks and are there any precipitating factors? Is there evidence of persistent airways obstruction such as a barrel chest or reduced respiratory function? Is growth impaired? Does the asthma affect his life style, for example by interfering with school attendance or restriction of activities? What is the child's reaction to an attack, is he frightened? What is the parents' reaction, are they overprotective or do they try to ignore it? What do they understand about asthma and are they competent in carrying out treatment?

Medical management

There is now a broad range of drugs available for the treatment of asthma. Success depends upon the child and his family being able to recognise symptoms early and being able to start treatment promptly at home. Thus they need confidence and expertise in the use of delivery systems such as inhalers or nebulisers. They need instruction in their use when they are introduced. Parents will also wish to discuss possible precipitating factors and measures which might be used to avoid them, for example an extra dose of a bronchodilator before exercise. Parents must also know that where there is no response to bronchodilators in an acute attack and the child's condition is worsening, that emergency expert help should be sought.

Drugs used in the treatment of asthma

Drug	Type	Route	Dose	Dose-interval	Side effects	Notes
Bronchodilator drugs						
Salbutamol	B2 ≫ B1 adrenergic stimulant	*Inhaled* aerosol	1–2 puffs	4–6 hours	Tremor	Useful for nocturnal cough
		powder (rotacaps)	200–400 µg	4–6 hours	Tremor	
		nebulised (respirator solution)	2.5–5 mg	4–6 hours	Tremor	
		IV/IM	4–6 µg/kg body weight	6 hours	Tremor	
		Oral tablets } syrup }	2–4 mg	6–8 hours	Tremor	
		spandettes	8 mg	At night	Tremor	
Terbutaline	B2 ≫ B1 adrenergic stimulant	*Inhaled* aerosol	1–2 puffs	4–6 hours	Tremor	
		nebulised	2–5 mg	4–6 hours	Tremor	
		Oral tablets syrup	0.75–3 mg	6–8 hours	Tremor	
		SC, IM, IV	10 µg/kg body weight	4–6 hours	Tremor	
Feneterol	B2 ≫ B1 adrenergic stimulant	*Inhaled* aerosol	1–2 puffs	4–6 hours	Tremor	
Rimiterol	B2 ≫ B1 adrenergic stimulant	*Inhaled* aerosol	1–2 puffs	2 hours	Tremor	Rapid onset short duration
Ipatropium bromide	Acetyl choline blocker	*Inhaled* aerosol	1–2 puffs	6 hours	Tachycardia	Value still to be proven

Drug	Type	Form	Dose	Interval	Side effects	Comments
Theophylline	Xanthine derivative	*Oral* tablets } syrup } slow	6–8 mg/kg body weight	6–8 hours	Nausea and vomiting	Blood levels recommended
		slow release tablets } capsules }	12 mg/kg body weight	12 hours	Nausea and vomiting	Blood levels recommended
Aminophylline	Xanthine derivative	*Oral* slow release tablet	100–200 mg	12 hours	Nausea and vomiting	Blood levels recommended
		IV	4 mg/kg body/wt. then 0.7 mg/kg body/wt.	initial then per hour	Nausea and vomiting	Blood levels recommended
Prophyllactic drugs						
Sodium cromoglycate	Mast cell stabiliser	*Inhaled* powder nebulised solution	20–40 mg 2 ml (20 mg)	6–12 hours 6–12 hours	occasional cough occasional cough	
Ketotifen	Mast cell stabiliser	*Oral* tablets } syrup }	0.5–1 mg	12 hours	Drowsiness	Value still to be proven
Beclomethasone diproprionate	Topical steroid	*Inhaled* aerosol powder	1–3 puffs (50–150 µg) 1–2 rotacaps (100–400 µg)	6–12 hours 6–12 hours	Oral candida Oral candida	
Systemic steroids						
Hydrocortisone	Corticosteroid	*IV*	100–400 mg	4–6 hours	None, in short term	For status asthmaticus
Prednisolone and prednisone	Corticosteroid	*Oral* tablets	Up to ½ mg/kg body weight	6–48 hours	Growth suppression. Fluid retention. Diabetes. Hypertension. Infection	Useful for status asthmaticus. Fewer side effects if given every other day for maintenance
ACTH	Pituitary hormone	*IM*	10–40 U	1–3 days	As above	? any safer of better than prednisolone

Mild and severe persistent asthma may be distinguished by the following characteristics (from McNicol & Williams, 1973)

	Mild asthma	Severe/persistent
Onset	Later childhood	Age less than 3 years
Frequency of attacks in initial years	Episodic	High
Evidence of persistent airways obstruction	No	Yes
Chest deformity	No	Yes
Growth impairment	No	Yes

One important decision to be made is when to institute continuous rather than episodic treatment. Continuous therapy should be considered in children who are never free of bronchospasm, children with attacks more frequently than once every 2 weeks, children who miss school on more than two occasions per term, and children with more than two admissions to hospital per year for asthma.

Other aspects of management

Dust control. Nocturnal attacks in a child who is well during the day are very suggestive of allergy to housedust mite. This can be confirmed by skin testing with the appropriate antigen. Measures aimed at reducing dust such as frequent vacuuming of the mattress and floor, and using a damp cloth for cleaning have been recommended but are probably of little help. In many households a nightly dose of a long acting bronchodilator has been found to be far more beneficial.

Exercise. Competitive sport is important to children for their self image and their standing with their peer group. Prophylactic use of bronchodilators or sodium cromoglycate is of great value. Breathing exercises may improve respiratory function, prevent chest deformity and increase voluntary control of respiration in circumstances where anxiety increases bronchospasm. Swimming is recommended for many asthmatic children: it seems not to induce bronchospasm and is a form of physical activity in which they can succeed.

Peak expiratory flow rate

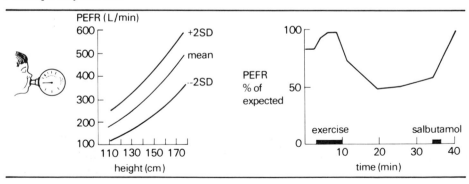

Emotional and family factors. Many asthmatic attacks appear to be provoked by emotional upset, indeed the pattern of attacks may follow the pattern of conflicts at home. In families with discord, regular treatment may not be possible.

In others, excessive anxiety or over-protection in the parents is communicated to the child thus frustrating the beneficial effects of religiously administered treatment. Counselling of the whole family is needed.

Educational aspects. Nearly all children with asthma should and do remain at ordinary schools. Teachers like parents, need to have explanations of the nature of asthma and the treatment that is being followed. Nearly all the children can follow a normal educational curriculum and partake fully in the social life of the school. Where this does not occur, more aggressive medical management is indicated rather than passive acceptance of a limited timetable and poor attendance.

A few children are easily controlled in hospital but not at home. Sometimes in this situation there is family discord or limited family ability or discipline so that therapy is not given as prescribed. For this very small group of children a residential school is the answer. There it may be possible to provide better medical control, greater emotional stability and the experience of success in education.

Career. Most children will be fairly unrestricted in their choice of occupation, but for children where therapy does not prevent attacks precipitated by dust, exercise or exposure to cold, avoidance of occupations involving these is clearly desirable. Also, as the natural history suggests that those who lose their symptoms in adolescence, develop them again later in adult life, career guidance away from manual occupations could be desirable on the basis of past medical history.

CYSTIC FIBROSIS

Cystic fibrosis affects 1:1800 of live births in Great Britain. It is inherited as an autosomal recessive condition with a gene frequency of about 1:25 of the population. The disorder is progressive. Although there is no treatment for the underlying defect, current medical management has greatly improved the prognosis so that 60–70% of children diagnosed early are still alive at age 14 and many survive to early adult life. Twenty-five to 30 years ago, the majority did not survive to school age. Primary prevention through detection of the carrier state or antenatal diagnosis is not available at present, though research is being directed at this in view of the severity of the condition. Genetic counselling is indicated for all families with an affected child.

Clinical features
Cystic fibrosis is a generalised condition of exocrine glands; its main clinical effects are seen in the respiratory and digestive systems. It may present in the neonatal period with meconium ileus or later with respiratory infection, diarrhoea and failure to thrive. Some are identified at an asymptomatic stage because of a positive family history and a sweat test, or through screening tests.

The pulmonary disease, which in the majority of cases is manifest in the first years of life, consists of recurrent purulent chest infections leading to progressive pulmonary damage with obstruction and emphysema and eventually pulmonary hypertension. There may be very little lung disease in some children and severe bronchiectasis in others.

The gastro-intestinal disorders due to pancreatic exocrine insufficiency give rise to malabsorption and failure to thrive with a distended abdomen with the passage of very offensive stools. The appetite is good and the children appear surprisingly alert.

The diagnosis is made by examining a sample of sweat for sodium, chloride or both. It should be considered in all cases of failure to thrive and recurrent respiratory infections.

Complications include heat fatigue in hot climates, rectal prolapse, nasal polyps, subacute abdominal obstruction (meconium ileus equivalent in older children), cirrhosis of the liver, diabetes mellitus, vitamin deficiencies and infertility in males.

Medical management

Any management programme will include postural drainage daily, physical exercise, antibiotics for infection, pancreatic enzyme supplements, low fat, high protein and carbohydrate diet, added vitamins, and added salt in hot weather.

Children need to be seen at regular intervals for clinical assessment and objective measurements of progress such as growth, pulmonary function, (peak flow) and X-ray changes. Over-reporting of symptoms is common with anxious parents as is under-reporting in those who deny symptoms or who get used to the chronic cough as 'normal'.

Immunisation against measles, influenza, diphtheria, tetanus, whooping cough and polio is strongly encouraged. Unimmunised children who are in contact with measles should be given protection with immunoglobulin as soon as possible after the contact.

Social and educational management

The chronic progressive disease and the need for daily and demanding treatment impose stress and restrictions on families who, over the years, will require considerable support, time, and explanation from medical and social services. Mutual support from other parents through such agencies as the cystic fibrosis research trust is valuable. Parents' attitudes to the child, his illness and treatment will vary greatly and will influence his progress. Some may be aggressive and uncooperative reflecting the guilt, anger and denial felt when the diagnosis is made. Others may be grossly over-protective and neglect other children. In certain families, the stress of dealing with cystic fibrosis has led to marital breakdown, but in many the parents have acquired a realistic acceptance of the disorder and great expertise in its management.

Children should be encouraged to attend normal schools and take part in a full educational curriculum. They should also take part in sport and social activities within their limitations. Teachers will need to know about the illness and treatments such as pancreatic extracts with all meals. As far as possible, the child should be responsible for his own treatment. With chronic pulmonary disease, part-time schooling, special education or a home tutor may be required.

Normal discipline is required at home. With confidence and consistent support from home and hospital the child learns to cope with hospital admission and the need for and restrictions of treatment. Older children when they begin to appreciate the severity of the disease and its progress may become seriously depressed. This might be helped by discussing the improving outlook, the wide range of severity and meeting other patients. A hopeful attitude should always be maintained and plans made for the future are often helpful. As the survival rate improves, youngsters with cystic fibrosis are leaving school for work in non-manual fields so that career guidance is needed. Some will marry, but the males are all infertile and the females have a reduced fertility.

Terminal care in cystic fibrosis should be anticipated and discussed with the parents in advance so that proper regard to their wishes for home care or easy hospital admission is made. Proper symptomatic relief and the abandonment of heroic and uncomfortable procedures, the support of all the family throughout and following the death of the child all need to be considered. Chapman & Goodall in 'Dying Children Need Help Too', gave a particularly moving account of the management of the terminal stages of two children with cystic fibrosis.

EPILEPSY

Epilepsy is not one condition but a series of conditions with some features in common. It varies widely in severity and thus in its significance with respect to education and career. Epilepsy carries with it a stigma out of all proportion to the clinical disability: it is frequently associated in the lay mind with madness, subnormality, 'possession by devils' and is widely feared. The diagnostic label is often applied loosely and without proper clinical evidence, and the label, (and a whole series of restrictions) may remain in force years after the last fit has occurred, and the child is off medication.

The figures from the National Child Development Study show that only 64 out of the total of 1043 identified as having seizures had established epilepsy. This underlines the need for care in making the diagnosis. One-third of the children with epilepsy were receiving special education, but this was necessary for backwardness rather than the epilepsy itself.

The findings from the National Child Development Study (Ross et al, 1980) showed that 6.7% of the 11 years old in the 1958 birth cohort had a history of seizures or other episodes of loss of consciousness

	total	No. per 1000
Established epilepsy	64	4.1
Reported but unsubstantiated	39	2.5
Febrile convulsions without later afebrile seizures	346	22.3
Febrile convulsions with later spontaneous afebrile seizure	20	1.3
Convulsions with meningitis or encephalitis	12	0.8
Breath holding attacks, faints, temper tantrums	280	18.1
Non-epileptic blank spells	7	0.5
Transitory afebrile convulsive episodes not occurring after age 5 years	307	20.6
Convulsions reported by parents but not to general practitioner or hospital	12	0.8

Clinical features

Taking as our definition of epilepsy 'recurrent paroxysmal disturbance of consciousness, sensation and movement primarily cerebral in origin, unassociated with acute febrile episodes', the following clinical types may be described.

Neonatal convulsions. About 12 per 1000 babies have a convulsion in the first month of life. They may be difficult to recognise at this age and be confused with apnoeic spells. Many occur in the first 24 hours of life when the main cause is brain damage due to birth asphyxia and the prognosis is poor. The drug of choice in this age group is phenobarbitone.

Febrile convulsions affect 3–5% of the age group of 6 months–5 years. Twenty-five per cent of children who have one febrile convulsion will have another and this is more likely in the very young child and where there is a family history of the condition. Parents should be taught how to lower the child's temperature in future episodes of pyrexia by skin exposure, giving aspirin or paracetamol and tepid sponging. Parents are frequently very frightened at the time of the convulsion and fear that their child is dying. They need reassurance. Prolonged convulsions do cause brain damage. There is an increased incidence of temporal lobe epilepsy following prolonged fits. If repeated and prolonged fits occur, then prophylactic sodium valproate may be indicated. In selected cases diazepam given rectally by the parents may be used to terminate a prolonged fit. The overall outlook for febrile convulsions is excellent.

Grand mal convulsions may be either idiopathic, or symptomatic of brain damage associated with another neurological disorder such as cerebral palsy or severe mental handicap. It is the most common type of epilepsy and is easily diagnosed, when there is a good history of aura, loss of consciousness, fall, tonic phase, and clonic phase. The outlook is good — 85% of children are free of convulsions at 20 year follow-up. Phenytoin and sodium valproate are the drugs of choice.

Petit mal is more difficult to diagnose on clinical criteria, but the EEG always shows classical three per second spike and wave discharges precipitated by hyperventilation. Petit mal is easily missed as 'day dreaming' in the classroom. Untreated or inadequately treated petit mal causes loss of vital information in lessons and impaired school performance. Eighty per cent of children are free of fits at 20 year follow-up. The drug of choice is ethosuximide.

Temporal lobe or 'psychomotor' epilepsy consists of attacks of impaired consciousness associated with strange sensations or complex semi-purposeful movements. The diagnosis may be difficult to make and the bizarre sensations or actions may be labelled as a behaviour problem or conduct disorder. There is an increased incidence of specific learning disorders, mental handicap and behaviour problems in children with temporal lobe epilepsy. Carbamazepine is the drug of choice.

Benign focal epilepsy occurs in primary school children and all go into permanent remission by adolescence. The convulsions are short and one sided, and the child does not have amnesia for the attack. Carbamazepine is indicated to prevent the individual seizures.

Anticonvulsant drugs

Drug	Dose	Indication
Phenobarbitone	3–6 mg/kg/day	Grand mal
Phenytoin	4–8 mg/kg/day	Grand mal, focal, temporal lobe
Sodium Valproate	20–40 mg/kg/day	Grand mal, petit mal febrile convulsions
Carbamazepine	10–20 mg/kg/day	Focal, temporal lobe, Grand mal
Ethosuximide	20–40 mg/kg/day	Petit mal
Clonazepam	0.05–0.2 mg/kg/day	Myoclonic Infantile spasms

Infantile spasms are a rare form of epilepsy carrying a poor prognosis. The attacks, consisting of sudden flexion spasms of the whole body commence between 3 and 8 months of age. Fifty per cent of children have an underlying neurological disorder such as cerebral malformations, perinatal brain damage, congenital infections and tuberose sclerosis. Normal development can be expected in 5% only with a better prognosis in those in the idiopathic group. Treatment is with steroids or ACTH in the early stages and later with nitrazepam or clonazepam.

Minor motor epilepsies like myoclonic attacks and drop attacks are commonly symptomatic of an underlying neurological disorder such as severe mental handicap. Treatment is with nitrazepam or clonazepam.

The following conditions, some of which are far more common than epilepsy and frequently confused with it, must be considered in the differential diagnosis, simple faints, breath holding attacks, temper tantrums, hysterical attacks (sometimes secondary to hyperventilation), nightmares, infantile colic and benign paroxysmal vertigo.

A detailed clinical history of an individual attack noticing particularly the sequence of events and the circumstances and antecedents of an attack is the simplest way of sorting these out.

Social and educational aspects of epilepsy

For many children with epilepsy, the problem is not the fits themselves but the educational and behaviour problems that might accompany them and the restrictions that these may place on their activities. Teachers and parents may be ill-informed about epilepsy; they may not know what to do if a fit occurs and their sense of panic and fear may be communicated to other children in the class. They may apply different standards of discipline to the child with epilepsy for fear of producing a fit. The school doctor needs to give the class teachers information about epilepsy so that they are confident in handling the child in the classroom. In one study of school children with epilepsy it was found that the teachers tended to hold off pressure as they regarded the children as being particularly vulnerable; others expected poor scholastic achievements to follow the diagnosis. Such predictions of children's potential tend to be self-fulfilling if they are not corrected. Teachers are anxious about the risks to the child of physical education, laboratory, wood and metalwork and thus the child's studies are restricted. Children should be permitted to participate in most normal activities and it is not reasonable to place uniform restrictions on all children who have fits as some school authorities have done. Decisions will depend on the degree of control, the amount of warning that the child gets and whether the fits only occur at night. Normal lessons should be possible for nearly all children and most should be able to swim with supervision. Most evidence suggests that supervised swimming carries a very small risk indeed. Cycle riding on main roads is not advisable for many children but again individual decisions must be made with the parent, depending on the history. It may well be that it is the parents, through fear of the child's death, who impose the restrictions rather than doctors and teachers. They might insist on escorting their children to and from school, restrict their social interactions and at night install a baby alarm or share the child's room. Anxiety in the parents and child is counterproductive and is associated with poor control. A good prognosis in social and educational terms depends upon medical cooperation and understanding between parents, teachers and doctors.

One-third of children with epilepsy will require special education because of mental retardation. One-third will have specific learning difficulties in reading, writing and arithmetic. Others will fail because of short attention span, overactivity, lack of expectation from teachers or poor school attendance. Delayed language development is associated with delayed reading and writing. These problems are more common in epileptic children with foci in the dominant hemisphere for language. Poorly controlled petit mal attacks which are not recognised easily lead to poor school achievement. Boredom in the classroom also increases the tendency to fits. Drowsiness due to drugs and other side-effects may also interfere with learning. Measurement of drug levels may be useful in preventing these effects. The educational problems are complex and must be assessed jointly by the teacher, doctor and educational psychologist for so many factors, medical, social and educational affect the school performance.

Behaviour problems may be a result of neurological impairment or be the reaction to failure at school or stresses at home due to anxiety or guilt feelings of parents. The children may be aggressive, impulsive and over-active; others may be apathetic, quiet, withdrawn and lacking in confidence. One can speculate that the anticipation or fear of abnormal behaviour (madness) in epilepsy increases its incidence.

Many children with epilepsy have none of these difficulties, are of superior ability and go on to excellent educational achievements.

Anticonvulsant drugs and their common toxic effects

Drug	Side-effects
Phenobarbitone	Irritability, hyperactive, rickets
Phenytoin	Cerebellar ataxia, gum hypertrophy, hirsuitism, rashes, rickets. toxic encephalopathy
Sodium Valproate	Drowsiness, nausea, thrombocytopenia, hair loss, hepatitis
Carbamazepine	Rashes, fatigue, dizziness, bone marrow depression, hepatic toxicity
Ethosuximide	Nausea, rashes, bone marrow depression
Clonazepam	Drowsiness, salivation

DIABETES MELLITUS

Diabetes affects more than one child in every thousand. It is a disease for which there is no cure, but which can be controlled by diet and insulin. The child and family have to learn to measure insulin, give injections, test urine, record results and monitor the diet; they have to be supported over times of stress when the necessary discipline may break down. Good control lessens complications such as blindness for which it is the commonest cause in this country in the age group 30–45.

Although we cannot cure diabetes, increasing knowledge of its aetiology raises the possibility of prevention. Diabetes seems to occur in vulnerable groups who may be identified by their HLA type. Infection of vulnerable individuals with a particular virus, for example Coxsackie B virus, gives rise to auto-immune responses resulting in pancreatic islet cell damage. If the mounting evidence for this hypothesis is substantiated an effective vaccine to Coxsackie B virus will protect susceptible individuals from diabetes mellitus.

The keys to diabetic care are a team approach and patient education and support. The development of the specialist diabetic health visitor is vital in this respect, for most of the care takes place in the patient's home.

It is important that the child and parents have an understanding of the following:

Diabetes and the relation between insulin, diet and exercise with blood sugar and the onset of symptoms like polyuria, hypoglycaemia. This is vital if the parents and child are to make sense of what they are doing, interpret urine test results properly and adjust insulin dose as needed.

Diet. They need to learn how to measure the amount of carbohydrate, and the importance of the timing, distribution of meals and carbohydrate exchanges. They can learn to judge portions by eye and are often able to eat a 'normal' diet with the other members of the family and school dinners.

Insulin. They must be taught how to measure the required dose, the technique of injection, and the rotation of injection sites to prevent induration, wasting and fat hypertrophy. Usually children are controlled with twice daily insulin injections. Short and medium acting insulins are generally used either singly or in combination. Purified monocomponent insulins may induce less reaction and be preferred.

Urine tests for sugar using clinitest and tests for ketones if urine is showing 2% or more sugar. Blood tests performed at home using capillary blood and portable blood glucose meters are being increasingly used in children as well as adults.

Crises. It is important that they know how to recognise hypoglycaemia and what action to take. They must also know to take extra carbohydrate to cover added activity.

Children with diabetes should be able to live a full life. Some parents are anxious and overprotective and prevent the child gaining independence in giving injections. Where there is family discord, inadequacy or just the normal stresses of adolescence, diabetes provides an excellent weapon with which the child can manipulate the family; he may go to the lengths of precipitating hypoglycaemia or ketoacidosis. Poor control increases complications, makes unhappiness for the child and his family and causes poor school performance. The emotional problems can usually be overcome by counselling and hospital admission for re-stabilisation. Occasionally, good control is impossible at home and a residential school placement is necessary to provide the stability that the child needs.

In addition to individual teaching, excellent handbooks are produced for children, parents and teachers by the British Diabetic Association and local diabetic clinics. The British Diabetic Association also organises local parents' groups and summer camps for diabetic children.

ECZEMA

Eczema is sufficiently common for one child with this condition to be seen in virtually every school medical examination and every well baby clinic session. Whilst most cases are mild (though even mild ones cause considerable discomfort to the child), severe cases require hospital admission and make heavy demands on parents in terms of treatment. Eczema is sometimes described as a disease in which 'one scratch is too many and a thousand is not enough'. Constant scratching by the child prevents any healing that may take place and the skin appears painful and weeping, with areas of lichenification and pigmentation. Secondary infection may occur. The child may find it difficult to straighten the legs because of flexural lesions, exercise is limited and perspiration may cause increased itching. Itching can prevent sleep and impair concentration on lessons. The appearance of the skin may frighten other children who may not want to sit next to a child with eczema or who may make unkind comments. The pupils, and the teacher may believe that the lesions are infected and for this reason isolate the child. If the child is also unlucky enough to have asthma and hayfever as well, then the extent of unhappiness is further increased.

The aetiology of eczema is multifactorial; inherited and allergic factors certainly play a great part. Food allergy may be especially important, cow's milk and egg sensitivity are the most common. Breast feeding until 3–4 months may protect susceptible infants from developing eczema but probably serves only to delay its onset. Emotional factors certainly also play a part; eczema becomes worse before exams and with other forms of stress. In 50% of affected infants the eczema resolves by the age of 6 years and 80% by 10 years.

Factors related to failure of the eczema to resolve in childhood include reversed pattern of distribution, that is involving extensor rather than flexor surfaces, discoid eczema with discrete discoid lesions, poor social circumstances, coexisting ichthyosis, Chinese origin, age of onset over 2 years and strong family history of atopy.

Management
Patients appear not to have the same respect for topical skin preparations as they do for other kinds of medication for they often apply them haphazardly and stop treatment abruptly. The keys to treatment are prevention of scratching by an oral antihistamine; avoidance of aggravating factors, for example known allergies, psy-

Heart murmurs

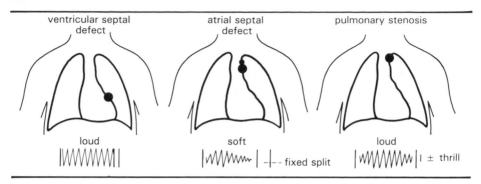

ventricular septal defect	atrial septal defect	pulmonary stenosis
loud	soft	loud

chological stresses; and a topical preparation, ointment for dry skins and cream for weeping lesions. Corticosteroid creams work and the weakest effective one should be used. Potent fluorinated steroids should only be applied over short periods as they cause striae and dermal atrophy. Dryness of the skin often instigates itching, emulsifying ointment in the bath helps to prevent this.

The parents, child and teachers all need counselling and information.

HEART DISEASE

Congenital heart disease affects up to 1% of live births. Some are incompatible with survival. Some present in the early neonatal period with breathlessness and cyanosis and require early treatment, others are discovered during routine examination of children who are entirely asymptomatic. Heart murmurs are most often innocent and can be heard in over 50% of children. Disease of the heart is a very emotive diagnosis, and much unnecessary anxiety is raised by the discovery or follow up of children with innocent heart murmurs. Some heart defects such as small ventricular, and atrial septal defects produce physical signs but no morbidity or mortality. So the children's activities must not be inappropriately restricted.

In particular, ejection systolic murmurs are very common, up to 90% in one series, in only 0.3% of which was there an underlying significant congenital heart disease. The features that suggest an innocent murmur are the patient is asymptomatic, the peripheral pulses are of normal volume and not delayed, the heart sounds are normal, the murmur is only systolic and does not radiate into the neck, and varies in intensity with position and respiration, and the chest X-ray and ECG are normal.

Clinical features

It is not within the scope of this book to describe the clinical features of every type of heart disease in childhood. Those that are asymptomatic and often found at routine medical inspection are illustrated. Children with symptoms would have come to medical attention earlier. The outlook without treatment is poor, 64% die without treatment in the first year. For those found subsequently there is no ground to restrict activities except for aortic stenosis, where there is a risk of sud-

Heart murmurs

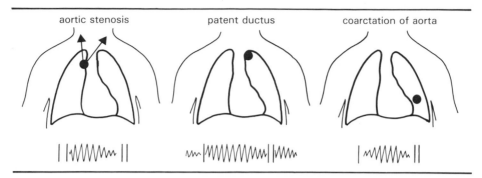

den death. It is important to give antibiotics prophylactically to cover dental operations and in other instances where there is a risk of bacteraemia.

Outlook

The development of cardiac surgery has made a dramatic difference to the prognosis for children with congenital heart disease. However, even after correction of the defects, there can be problems, which must be borne in mind when discussing the career prospects of children with 'corrected' congenital heart lesions. There may be muscle damage leading to subendocardial fibrosis, or pulmonary vascular disease due to irreversible pre-operative changes resulting in narrowing of vessels and impaired growth of vessels. Loss of exercise tolerance and haemoptysis may result. Arrhythmias may result from the original defect or from surgical interference with conducting tissue. There may be incompetence or stenosis or endocarditis of prosthetic valves.

BLOOD DISORDERS

Sickle cell disease

Sickle cell disease, the commonest abnormality of haemoglobin, is a genetic defect in haemoglobin structure which results in sickling of cells at the O_2 tension normally found in venous blood. In some areas of Central Africa the incidence of carriers of the gene is 40%, in the West Indian negro it is 10%. The gene is also found in people originating in the Mediterranean area and Western Asia. It closely follows the distribution of malaria.

The heterozygous condition (carrier) is sickle cell trait. Such individuals are asymptomatic and are not anaemic. They carry up to 35% of abnormal haemoglobin; however, hypoxic conditions can cause sickling and splenic and renal infarcts, and therefore they need to be identified prior to any procedures involving anaesthesia. Routine tests of school children in susceptible racial groups is carried out in many areas.

In the homozygous condition, 80–95% of the haemoglobin is HbS. The severity of the condition varies widely, some children having minimal symptoms. Problems such as pallor and jaundice associated with splenomegaly usually begin between 6 months and 2 years of age.

Painful crisis. This is much the most common initial presentation and is caused by infarction either in a bone or spleen. The haemoglobin does not fall. Infection may be present.

Aplastic crisis. This is usually associated with an infection. The haemoglobin falls and there is not reticulocytosis. Blood transfusion, fluid and antibiotics are normally required.

Megaloblastic crisis. This is due to associated folic deficiency.

Haemolytic crisis. In this reaction the haemoglobin falls but the reticulocytes are high.

Hepatic crisis. This is rare. Severe obstructive jaundice develops which seldom remits.

Other clinical problems include persistent ulceration around the ankles, infection with tetanus and salmonella which may cause osteomyelitis, and persistent signs of pneumonia which are probably infarctive in origin.

There is no specific treatment for sickle cell crises. Management consists of adequate fluids, warmth, antibiotics and analgesia. Blood transfusions are only needed if the haemoglobin falls, which it practically never does, during painful crises. Both anoxia and acidosis cause sickling, and so treatment should be aimed at preventing both. Apart from painful episodes, it should be possible for people with sickle cell anaemia to lead a fairly normal life. Splenectomy is not indicated and indeed recurrent infarcts in the spleen reduce its size so that it may be impalpable by mid childhood. The sickling episodes are often followed by a transient jaundice and occasionally lead to an aplastic crisis when blood transfusions may well be required.

General management includes genetic counselling for the parents, prompt treatment of infections, especially respiratory infections which could give rise to hypoxia, and folic acid supplements. Most children now survive to adult life. Children with sickle cell anaemia can usually attend ordinary schools and follow an unmodified timetable. Teachers need explanation so that they know when to request prompt medical help. Exercise tolerance may be limited by anaemia, leg ulcers or bone pain. Acute crises do not seem to be precipitated by physical activity. In theory at least, sickle cell anaemia is a preventable disorder. However, the carrier state is so widespread that the provision of a counselling service for such a large number of people will be an enormous task.

Thalassaemia

Thalassaemia is less common than sickle cell anaemia in the UK. It is an inherited disorder. The gene is widely distributed in the Middle and Far East and Africa, but is most commonly found in the countries bordering the Mediterranean with the highest incidence of 20% in Turkey and Greece. In β- Thalassaemia the homozygotes have thalassaemia major and develop severe anaemia after the first 6 months of life. Fetal haemoglobin does not contain β-chains and hence the disease is not manifest in early life. The spleen is always enlarged. The heterozygotes have thalassaemia minor. They are usually asymptomatic but may show a mild anaemia. Treatment of the homozygous condition is by regular blood transfusion to keep the haemoglobin above 10 g/dl, which minimises constitutional symptoms and skeletal changes and improves the growth of the child. The main problem is iron overload giving rise to haemosiderosis. Daily desferrioxamine given intramuscularly or by subcutaneous infusion is usually prescribed. With this management children now survive to adult life. They must, however, learn to live with the problems of monthly or 6 weekly transfusions and daily injections.

Prevention of thalassaemia is possible through a combination of health education, routine screening by haemoglobin electrophoresis and genetic counselling. The results of such a programme have recently been reported from Cyprus.

Haemophilia

Haemophilia is the commonest of the inherited coagulation disorders with an incidence of 1: 30 000. It is inherited as an X-linked recessive condition so that half the male children have the condition, half the female children are carriers and the rest are normal. As in other chronic disorders success depends on patient education and appropriate lifestyles.

Acute bleeding episodes may take the form of soft tissue haematomas, muscle haematomas, haematuria, bleeding in the tongue and most commonly haemarthrosis. The parents need to be able to recognise these situations and have prompt access to the local haemophilia centre or other hospital department dealing with the child. Treatment involves the giving of cryoprecipitate or factor VIII concentrate. Treatment, particularly for haemarthrosis needs to be prompt. Home transfusion with Factor VIII concentrate is now available. Parents in suitable cases need to be instructed in the technique of venepuncture.

Repeated haemarthrosis leads to chronic arthropathy affecting mainly the knees and ankles. The joints can become grossly deformed with muscle wasting and contracture. Treatment is aimed at pain relief, anti-inflammatory drugs, regular physiotherapy and swimming to maintain muscle strength and joint movement. The child with haemophilia should be restricted in physical activity (although this will vary with the severity of the disorder), in order to minimise the crippling effect of arthropathy. Likewise, their education should direct them towards non-manual occupations. Some children may need special residential schooling because of excessive acute episodes at home and at school. The children should carry an identity card giving the diagnosis and details of blood group and treatment centre. Regular prophylactic dental care is important to avoid the bleeding complications of extraction. Prophylactic fluoride is also of great value.

Genetic counselling should be available for the family including sisters and cousins. If a female is presumed to be a carrier, amniocentesis and termination of pregnancy for male fetuses is offered.

Leukaemia

Leukaemia is the commonest childhood cancer; the diagnosis is made by examination of peripheral blood and bone marrow. Further determination of the cytological type provides a guide to prognosis. The prospects for the long term survival are better in acute lymphoblastic leukaemia than myeloid leukaemia, although children with this disorder respond better than adults. Children who are white, with null cell leukaemia (that is have the characteristics of neither T nor B lymphocytes), with lymphocyte counts below 20 000 and with little enlargement of liver or spleen and no mediastinal masses have greater than 50% 5 year survival.

Treatment consists of three stages.

Remission induction. In this phase intensive chemotherapy is used with the aim of removing clinical signs, reducing the peripheral blood count to normal levels and reduction of blast cells in the marrow to less than 5%. Rapid lysis of cells can give rise to high uric acid levels and stone formation. This is prevented by adequate fluids and allopurinol.

CNS prophylaxis to prevent meningeal leukaemia. This consists of cranial irradiation and intrathecal methotrexate to prevent CNS manifestation of the disease. In spite of this 5–10% develop CNS leukaemia.

Maintenance therapy. This can be continued as an out-patient using cyclical courses of cytotoxic drugs. Such treatment would need to be continued for 3 years with regular monitoring of the blood count. There is no evidence that results are improved by continuing treatment beyond this time.

The diagnosis of leukaemia places enormous stresses upon the resources of the family. They benefit from continuing support as they adjust to the reality of the diagnosis and the need for regular and intensive therapy. Repeated lumbar punctures, venepunctures, transfusions and hospital admissions place heavy demands on the parent as well as the child. Immunosuppression brings increased susceptibility to infection, which requires careful surveillance and intensive treatment when present. Immunisation with live vaccines such as measles and polio is contraindicated. Immunoglobulin is available for children who are in contact with the ordinary infectious diseases of childhood such as measles. Cytotoxic drugs also frequently produce unpleasant side-effects such as loss of hair, nausea, vomiting and abdominal pain. Cranial irradiation can produce excessive drowsiness and irritability. Time is needed to discuss feelings and answer questions as well as to give the details of treatment. Parents appreciate honesty in answering their questions and being given accurate information on the progress. With improved treatment, children survive to adult life and the question of fertility following irradiation

Age distribution of cancers in childhood (from OPCS 1982 No. 37)

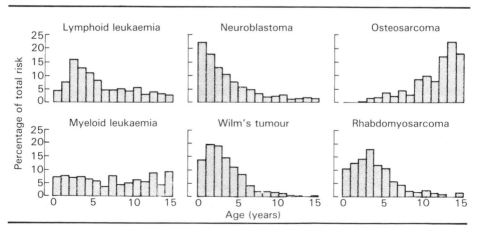

undoubtedly arises. This is impaired, especially in the boys, many of whom will have received testicular irradiation. Due to the stresses of the disease and its management, psychiatric problems affect as many as one-third of the children and their families.

Most children with leukaemia will attend ordinary schools and follow a normal curriculum. Explanations about the disorder, and information on hospital attendances and admissions must be given to the teachers, who should treat the child like any other in the class.

URINARY TRACT INFECTIONS

Urinary tract infections differ from the other chronic disorders described in this chapter in that many of them are asymptomatic. An incidence of asymptomatic infection in girls aged 4–16 of up to 2.5% has been reported. Except in the neonatal period, girls are more frequently affected than boys. Urinary infection is clinically most damaging in children under 4 years when, in association with gross vesico-ureteric reflux, there is intra-renal reflux. Renal scarring may occur with impaired renal growth and the potential for impaired renal function. Scarring that develops before 4 years can progress after this age if infection is not controlled. Thirty-five per cent of children with urinary infection show some degree of vesico-ureteric reflux and 12% have scarring.

Clinical features
In the pre-school child urinary infection presents with non-specific symptoms of fever, malaise, vomiting or failure to thrive. Older children may present with enuresis or specific symptoms related to the urinary tract. Often infections or re-infections may be clinically silent so a high degree of suspicion of urinary infections should be maintained throughout childhood. Just as clinical evidence of urinary infection is difficult in childhood, so is bacteriological proof. The collection of clean urine specimens from children requires time and patience!

In the child health clinic where delay may be experienced between collection of urine and setting up culture, the dip-slide technique is very suitable.

Management
Following diagnosis, the infection should be eradicated with a 7–10 day course of antibiotic, chosen according to the sensitivity of the organism. Co-trimoxazole or amoxycillin which give high concentrations in the urine are frequently suitable. Investigations include radiography to detect reflux, scarring, abnormal renal growth and other anatomical abnormalities. Children with reflux or recurrent infections are given regular prophylactic antibiotics to prevent further infection and renal damage. Double micturition is also useful in preventing reinfection. Follow-up includes repeated examination of the urine to detect further infections, measurement of growth and blood pressure to monitor general health and renal function. The natural history in the majority of children with reflux is for resolution; however, surgical reimplantation of the ureters is considered if there is failure to prevent infections, the development of fresh renal scarring, or gross reflux in a young infant with abnormal kidneys.

Orthopaedic problems found at birth in the National Child Development Study (Davie et al, 1972)

	Incidence per 1000 births
Talipes	4.1
Congenital dislocation of hip	1.1
Other bone and joint	2.1

ORTHOPAEDIC PROBLEMS

Orthopaedic problems are common in both the pre-school and the school child. At birth they account for more than 35% of the congenital abnormalities notified. The severity varies widely from mild talipes to severe defects of the spine and limbs. However, children with orthopaedic abnormalities survive into school and adult life more frequently than children with other types of congenital malformation.

Children with orthopaedic conditions may have decreased mobility and restrictions in activity caused by the disorder or its treatment, periods of immobilisation in hospital, both of which can influence educational and social development.

Congenital dislocation of the hip

The incidence of congenital dislocation of the hip is reported to be from 0.75 to 1.5 per 1000 births. The incidence of unstable hips at birth, many of which will resolve spontaneously, is variously reported from 2.6 to 21.8 per 1000 births. Early detection of the true dislocation is necessary in order to avoid the long lasting disability caused by late diagnosis and treatment. However, the clinical tests to detect dislocation require considerable experience in their execution, and the rate of missed dislocations has been reported from 0.04 per 1000 births to 1.12 per 1000 births. Some may argue that a proportion of the 'missed dislocations' are not present at birth or cannot be detected at this time. The other aspect of the clinical problem is that splinting of hips can cause damage to the femoral head; this risk and the high incidence of spontaneous resolution of unstable hips needs to be carefully balanced.

There is a strong case for the meticulous review of children at high risk.

Examination of the hip for dislocation can only be properly learned by practical teaching with the demonstration of positive and negative findings reinforced by experience. Barlow's modification of Ortolani's test is used, the test is divided into two parts.

The epidemiology of congenital dislocation of the hip is interesting, not all the findings can be adequately explained

C.D.H. is more common in:	
Girls	8 : 1
Where there is a family history	20% of cases
Breech delivery (or late version) / Caesarean section for breech	25% of all cases
Left hip/right hip	2.3 : 1
Delivery in winter	1.5 : 1
Oligohydramnios	
Foot deformity	

The baby must be relaxed and lying supine on a firm surface, with the legs pointed towards the examiner. The hips and knees are flexed to a right angle. The legs are grasped with the middle finger of each hand over the greater trochanter and the thumbs on the inner aspect of the thigh opposite the lesser trochanter. With one hand stabilising the pelvis and opposite hip, each hip is tested in turn. In the first part of the test, the hip is moved into mid-abduction and forward pressure is exerted behind the greater trochanter. If the hip is dislocated it will be felt to slip back into the acetabulum. In the second part of the test, backward pressure from the thumb over the inner aspect of the thigh will cause the dislocatable femoral head to slip over the posterior lip of the acetabulum and return when the pressure is relaxed. This test cannot be applied if the examiner's hands are too small, or the baby's thighs too big to secure the necessary grasp. Limited hip abduction is an important physical sign in the older child and in those with a fixed dislocation which cannot be felt to move in and out of the acetabulum in the Barlow's test.

Reasons for failure to identify the dislocated hip include: the examination may not be carried out for example, home delivery, sick neonates; attempting to examine a poorly relaxed baby; failure to examine the baby on a firm surface; failure to recognise the significance of restricted abduction; inexperience and poor instruction in the technique of examination and failure to re-examine hips at examinations other that at birth.

With early diagnosis the outlook for children with this condition is excellent.

Management of the unstable hip; a reminder. Double nappies have a doubtful place in management; follow-up for all suspected hips is essential

	Clinical findings	Management
I	Hip stable Abducts fully No click	Nil
II	Hip stable Abducts fully ligamentous click	Check at 3 months for full abduction. If doubtful, X-ray
III	Hip stable Limitation of abduction	Initially passive stretching to improve abduction. Adductor tenotomy for those that fail to improve. Clinical and radiological follow-up
IV	Hip dislocatable by Barlow's test	Initial: double nappies for one week (in view of high spontaneous resolution rate and risk of incorrect splinting If unstable at follow-up — Abduction, splint, e.g. Von Rosen or Craig. If normal at follow-up — clinical and radiological follow-up until walking
V	Hip dislocated at rest but can be relocated by abduction	Reduction of the dislocation and retaining it in the reduced position by an abductive splint for 3 months If normal at follow-up — clinical and radiological follow-up until walking
VI	Fixed dislocations	Often associated with other congenital abnormalities. Will need surgical reduction

Removable splints, which might not be correctly applied by parents are probably not as suitable as those that are applied by properly trained staff.

Osteochondrosis

Osteochondrosis is a condition of focal ischaemic aseptic necrosis at centres of ossification. The clinical consequences of the disorder vary widely from minor disorders requiring no treatment, such as Osgood-Schlatter's disease of the tibial apophysis to potential severe joint damage such as Perthes' disease of the hip. Treatment at some sites is controversial. The condition is also riddled with eponyms.

Juvenile chronic polyarthritis

Juvenile chronic polyarthritis comes into the differential diagnosis of many other disorders in view of its protean joint and systemic manifestations. In its initial presentation it may be confused with such conditions as leukaemia, infections, ankylosing spondylitis, osteochondrosis, and systemic lupus erythematosis. The diagnostic criteria generally accepted for juvenile chronic polyarthritis are: an onset before the age of 16 years; four or more joints involved for a minimum of 3 months; if less than four joints are involved; synovial biopsy must show histological evidence of rheumatoid disease; and other causes of arthritis excluded (Ansell & Bywaters, 1959).

Three sub-divisions of juvenile chronic polyarthritis are described. The early onset type is the most severe with prominent constitutional disturbance and some mortality resulting from amyloidosis. Twenty-five per cent of this group will have severe joint destruction. The late onset group is predominantly arthritic in presentation and carries a much better prognosis. The monoarticular group may progress to polyarthritis.

The arthritis typically involves interphalangeal, temporo-mandibular joints, wrists, ankles, and hip joints. There may be lymphadenopathy, splenomegaly (50% of the early onset group), pyrexia, rashes, nodules on tendons and bony prominences, growth retardation, carditis (rare), and iritis.

Treatment requires careful clinical judgement and a proper balance between the benefits of rest and immobilisation (relief of pain and swelling) and the risks (muscle wasting, loss of joint movement, emotional, educational). The three elements of treatment are drugs, physiotherapy and surgery. Aspirin in high dosage is a first line treatment, steroids are only given if carditis or iritis are present. Second line drugs include indomethacin, gold, chloroquine, naprosyn, ibuprofen and penicillamine. Physiotherapy is given to ensure full movement and with splintage to rest affected joints.

Eighty per cent of children with chronic juvenile polyarthritis enter adult life with no significant disability. Severe joint destruction is much more common in those with early onset disease and in 50% of those who are sero-positive for rheumatoid factor.

Scoliosis

The incidence of scoliosis requiring treatment in the school population is 3–4/ 1000. It is an important condition to recognise early because progression leads to cardiovascular and respiratory embarrassment and death in early adult life. Most

Types of scoliosis

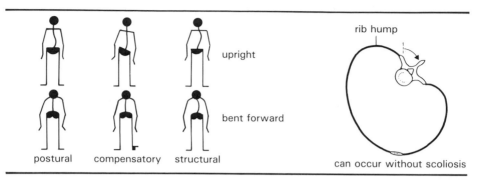

upright

bent forward

postural   compensatory   structural

rib hump

can occur without scoliosis

cases at presentation are so advanced that only major surgery is helpful. Children diagnosed early through school screening can be treated successfully by bracing. There are no symptoms until scoliosis is advanced.

Postural scoliosis results from poor standing habit. compensatory scoliosis is secondary to unequal leg length. Both of these disappear when the child bends forward. Structural scoliosis which does not disappear with bending forwards, is not a single entity.

Only a small number of those in the infantile group will progress. Current school screening programmes are aimed at identifying the juvenile and adolescent type.

School screening programmes. This can be done by trained school nurses or by PE teachers by simply looking for a spinal curvature that does not disappear when the child bends forward. The detection of a rib hump on its own is not adequate as 10–15% will not have a scoliosis. School screening programmes have shown that asymmetry of the spine is common in healthy children and only a small proportion have curves that will progress or require treatment. Our present knowledge of the natural history of the condition and the clinical features of those that will progress gives this screening procedure a low specificity.

Management of scoliosis. The brace may be the unsightly but well tried Milwaukee brace as illustrated, or a plastic corset

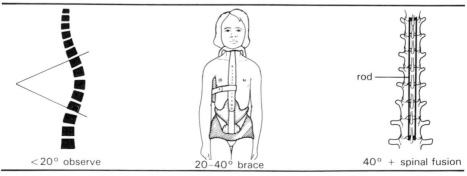

< 20° observe   20–40° brace   40° + spinal fusion

rod

Treatment. Without knowledge of the aetiology of scoliosis, treatment follows the empirical rule, 'If it is bent, straighten it'. Assessment involving measurement and X-ray of the spine to determine the severity of scoliosis (the angle of spinal curvature) is undertaken to determine the type of treatment required.

REFERENCES AND FURTHER READING

Bower B 1978 The treatment of epilepsy in children. British Journal of Hospital Medicine 19: vol. 8–19

Catford J C, Bennet G C, Wilkinson C 1982 Congenital hip dislocation: an increasing and still uncontrolled disability. British Medical Journal 285: 1527–1520

Dickson R A 1983 Scoliosis in the community. British Medical Journal 286: 615–617

Editorial 1983 Prevention of insulin dependent diabetes. Lancet 104–105

Editorial 1981 School Screening for scoliosis. Lancet 345–346

Farquhar J W, Campbell M L 1980 Care of the diabetic child in the community. British Medical Journal 281: 1534–1537

Forfar J, Arneil I G C 1978 Textbook pf Paediatrics. Churchill Livingstone, Edinburgh

Godfrey S 1977 Childhood asthma. British Journal of Hospital Medicine 17: 430–441

Gordon N 1982 Duration of treatment of childhood epilepsy. Developmental Medicine and Child Neurology 24: 84–87

Lee D A, Winslow N R, Speight A, Hey E N 1983 Prevalence and spectrum of asthma in childhood. British Medical Journal 286: 1256–1258

Martin A J, Landau L I, Phelan P D 1982 Asthma from childhood at age 21: patient and his diseases. British Medical Journal 284: 380–382

McNicol L N, Williams H B 1973 Spectrum of asthma in children. Clinical and physiological management. British Medical Journal 4: 7–11

Milner A D 1980 Treatment of infants and children with asthma. Prescribers Journal 20: 33–39

Pearn J, Bank R 1978 Drowning risks to epileptic children: a study from Hawaii. British Medical Journal 2: 1284–1285

Ross E M, Peckham C S, West P B, Butler N R 1980 Epilepsy in childhood: findings from the National Child Development Study. British Medical Journal 207–210

Ross E M, Kurtz S, Peckham C S 1983 Children with epilepsy: implication for the School Health Service. Public Health 97: 75–81

Speight A, Lee D A, Hey E N 1983 Underdiagnosis and undertreatment of asthma in childhood. British Medical journal 286: 1253–1255

14
Physical Handicap

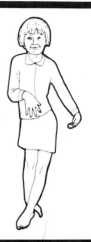

Severe physical handicap places heavy and continuing demands upon a broad range of professional services as well as on the parents and children themselves. Lesser degrees of handicap make fewer demands in terms of special resources but the children and their families still require the same quality and continuity of care. Although we may classify the child's disorder in broad terms according to aetiology or the pattern of motor disability, each child is an individual and has his own special needs. For this reason generalised statements may be of little practical value for an individual child. Often there are associated problems like epilepsy, mental handicap, vision or hearing problems or specific learning difficulties.

EPIDEMIOLOGY

The incidence of physical and multiple handicap amongst primary school children is approximately 12 per 1000. The commoner ones include cerebral palsy at 2.5 per 1000, spina bifida 1 in 1000 and muscular dystrophy 0.2 per 1000. The large remainder consists of a wide range of rarer central nervous system and ortho-

Diagnosis and management of 114 children age 4–19 in a school for the physically handicapped

Diagnosis :	Spina bifida	45
	Cerebral palsy	39
	Muscular dystrophy	11
	Others	19
Management :		
Physiotherapy		104 (91%)
Speech therapy		35 (31%)
Assistance with feeding		16 (14%)
Toileting — needing assistance		36 (32%)
— in nappies		24
— indwelling catheters		17
— penile appliance		13
— urostomies		10
— colostomies		1

Estimated number of physically handicapped children in a population of 250 000

Cerebral palsy	150
Spina bifida	50
Duchenne muscular dystrophy	8
Other (neuromuscular and orthopaedic)	40

paedic abnormalities. Cerebral palsy is twice as common in the children of un-skilled workers as in the higher social classes; 55% of lesions are thought to be prenatal, 40% perinatal and 5% postnatal. The incidence of physical handicap has dropped considerably over the last 20–30 years.

HOSPITAL AND COMMUNITY CARE

Traditionally the care of the handicapped child has been practised in two areas — the hospital assessment unit and the special school. The advent of District Handicap Teams and a broad based approach to services for handicapped children has lead to a blurring of these boundaries and the growth of an integrated service. Although the hospital can concentrate the resources for the specific assessment and management of the handicapped child, the hospital is not the environment in which the child lives. For this reason evaluation and management programmes must be placed in the context of the home and school and ideally involve the same professionals in all three settings.

Inevitably many agencies and individuals are involved with a multiply handi-capped child and the turnover of staff within these agencies is often high. It is not surprising that parents become confused and bewildered by their various specialist roles and the number of people involved. Someone should have an over-view of the total care and progress of the child and provide continuity through-out childhood. The professionals who are able to fulfill this role are the hospital consultant paediatrician, the community paediatrician, the general practitioner, the health visitor, and the head teacher of the school. Parents rightly appreciate the continuity and the familiarity with themselves and their child which an individual can provide. They are distressed when they have to piece together the various bits of professional advice or face a complete stranger who has hurriedly thumbed through three thick volumes of out-patient notes.

Teamwork

Close multi-disciplinary teamwork between the health, education and social work-ers, has become the cornerstone of management of the physically and multiply handicapped child. With the sharing of professional skills and good communi-cation this can be highly effective.

Initially the team will be concerned with assessment and the formulation of recommendations for management. The results need to be made known to parents in a written as well as a verbal statement. They should be available to all those who deal with the child and family. Following initial assessment, periodic reviews

Agencies involved

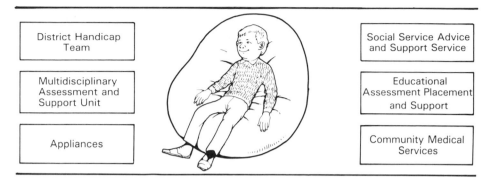

District Handicap Team		Social Service Advice and Support Service
Multidisciplinary Assessment and Support Unit		Educational Assessment Placement and Support
Appliances		Community Medical Services

are required to monitor progress, update recommendations and deal with new problems as they arise. Some team members will be involved in the day to day management and therapy and a familiar person must always be available when parents request help.

The role of the community paediatrician

A paediatrician working in the community can help handicapped children and their families in many ways. Working within special schools, day nurseries or child health clinics, he is in an ideal position to know the local resources and collate the information received from agencies dealing with the child. Many have a joint role, and are able to bridge the gap between hospital and community services.

Contributing towards assessment and reviews. Observations of behaviour and functioning at home and at school of the child and family may bring to light problems and abilities that are not apparent in the hospital clinic and thus contribute towards the original assessment and subsequent reviews. Recording growth, vision, and hearing, social and educational progress are important measurements of the child's functioning which the community services provide.

Explaining the child's medical condition to other professionals. Staff in nurseries and in schools do not have direct access to the child's medical records. Explanation and reassurance from the paediatrician will greatly ease the task of the teacher and provide an appropriate regimen for the child.

Providing required resources within the community. Although the number of professionals involved with a handicapped child may be large, they are sometimes not present in the right place at the right time. For example, the school might seek advice on seating from the occupational therapist or the nursery might approach a speech therapist to deal with particular problems that arise in that setting. Alternatively the need may be not for professional help but for additional physical resource at home or in school in terms of special equipment, transport, finance or aids. The paediatrician can play a part in ensuring that the limited resources are put to optimal use.

Dealing with day to day problems. The community paediatrician needs to be available to deal with problems as they arise in the home or school. These may be related to infections, skin problems, constipation, medication, fluctuations in the child's condition or arranging relief for parents at times of crisis or added stress. The parents, teachers, school nurse and health visitor are obviously vital links in identifying these changing day to day needs.

Innovation. The paediatrician also has a role in assessing needs within the community and providing new resources where they are required. This may mean setting up a teaching and support group for nursery nurses dealing with handicapped children, providing a toy library, helping to set up a local parents' group or encouraging local play groups and mother and toddler groups to accept the physically handicapped child.

An advocacy role. Parents may not always find it easy to obtain the necessary help that they require. They may also not have the necessary skills to locate and obtain special sources of help. The doctor therefore may be of help in dealing with local authorities, housing departments, social services and in obtaining help for such things as telephones, washing machines, and holidays from sources such as the Family Fund.

Counselling parents. Counselling is a major task for anyone dealing with the handicapped child and his family. It is much more the art of listening patiently than of giving advice. The priorities for the family may not be the same as the priorities for the professionals. The families should not be so overwhelmed or over-awed that they do not state their own views or needs. The potential complexity of handicap may leave the parents' understanding of cause and treatment well behind and the parent can become a technician in carrying out the instructions of the professionals rather than a partner. The day to day demands of looking after the child, the restrictions that are placed upon the parents and their own grief and disappointment are subjects that require discussion.

Continuity in this role is vital; knowledge about the child over an extended period of time encourages growing mutual respect. It is essential to be unhurried, and to have humility, and to have patience as the parents repeatedly discuss the same issues. The counsellor may need to absorb the parents' anger. Dealing with the emotions that arise in the family of a multiply handicapped child can itself provide stress for the professionals, so they need support too.

Certain questions help tease out particular problems that might not be easily identified. What is the biggest problem about living with him? What are you most afraid of? If he could speak what would he say his biggest problem is? Do you think about what will happen when he grows up? Who plays with him most? This helps identify whether the task of care is falling predominantly on one person. Are you getting a holiday this year? Families with handicapped children often miss out on holidays and the sorts of day to day recreation that others take for granted.

It is important to realise the needs of the whole family. Although one parent may be the one who commonly brings the child to clinic or to school, it is necessary to meet and enquire about the health and wellbeing of both parents and siblings. The question of another child in the family or the neglect of the parents' or other children's needs are issues which often need to be aired.

THE EFFECTS OF PHYSICAL HANDICAP

Before considering the roles of the various professionals involved in the management of physical and multiple handicap, it is useful to discuss the overall effects. Students in some medical schools have some of these problems brought home to them by spending a day in a wheelchair, and experiencing for themselves the limitations and frustrations. Limited mobility makes stairs difficult or impossible. Access to many public buildings and to public transport may also be impossible. Much movement is dependent upon external help. The children's natural wishes to explore, to be independent, and even to misbehave are restricted. Aspects of personal life, such as using the toilet, dressing and washing often cannot be accomplished independently and with privacy. Not only is the child's self-image damaged but also the way he is treated by others. The title of a series of radio programmes 'Does he take sugar?' nicely summarises the attitude of many towards physical handicap. Questions are addressed to the one who pushes the wheelchair and not the one in it.

Although numerous benefits are available for the physically handicapped child and his family, increased expenditure, restriction of family's earning capacity because of the time required to care for the child, and later his limited ability to earn, all lead to limitations in finance compared to other families.

A happier meaningful life means not only meeting the needs of therapy and day to day care, but also covers friendships and recreation. These needs are no different to those of anyone else though they are more difficult to meet. Shopping, sport, parties, pop culture, going to the cinema or park, travel, planning holidays are just as important for the physically handicapped as for any other child.

PHYSIOTHERAPY AND OCCUPATIONAL THERAPY

Physiotherapy and occupational therapy are essential in the assessment and treatment of physically handicapped and multiply handicapped children. The skills of physiotherapists and occupational therapists overlap. Often they work together as a team, borrowing each other's skills and techniques and referring children back and forth. There are a large number of treatment methods available, for example the Bobath, Peto, Fay-Doman systems. Many therapists are eclectic in style, using bits of different methods according to the needs of individual children.

Therapists work directly with the children and perhaps more importantly through parents, nurses and teachers guiding them in play, daily handling and outside leisure activities appropriate for the child. They also perform a valuable support and advice role, not just for parents but for teachers — particularly when physically handicapped children are in ordinary schools. Much of the therapist's time therefore may be spent outside the hospital or handicap centre, making home visits, going to day nurseries, schools, and clubs.

Therapy at hospital is important too. Hospital centres can concentrate a lot of resources, for example a 'bank' of aids which the child can try. A parents' 'club' held informally during clinic time can provide social support. Also at some points in many children's development parents find it hard to give the needed therapy themselves and it has to be done by the therapist. However, it is essential to remember the financial cost to the family of repeated hospital visits and the inevitable waiting for transport at home and hospital.

The child is not a passive recipient of therapy, but an active partner, trying to develop his own independent skills. The relationship of the child and therapist and their personalities are important variables in determining progress.

The aims of therapy

Promoting motor development. Therapists aim to take children through the normal sequence of motor development. For multiply handicapped children this is not necessarily an automatic process. All the individual stages have to be worked out and learnt. In cerebral palsy the child will usually have to combat persisting primitive reflexes, dystonic movements and spastic reflexes. These can interfere with every skill from sitting to feeding. The child and parents work with the therapists to inhibit these reactions. Correct handling of the child is crucial. Because of their lack of automatic protective reactions (righting responses, parachute reactions, etc) cerebral palsied children can be very scared when learning to be mobile. They particularly need to be made to feel safe and secure.

Promoting functional development. As well as normal motor development the handicapped child has to learn normal social and self-help skills, like eating, washing, toileting. Therapists have a major task in promoting these developmental skills.

Preventing deformities. For a number of reasons physically and multiply handicapped children often develop physical deformities. Muscle imbalance, persistent primitive reflexes, immobility and unsatisfactory posture determine many of these. The most profound is the 'wind-swept' deformity of the severely cerebral palsied child. Equally crippling may be the kypho-scoliosis of the child with spina bifida or muscular dystrophy. Once established these deformities are hard to correct and the therapists have a crucial role in preventing them. Correct seating is paramount.

AIDS

When considering an aid two groups of people must be involved, the child and family, and the therapists and teachers. An aid that the child or family is not committed to will not be used. Some aids, especially splints, supports and seating, can even worsen the handicap. There is no such thing as the all-purpose aid that fits every handicapped child, and it is impossible to know how an individual aid is going to work out and so an 'aid-bank' or resource centre full of aids that can be tried out is essential. For aids that have to be individually made, like seating, the closer the maker is to the child the better. Parents with odd-jobbing or carpentry skills are invaluable. Children outgrow aids and this has to be anticipated. Many individual aids which have to be ordered take too long to arrive. Happily there are now aids which are designed to be bright and attractive to the children. Imagination combined with the skills of the toy designer have produced equipment which not only meets the need but is useful, fun and also teaches cognitive skills.

Aids that prevent deformities and allow development

Seating. Correct seating can both open up the handicapped child's world and prevent deformity.

For the multiply or physically handicapped child very soft seating is perilous and bean-bags are absolutely contraindicated as they lead to the wind-swept deformity. Seating must be firm and promote an upright posture. Some useful seats are: corner seats, moulded seats, activities tables with inset, saddle seating for adductor spasms, self propelled chairs and Matrix body supports.

Prolonged seating keeps a child's hips flexed for too long a period. Some time spent standing is useful and is achievable in all but the most handicapped child by use of a Flexistand. It would however be wrong simply to select a chair from the above 'shopping list'. Each child needs individual assessment by a therapist. When placing a child in a seat his posture must be considered critically, particularly that of the hips and spine. A fixed deformity may need surgical intervention before adequate seating is achievable.

The seated child's feet should be flat to provide security. They are also vulnerable to deformity, especially when the child is beginning to stand. For younger children firm slippers (e.g. Shoos-Shoos) and for the older child Piedro boots are useful.

Example of appliances for posture

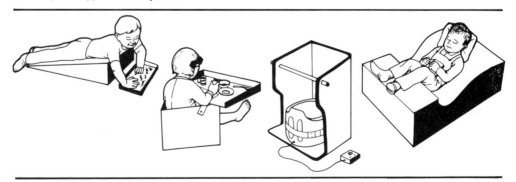

Splints and Supports. Ankle-foot and knee ankle-foot orthoses are useful in holding joints in positions which are not possible naturally due to spasticity or weakness. Although they appear simple in design, their use is a highly specialised subject. Some centres are now using rigid plastic orthoses which are cosmetically much preferable to the older metal braces. Much more straightforward are gaiters which will keep arms, legs or bodies straight, they are especially useful for arms that insist on flexing back towards the child.

Wedges and rolls are excellent in helping the floppy child develop spinal and head control.

Mobility aids. The handicapped child's world opens up when he becomes mobile. Any number of aids are available. Some useful ones are: Cell Barnes Walker, crawlers, trundle toys, rollators, prone boards (for very floppy children).

Wheelchairs. There is no perfect buggy or wheelchair, again individual assessment by a therapist is essential. The advantage for the parent or child is that they get you quickly and efficiently from A to B. Unless, of course getting from A to B involves climbing into a bus or car. Buggies and wheelchairs are bulky.

Example of appliances for mobility

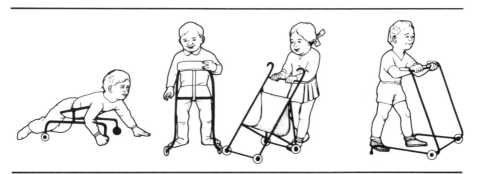

Aids that help with skills

Feeding. Dycem mats (sticky mats that stop plates sliding about) are extremely useful. Feeding dishes and beakers have been designed for children with poor motor-skills. 'Prior and Howard' spoons are plastic but malleable such that they will not break even with children who have pronounced bite reflexes. Heated dishes (from Boots and Mothercare) into which hot water is put before feeding are valuable. They are heavy enough not to slide about and keep food warm during long feeding sessions.

Bathing. Bathing the handicapped child always seems perilous but can be helped by a number of aids. The Western Medical Bath seat which is like a baby-relax but waterproof and sits in the bathwater, is good for babies. Non-slip bath-mats increase safety, as do whole bath inserts which reduce the depth of water and the parents do not have to bend double over the side of the bath. For older children the Safa-bath seat and Suzy-Air chair both fit inside a normal bath.

Toileting. For any success at toileting it is essential that the child feels secure on the toilet. A number of aids are available. For babies there are built-up potties. An older child can use the Watford Potty chair or insert seats into the family toilet. Most mobile physically handicapped children over 5 will need substantial home alterations including a toilet with handrails, and provision for a wheelchair if necessary. Such substantial aids need a lot of forward planning with therapists and parents.

How to get an aid

When all the relevant parties have decided on an aid, and preferably when a short-term loan has demonstrated its usefulness, it then needs to be procured. Usually the therapists will be known in local channels but they may need medical support for an application. Where to apply and who pays will depend on the aid itself, the age of the child and where the aid is to be used. For the more expensive items a number of options often have to be explored.

Department of Health. The Department has rulings over the substantial aids it will and will not supply. For example at the time of publication it will not pay for the ortho-kinetic wheelchair, charitable bodies have to provide these. Many aids however are in a 'grey' area and it is always worthwhile applying.

Handicap/Rehabilitation Centres often have a certain number of aids for loaning out, especially if they have an aid 'bank'.

Social Services Departments will provide many home and personal aids. Contact the social services department's occupational therapists who also can advise on home alterations.

Local Education Authorities will provide aids for educational purposes. How broadly this definition is interpreted depends on the authority. Most will allow such aids to go to the home, but often this is not practical, e.g. with bulky wheelchairs.

Local charities if approached will sometimes pay for aids, and will welcome guidance as to what is needed.

Businesses. Some companies producing aids will loan out equipment on a short or long-term basis.

Family Fund. When other channels have failed this government financed agency can help out for substantial items.

Manpower Services Commission. This will sometimes provide an aid (e.g. typewriter) if it will enable a person to gain employment. Enquiries should be made to a disablement resettlement officer.

The family. Parents and extended family members can be very resourceful in providing home-made aids. This is to be encouraged as they know their child's needs best. However, they should not be expected to pay out large amounts for the financial burden of a handicapped child is considerable.

COMMUNICATION FOR THE PHYSICALLY AND MULTIPLY HANDICAPPED

Delay in the development of language and communication skills is a critical problem in the care of the handicapped. Lack of understanding of expressive language raises barriers to further learning with immense frustration for both parents and children.

Language development programmes demand careful observation of the child to record current abilities. This means paying attention not only to comprehension, expression and articulation but also to other more basic skills of symbolic understanding and attention control. Based on these initial observations an in-dividual language programme can be constructed, based on the child's ability. Each step in the programme is structured so that the progress of the child can be easily monitored. Opportunities to acquire language skills should be available throughout the day as well as concentrated in therapy spells. The use of carefully chosen toys to encourage growth of attention, and symbolic understanding is most useful.

The role of the speech therapist

The specialised speech therapist is essential to the team assessment of the child and in directing therapy. They must be involved early and not just as an after-thought because speech has failed to develop. The speech therapist has a number of roles, the first begins very early in the handicapped child's life. In their initial assessment they evaluate tongue, palate and mouth movements and advise over feeding problems. At a slightly later age they can assess the child's inner language, the essential prerequisite to expressive language. They will see what concepts of language have developed and how this development can be enhanced through play. The therapist will not be confined to verbal communication but will concentrate on functional communication by all means so that the child's needs can be met.

In the pre-school years the therapist works with and through the parents and carers of the child (e.g. nursery nurses in a day nursery). As in physical devel-opment, the development of communication may not be automatic. Often a con-siderable amount of therapy through play is necessary. Hence it is doubly important that parents and carers understand concepts of early language devel-opment and enact the development programmes themselves. Once at school the child's communication therapy is again more likely to be directed by the speech therapist via the work of teachers and parents than given directly. The therapist will advise on alternative communication systems. Throughout the child's life the therapist and community paediatrician will check his hearing.

Alternative communication systems

Multiply handicapped children often have considerable communication problems which can result in frustration, social withdrawal and under-estimation of their abilities. Physically handicapped children also can have problems if their speech or hand function is affected. The possibility of using alternative communication may therefore arise. Either a communication signing-system like Makaton, or communication equipment such as an electric typewriter may be used. Parents are often afraid that using an aid may inhibit normal speech development and as a result they tend to be introduced too late rather than too early. On the whole, alternative systems and aids encourage rather than inhibit language development. Sometimes they are used at a young age and abandoned later as natural com-munication takes over. In practice aids are helpful in a minority of multiply handi-capped children only. It is not easy to decide which children will benefit.

Three questions should be asked.

What is the child's ability and motivation? The child needs to want to com-municate and to have a cognitive ability of at least 12 months, preferably 18 months. Sometimes verbal comprehension is the only means by which one can assess the child's cognition. If the child has severe mental handicap chronological age is rarely important.

How is the child communicating already? If the child is already communicating all his needs as much as he apparently wants, an aid will not be successful. However if he is not, the type of communication he and his parents are using will give a clue to what sort of aid is appropriate. Is the child using any speech and if so how much? Is he using direct pointing or associative pointing, that is pointing directly to food or to a plate meaning 'I'm hungry'. Is the child using symbols like pictures in a book? Can the child cope with delay in communication? Is he using gesture or mime?

What are the limitations for the parents/carers/school? For any aid to work the parents have to be committed to it, the school similarly. If a family takes on an alternative system all or almost all those dealing with the child have to use it, which can be a considerable strain. Families often cope very well but schools and other institutions have problems if only one or two children are using a particular sign system.

Types of alternative communication systems

Sign languages. These have the advantage over other systems in that they are immediate in their communication. Their disadvantages are that they demand a lot of parents and school staff and require a certain level of hand function.

British sign language for the deaf. This was developed from spontaneous gestures into a formal language. The gestures are equivalent to ideas *not* spoken language and it has its own grammar. There is a finger-spelling supplement and communication is aided by facial expression and body language. It is rarely suited to the multiply handicapped because it needs good cognition and reasonable two handed function. Details are available from the RNID, 105 Grosvenor Street, London WC1E 6AH.

Makaton vocabulary. This takes 350 of the most useful and easier hand signs from the British sign language. It was developed for the deaf, severely mentally handicapped and is now used widely by severely handicapped children and adults in schools and adult training centres. Parents and carers talk while they sign. It is possible to start with a few basic signs and build up to a larger collection. Makaton is less successful for children with severe motor problems as two-handedness is needed.

Paget-Gorman. This needs more cognition than Makaton and the hand movements are complex. Parents often find it hard because of its complexity. It is a translation of spoken English and you talk as you sign. Hence it is much used in schools for the speech impaired.

Total communication. This is a manual, auditory, and oral system of communication, recognising signs as an essential reinforcement to oral and auditory aspects of communication for deaf persons. While it is rarely formally used for multiply handicapped children many parents are naturally using all those modalities of communication.

Non-sign languages

Direct pointing picture or word boards. The BLISS symbol board was developed in Canada and uses a mixture of pictograms, abstract symbols and ideograms usually representing an idea or concept rather than a 'word'. Arrays of symbols are displayed on a board or TV screen for children to point to. The English equivalent words are displayed above each symbol so training is less necessary. Details of courses are available via BLISS Symbolics Communications Resource Centre (UK). Children need only limited motor skills for this system. It is rather laboured for the parents and the child needs cognition above a 2.5 year level.

Physical aids

There are a variety of these being developed in parallel with advances in microelectronics. But as yet few are available widely. There are: 'Direct accessing' aids, for example head pointing apparatus for those with poor hand function and specialised typewriters for those with limited but usable hand function. 'Indirect accessing' aids like scanning devices that run a pointer or light over a list of letters, symbols or words and the child halts the scanner when he chooses, are also being developed.

Many of these aids are heavy and are often only usable in one place, thus a child using a computer can only communicate where that aid is located. There are currently problems getting these aids supplied and paid for. The DHSS only recognises the POSSUM and PET computer and children must be assessed by a DHSS representative before they are issued. Education Authorities may pay for adapted typewriters if it can be proved they are essential to education; usually the typewriters are restricted to the school and cannot be used at home.

SEX EDUCATION FOR THE HANDICAPPED

Sexual relationships are as important to handicapped adults as to ordinary people. Handicapped adolescents are in a poor position to gain knowledge and experience. Few of them have girlfriends or boyfriends. In special schools sexual knowledge is less likely to come from other adolescents. Society's attitude appears to be that the handicapped should not be aware sexually. A high proportion of handicapped adults suffer emotional and physical sexual problems.

There is a need for careful teaching and counselling of the adolescents. This is best done in the home and in the school. Some group work is useful but is no substitute for individual counselling. Physically handicapped adolescents often have fears of sexual dysfunction which may be real due to neurological impairment and fantasies of 'passing on' their handicap. Teaching needs to include general relationships and responsibilities as well as biological information and contraception.

The mentally handicapped present particular problems, and need to be taught what is and is not acceptable behaviour. Girls can be very upset by menstruation unless it is explained to them.

Teaching a sex education programme for the handicapped is particularly challenging as it runs contrary to society's attitudes. Parents should be involved, a few will object and many will wish teachers, doctors and the school nurse to take on this responsibility. Some staff will find it very hard and full discussions should take place before embarking on any programme.

SCHOOL LEAVING

Leaving school is often a time of crisis for the family with a handicapped adolescent. Support and care for the young handicapped adult and his family are usually less than for the adolescent in school. Parents are getting older and may find it harder to meet the needs of the more handicapped; the age between 16 and 20 represents the peak age for admission of severely mentally handicapped people into residential care. There is a change in the agencies for the family, from education to social services and from paediatric to adult health services. Many handicapped adolescents make this transition smoothly, particularly the mildly handicapped. If jobs are available, leavers from ESN (M) schools may gain employment in manual professions. Less severely handicapped children in ordinary schools will also find jobs, perhaps using the specialist careers officers or the disablement resettlement officers (DROs) in job centres. But for the more handicapped adolescent the transition is rarely smooth and all handicapped children should have a re-assessment of their needs. This ought to start 1 to 2 years before school leaving so that the transition can be taken in a series of small steps. The school is the best venue for the process. Special schools are usually more used to the procedure. Special efforts must be made so that it is also available to the handicapped child in an ordinary school.

The assessment of needs is multi-disciplinary, the necessity to involve the adolescent and family is paramount.

The following should be reviewed.

Home living. For the physically handicapped this is an opportunity to review home aids at a time when further physical growth is unlikely. The local authority OT must be involved and identified for the family.

Finances and benefits. At 16 the mentally or physically handicapped adolescent who is unlikely to work becomes entitled to the non-contributory invalidity pension (NCIP) whether he is still at school or not. DHSS offices are often willing to send representatives to the school to explain the situation to parents and professionals.

The handicapped adult is entitled to many benefits, for example transport concessions, 'disabled sticker', and help with holidays. These are all available via the local authority social services. It is not necessary to register as disabled with the social services to receive any of the benefits but since the disabled register is used by social services to plan for local needs all handicapped adults should be encouraged to register at 16.

Continuing medical care. The medical needs of the handicapped rarely decrease with age, usually they increase. It is important that medical responsibility be clearly identified for each young adult. A number of options is available depending on the handicap, local resources and preferences, e.g. specialists in rehabilitation medicine, neurologists, specialists in mental handicap.

Where to go after school? It is not a satisfactory option for severely mentally or physically handicapped adults to stay at home all day with their parents. The support given to the adolescent and his family by the school, social workers, and physiotherapists must be maintained after leaving school, despite the change of agencies. There are a number of options according to the handicap and local resources such as day centres, adult training centres, sheltered workshops, or specialist further education courses. Deciding on which, requires careful counselling over a period of time.

BENEFITS

A handicapped child in a family usually results in more expenses. The family is also likely to be earning less, most often because mother is not able to work. There are a number of benefits which attempt to reduce the financial strain. For a variety of reasons uptake of these benefits is poor. It is important that professionals advise families that these benefits are a 'right' and not 'charity'. Unfortunately the rules and regulations governing the individual benefits are complex, often the family will be in doubt whether a particular benefit applies to them. If in doubt apply.

Attendance allowance is a cash allowance given to any parents whose child needs more attention than the ordinary child. It is available from 2 years of age, but it is worthwhile applying from 21 months. If there is uncertainty the parents should be encouraged to apply. The allowance is paid at two rates according to whether the child needs extra attendance day and night or just during the day. The rate of £26.25 and £17.50 per week respectively will be reviewed in November 1983. To apply parents have to get a form (N1205) from the Post Office, Social Services or DHSS Office, complete and return it to the DHSS Office. After applying, an independent doctor (usually a GP) comes to visit the family at home. If the family is not given the allowance which they think they need, they should then appeal. The allowance is given irrespective of the family's resources and is non-taxable.

Mobility allowance is a cash allowance given in addition to the attendance allowance if the child is unable or virtually unable to walk. It can be claimed from the age of 5 years. Apply on form NI211 as for the attendance allowance. At present there is a debate taking place on the eligibility of children who need constant supervision when getting from place to place, but are technically mobile. So far their families cannot get this allowance. The rate up to November 1983 is £18.30 per week. As for attendance allowance, mobility allowance is not means tested, is non-taxable and there is a right of appeal.

Motability scheme. In this the monthly mobility allowance is forfeited in exchange for help in leasing or buying a car but it will not cover alterations to the car.

Road tax. Those who have attendance allowance (even if under 5) or mobility allowance, can apply to be exempt from road tax. For the 2–5 year age group the qualification is being unable or virtually unable to walk. The parents need to write to DHSS Disablement Services Branch, Artificial Limb and Appliance Centre, Cardiff, or in Scotland to the Scottish Home and Health Department.

Family Fund. This is funded by a grant from the government but is administered by the Joseph Rowntree Trust. It is for children under 16 years with multiple or very severe handicap and it specialises in block grants for specific items which are not available through statutory channels. More imaginative items are often successful. The sorts of items are washing machines, road tax insurance, driving lessons and holidays. The fund does not like retrospective payments and generally only gives one grant per family per annum, though one grant may include a number of items, e.g. clothing, holiday, washing machine. Most social services offices have application forms or write to; The Family Fund, PO Box 50, York, Y01 1UY. Application is followed by a Rowntree Trust Social Worker visiting the home. They make the necessary assessment and recommendation and may approach doctors for medical details.

Rate rebate. The Rating (Disabled Persons) Act 1978 made provision for rate relief for disabled people. This can apply if they have made alterations, or additions to help cope with the disability, or have moved house for extra space or special features needed because of the disability. This can include extra rooms, garage or car space. Families should ask their local council for an application form and discuss any alterations with the social services occupational therapist.

Disabled car sticker. There is no lower age limit for this sticker. All car-owning families who have mobility problems with their handicapped child should have one. They are available via social services occupational therapists.

British railcard. As for ordinary children, handicapped children travel at half-price on the railways. If they have a Disabled Railcard bought for them there is no further reduction but an accompanying adult travels at half-fare. There are exceptions, for example all London Transport, and Motor Rail. All children having attendance or mobility allowance can have the Railcard. Leaflets are available from British Rail.

Building extensions for the handicapped. Councils may be able to help with a cash grant. Families should contact the social services occupational therapist or home improvements grant sections of councils.

Housing transfers. These can be given priority for handicapped children. Families need to write to the council housing department. Social workers can also make priority recommendations on social grounds.

Short term relief. This is available in most areas. It is not necessary for the child to go into care which, understandably, parents find distressing. The child is cared for for an evening, a weekend or a few days in social services premises such as a children's home or residential nursery. Some social services departments insist on going through voluntary care proceedings! Short term relief can be offered under provisions in the National Health Act 1977 without the child going into care.

Financial Benefits at 16. At 16 the physically or mentally handicapped adult is entitled to the non-contributory invalidity pension (NCIP) if they are unlikely to be able to work. This is a non-means tested, untaxed pension worth £19.70 per week. It is in addition to any attendance or mobility allowance and is paid whether or not the person is still in school or college, so long as he is not following an ordinary school curriculum. For example, an adolescent doing a 'Preparation for Life' syllabus would receive NCIP whilst a less mentally handicapped person doing A-levels might not. If the adult is unable to manage the money it is paid to the parents. The NCIP is still claimable if supplementary benefit is being claimed though the situation becomes more complex. It is worth consulting a DHSS office (through whom the pension is claimed) or a specialist social worker.

It is difficult to keep up with all these benefits plus schemes run by the voluntary agencies. One way for families or professionals is to listen to the Radio 4 programme 'Does he take sugar', for all handicaps, and 'In Touch' for visual handicap.

Useful booklets include 'Aids for the disabled.', 'Which benefit?' 'Help for handicapped people' all from DHSS Offices, and 'Door to Door' — a Guide to Transport for Disabled People' from Social Services or from the Department of Transport.

Disabled registers

Two registers exist. One is held by the Social Services. It is not necessary to register to receive any of the benefits but since the disabled register is used by social services to plan local needs all handicapped adults should be encouraged to register at 16.

The other is kept in the disablement resettlement offices and has two levels of severity. There is a poorly enforced requirement for all businesses to have 3% disabled employees. If employment on the open market is feasible then the handicapped adult should be encouraged to register via a job centre.

INTEGRATION

It is recommended that, wherever possible, handicapped children should be integrated within ordinary schools. This gives them access to a broader based curriculum and permits social contacts with non-handicapped children. The decision to send the child to the local school depends upon the level of handicap of the child, the learning ability of the child, the special resources that are needed, the geography of the school building which should permit easy access for the child with limited mobility, the wishes of the child and parents and the attitude of the health authority, education authority and the individual school. Work needs to be done within the school to ensure that the other pupils accept the handicapped child within the peer group.

For some children where the ordinary school does not have all the required resources, partial integration may be possible. An example would be children attending an ordinary school for most of the curriculum but visiting the nearby school for the physically handicapped for physiotherapy.

The arguments for integration are strongest in the case of children who are

Integration into school

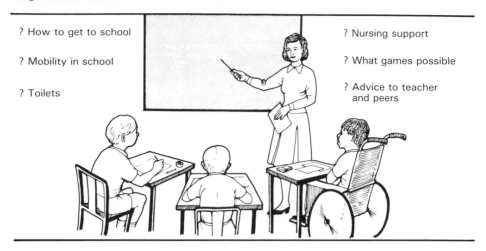

? How to get to school

? Mobility in school

? Toilets

? Nursing support

? What games possible

? Advice to teacher and peers

physically handicapped but intellectually normal. But even for them integration is not always successful. The children who are likely to succeed in ordinary school are primarily those with good learning ability but it is also important that they have outgoing personalities and both the parents and the school are committed to integration.

When a handicapped child is in an ordinary school, he should not be deprived of the services and facilities supplied by the special school, for example specialist counselling, school leaving arrangements and medical and physiotherapy supervision. This is undoubtedly harder to organise with a number of children spread through ordinary schools rather than focused in special schools.

CEREBRAL PALSY

Cerebral palsy is a persistent but not unchanging disorder of posture and movement appearing in the early years and due to a non-progressive disorder of the brain. It is the commonest cause of physical handicap in childhood with a prevalence of 2.5 per 1000 at 5 years of age. Although the definition relates only to motor disability, other associated features are usually found. Most have language or articulation problems, a third have epilepsy and a quarter have visual disorders. A quarter will also have hearing losses which are usually conductive. High tone sensori-neural hearing losses are common in children with athetosis. A third of children with cerebral palsy will have mental handicap, a third will be borderline and a third will be of average or above average intelligence. Behaviour problems are common. Multiple handicap is therefore the rule and there is enormous individual variation in the pattern of disability.

Early diagnosis is not easy; up to 80% of babies with neurological abnormalities in the neonatal period were found to be normal at follow-up. In view of this and the wide variation in normal motor development, it is important not to rush into an early and incorrect diagnosis. On the other hand persistent abnormalities and failure of developmental progress should not be ignored. Cerebral palsy may also present in infancy as feeding difficulties, seizures, or apathy. Once the diagnosis has been made, appropriate medical, educational and social programmes need to be set up following a multi-disciplinary assessment. Nearly all children with cerebral palsy survive into adult life.

Patterns of involvement
Cerebral palsy may be classified according to neuromuscular tone; spastic, hypertonic, rigid, hypotonic, athetoid, ataxic or dystonic, and, according to the pattern of the limbs affected, monoplegia, hemiplegia, diplegia, quadriplegia and bilateral hemiplegia. It is important to realise that these patterns are not static and that in the course of neurological maturation, children may go from a hypotonic phase through a dystonic phase to a spastic phase.

Initial assessment
Clues about aetiology may be obtained from the antenatal, perinatal and postnatal history. A family history is also relevant. Physical examination will show delay in motor development. Tone may be increased or decreased according to the patterns described above and primitive reflexes may be unduly persistent. Tendon reflexes are often very brisk and increases or imbalance in muscle tone may cause abnormal posture or deformity. Voluntary movements are poor and lack precision. Where the cause is not obvious, further investigation is indicated. This may include investigations to exclude congenital infection (rubella, cytomegalovirus, toxoplasma, herpes simplex), aminoacid chromatogram, skull X-ray, CT scan and chromosomal analysis.

Management problems

Eyes may be affected in a variety of ways. There may be partial sight, refractive errors, hemianopia and other field defects. The latter may impair left right sequencing in reading or writing.

Teeth. Dental disease is common because of difficulty in brushing teeth and excess sugar in the diet. Preventive dental care is therefore important and any necessary dental surgery should be carried out by a senior dentist and may often require general anaesthesia in hospital.

Arms. Loss of sensation often affects areas where there is motor involvement. In some cases whilst the sensory loss is incomplete the child may carry the limb as if it did not exist.

Obesity. Obesity may occur but more often growth is below average. Obesity will cause difficulties in independent mobility and handling by others.

Leg mobility. About 75% of children with cerebral palsy will eventually walk. If the child is sitting by the age of 2 he will probably walk eventually, whilst if he is not sitting by the age of 4 he will probably not.

Deformities are common but are often preventable when they result from muscle imbalance, immobility and incorrect positioning.

Circulation to arms and legs is sometimes poor, making them susceptible to cold injury.

Toilet training. Continence is delayed but can almost always be achieved. Firm comfortable seating in which the child feels secure is vital and training is easily upset by anxiety or stress. Behavioural approaches described in the chapter on mental handicap are often useful.

Constipation. Constipation is often a problem because of low fibre diet, poor autonomic function and immobility. Appropriate use of a high fibre diet, stool softeners and a bowel stimulant should remove the need for more drastic measures such as enemas.

Nutrition. Deficiencies, for example of iron, can occur on liquidised diets. Feeding difficulties can cause the growth of many children to be poor.

Persisting primitive reflexes. Persistent primitive reflexes, particularly the asymmetric tonic neck reflex and the tonic labyrinthine reflexes may interfere with postural reactions and the development of voluntary hand movements. Central head positioning is vital in inhibiting these reflexes.

Deafness. Both sensori-neural and conductive deafness are more common than in other children.

Perceptual problems related to identification of shapes, directions in space and body image produce practical problems in self-help such as undressing and in acquiring basic reading and writing skills.

Epilepsy. This is common and the side-effects of anticonvulsants should be actively looked for.

Behaviour problems are common and may affect relationships at home, in school, with therapists and may indeed be the major obstacle to be overcome.

Play and toys

The normal child through play acquires fine motor and gross motor skills and knowledge of the world around him. The child learns through imitative play such as domestic mimicry and through imaginative play he is also able to explore

District handicap team

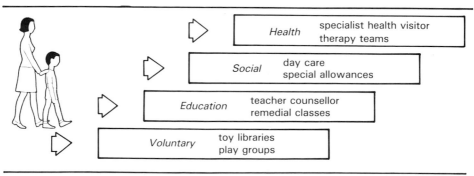

his environment. Diminished mobility may deprive the child with cerebral palsy of the pleasure of discovering that he can open and empty a cupboard of its saucepans. Through play the child also learns to socialise and to engage in cooperative play with other children. The child with cerebral palsy should not be denied these important opportunities. Although children learn through play, play is primarily for pleasure and this basic fact must never be forgotten lest it become yet another exercise.

Manipulative skills may be acquired by such activities as play dough, large building bricks, finger painting, play with sand and water and cradle play toys. Ideas of shape, size, texture and orientation may be obtained from posting boxes, form boards, jigsaws and a feely bag. Gross motor skills may be practised within the context of play with balls, hoops, construction of obstacle courses and through action songs. Items such as a Wendy house, a toy telephone or dressing up encourage imaginative play. Many useful ideas and information are obtained in the ABC of toys published by the Toy Libraries Association.

Outdoor activities such as swimming and riding should not be forgotten. They encourage self confidence and independence.

Education of the child with cerebral palsy

Schools need to provide for the medical as well as the educational needs of the child. Thus in addition to teachers the staff will include physiotherapists, occupational therapists, speech therapist, nurses, nursery nurses and doctors. Classrooms are designed for teaching of basic skills and also home economics, crafts and science activities for older pupils. Many have swimming pools for hydrotherapy, all will have physiotherapy rooms and a bank of aids. For some children progress will be slow, the child may be distractable and skills which other children pick up spontaneously may need to be specifically taught. Important principles to be followed are that the tasks should be interesting, that goals are set based upon initial observation for the child and that these goals are broken down into smaller steps. The child's progress needs to be monitored and recorded and praise and encouragement should be given for progress. Teaching takes place in small groups because of the many individual needs of the children. Early entry into school at the nursery stage is encouraged. Accurate observation and assessment of perceptual difficulties which are often associated are important in ana-

Help for the handicapped child

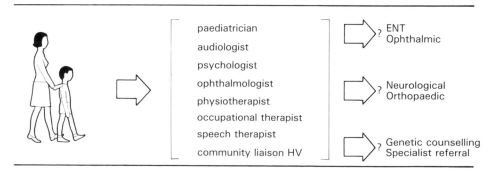

lysing difficulties, for example in recognising letters. For children with speech and language problems, communication aids may be vital, and for children with poor hand coordination, typewriters or other aids may be needed. Children with spastic quadriplegia need proper seating at school to ensure sufficient stability for school-work and to inhibit unwanted movements. Children with spastic diplegia are often of normal intelligence and may do well in a normal school if the problems of mobility can be overcome. Children with hemiplegias are often also managed within ordinary schools though perceptual difficulties and visual field defects need to be carefully looked for. The child with athetosis, because of speech problems and involuntary movements, often presents the greatest challenges to education. The use of new electronic aids may be of great benefit.

Best results are achieved in education where the child has good drive, persistence and resilience, the parents are supportive, appropriate special help and physical resources are available and the educational programme expects a realistic level of independence for the child.

SPINA BIFIDA

The number of children with very severe handicap due to spina bifida has fallen since the introduction of selective surgical management. In the UK there is currently a natural fall in the incidence of the condition; this, with the introduction of the alphafetoprotein screening programmes and the greater availability of genetic counselling has greatly reduced the number of infants born with the condition. The possibility that periconceptional multivitamin supplementation may prevent or partially prevent the abnormality, is very attractive.

The individual needs of children with spina bifida depend upon the level and extent of the spinal lesion and the degree of CNS abnormality secondary to hydrocephalus. As with other causes of physical handicap, a multi-disciplinary approach is important. Coordination is sometimes more difficult with spina bifida as the professions involved — neurosurgeons, orthopaedic surgeons, physiotherapists, nurses, doctors, paediatricians, paediatric surgeons and teachers — work in different centres.

Management problems

Mobility. With lesions above T12 there is little hope of walking. Between L1 and L3 walking may be achieved but only by extensive use of calipers and tremendous muscular efforts of arms and trunk. However because of its general inefficiency most resort to the use of a wheelchair as this enables more dignity, mobility and independence to be achieved. Much work is required to enable the child to manoeuvre the wheelchair in difficult situations over kerbs, across roads, in and out of cars, toilets and awkward passages. With lesions between L3 and S1, children usually manage with short calipers with or without aids. Children with lesions at S2 or lower can manage without calipers but muscle imbalance may require orthopaedic operations to the feet to ensure good function. For younger children a variety of trolleys in which the child sits with legs extended on a base, may be useful.

Urinary incontinence. This occurs in 85% of children with myelomeningoceles. In some children this is a flaccid paralysis of the bladder and in others there are strong uncoordinated bladder contractions likely to produce back pressure. Possible approaches towards urinary continence are toilet training where possible, bladder expression, a penile appliance for boys, intermittent catheterisation which is being increasingly used, ureterostomies and ileal loop diversions.

Bowel incontinence. Only 50% develop reliable bowel continence. Twenty-five to thirty per cent have occasional accidents and 10–15% have severe problems with sudden expulsion of faeces without warning. The use of suppositories and enemas may be of value.

Hydrocephalus and shunt. Of those children who develop hydrocephalus one-third will arrest spontaneously and two-thirds will require shunt procedures. Shunts may become blocked or infected and this may be suspected by changes such as drowsiness, pyrexia, personality or visual changes. When this occurs rapid action is essential.

Orthopaedic problems. Kyphosis and scoliosis are common and surgery may be required. Likewise immobility may give rise to dislocation of the hips and leg and foot deformities.

Puberty and adolescence. Menarche is often very early in girls with spina bifida. It can occur as early as 9 years. A combination of immobility, incontinence and menstruation may cause considerable distress. Older children with spina bifida need to be counselled as their offspring have a high risk of inheriting the condition. Anxieties about sex and fertility are common and counselling needs to be provided.

Educational problems. Learning difficulties are common in children with spina bifida. Characteristically many of the children get 'cocktail party' speech in which the child has deceptively precocious expressive language but very poor comprehension. Similarly the children may have specific difficulties with mathematics. On testing there may be identified defects in visual perception and also of fine motor skills sufficient to impair accuracy and speed in handwriting.

DUCHENNE MUSCULAR DYSTROPHY

Muscular dystrophy is a generic term covering a variety of types of muscle disorder. The most common form is Duchenne muscular dystrophy (incidence 0.3:1000 boys) and in the lay mind this is synonymous with 'muscular dystrophy'. The condition should be suspected in any boy with progressive difficulty in walking. Prominent, hypertrophied but weak calf muscles are also an important sign. Diagnosis is by a blood test for a muscle enzyme, creatinine phosphokinase, electromyography and muscle biopsy. Even allowing for individual variation the disease is relentless with motor skills being lost progressively. The boys are rarely walking unaided beyond 12 and death from cardio/respiratory failure usually occurs before 25.

Inheritance is by an X-linked recessive gene with a considerable number of

Steps in the progress of sex linked Duchenne muscular dystrophy. The age is only approximate

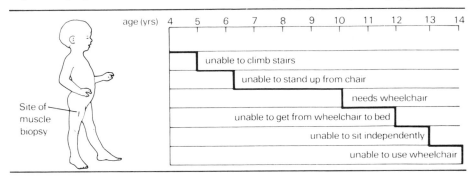

spontaneous mutations. Carrier mothers and aunts can be detected once a case is identified. Hence genetic counselling for the family should be strongly recommended as soon as diagnosis is made.

Educational implications

With a lot of help most boys are able to start in an ordinary school. But as they get older and the handicap progresses, more help is needed with toileting, dressing and mobility. Many secondary schools are built on two or more levels and are not designed for wheelchairs, though hopefully this will not be the case in the future. Some schools have provided the means to get round all these difficulties and boys have been educated with their peers throughout their school life. However, integration is not the ideal for every boy, each case has to be considered individually. Some boys become more depressed at the gap in ability between them and their peers. Loneliness is common. These two problems may be expressed aggressively. The boys may be happier in a physical handicap (PH) school where there are other boys with similar problems and in such a physical handicap school the 'Duchenne' boys often stick together.

In the special school awareness of long term prognosis often leads to depression, especially following the death of one of the boys. Such an event affects the staff as well as the boys. Treatment facilities and expertise are more readily available in a special school, but the school itself may not be near to home. For rural children the nearest school may be many miles away and boarding is the only option. A normal part of adolescence is 'kicking over the traces' of adult control, like the boy sneaking into an 'X' film or buying some cigarettes. This is much harder to do in a wheelchair and can lead to a lot of frustration. Some special schools have found ingenious ways round this.

This disease has such a relentless and predictable course that it is quite easy to predict future needs of the boys and their families; house conversions, ramps for wheelchairs, adjustable beds for night-turning, toileting aids, lifting facilities. Delays abound. It is vital for professionals and parents to anticipate the needs and develop a relationship with the local authorities so that facilities are provided when they are needed.

REFERENCES AND FURTHER READING

Bowley A H, Gardener L 1980 The Handicapped Child. Churchill Livingstone, Edinburgh
Brocklehurst J C 1976 Spina Bifida for the Clinician. SIMP (Spastics International Medical Publications), London
Cavanagh N 1981 A Scheme of Paediatric Neurological Investigation. Geigy Pharmaceuticals
Dubowitz V 1980 The Floppy Child. SIMP, London
Equipment for the Disabled 'The Disabled Child', 'Communication' and 'Wheelchairs'. Available from Equipment for the Disabled, Mary Marlborough Lodge, Nuffield Orthopaedic Centre, Headington, Oxford OX3 7LD.
Finnie N 1974 Handling the Young Cerebral Palsied Child at Home. Heinemann, London
Hewitt S 1970 The Family and the Handicapped Child. George Allen and Unwin, London
Jeffree D M, McConkey R 1976 Let me Speak. Souvenir Press, London
Jeffree D M, McConkey R, Hewson S 1977 Let me Play. Souvenir Press, London
Levitt S 1982 Cerebral Palsy and Therapy. Treatment of Cerebral Palsy and Motor Delay, 2nd edn. Blackwell Scientific Publications, Oxford
McGovern S 1982 The Epilepsy Handbook. Sheldon Press, London
O'Donohoe N 1979 Epilepsies of Childhood. Butterworths, London
Riddick B 1982 Toys and Play for the Handicapped Child. Croom Helm, London
Russell P 1978 The Wheelchair Child. Souvenir Press, London
Smith D 1976 Recognisable Patterns of Human Malformation. W B Saunders, London
The Good Toy Guide 1983 Toy Libraries Association and Inter-Action, Inprint

15
Vision, Hearing, Speech

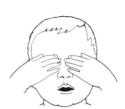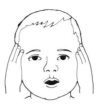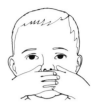

VISION

Visual disorder is common. All doctors working within the community child health services will meet many children who, on routine testing, will be found to have reduced visual acuity. However, severe visual handicap requiring special education is rare. In the UK there are fewer than 3000 children attending special schools. In tropical countries, blindness is a more common condition. Causes include keratomalacia secondary to vitamin A deficiency, often exacerbated by measles and trachoma. Children with severe visual handicap are registered either as blind or partially sighted. If the visual acuity is 3/60 or less in the better eye, children are registered as blind. Children with a corrected visual acuity in the better eye of 4/60 to 6/24 are registered partially sighted. The overall reported incidence in the UK is in the order of 1 in 2500 children. However there may be considerable under reporting because some partially sighted children attend ordinary schools and those with other associated severe handicap may not be registered.

The recorded incidence of children with visual defects, squints, myopia, etc rises with age. This is partly due to abnormalities not being detected but also in part due to the effects of growth of the eye. Muscle compensation will act to postpone diminished visual acuity due to of an error of refraction. For this reason vision testing in children cannot be a once and for all process. A significant proportion of those found to be normal on testing at age 7 and 11 had severe unilateral or bilateral problems by the age of 16.

Ophthalmic services

The school eye service is generally staffed through the hospital eye service. It provides diagnostic and treatment facilities for school children and children referred from child health clinics. Through the clinics the educational performance of the child can be related to the visual problem detected. In the UK there is no fee for prescription or eye testing in children.

Ophthalmic services

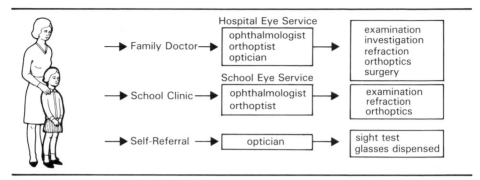

Visual screening

For toddlers there are not, at present, any generally available rapid and reliable methods of vision testing. Accurate assessment in this age group requires time, patience and considerable expertise. Some advocate that orthoptists should be responsible for primary vision screening in preschool children, in view of the level of expertise required. Others suggest, in view of the limitations of simple clinical and observational methods, that refraction should be used as the standard screening technique. However, as there is a wide range in the normal development of visual acuity it is difficult to decide the cut off point for referral. Even if they are identified, there are still problems with very young children, for they are not amenable to strategies such as orthoptic training or wearing glasses. The need for correcting lesser degrees of impaired acuity for educational purposes does not arise until school children are required to cope with progressively smaller print. It could be argued that early objective screening is required to prevent amblyopia. As 50% of children who develop amblyopia do not have a squint, this clinical finding cannot be relied upon for early detection.

Some children are at a particularly high risk of visual abnormality and may require special attention. These include children with a family history of squint or amblyopia, and children with other handicaps, such as mental subnormality, behaviour problems and clumsiness. Those who require intensive care in the neonatal period are particularly at risk.

Development of visually directed behaviour

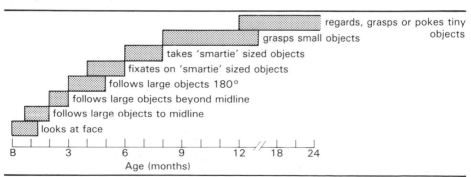

Vision testing. If the child is unable to do a test which she clearly should be able to according to her age, it is desirable not to record her as 'uncooperative' but to explain these findings in terms of either a genuine visual loss or a behavioural or developmental problem which causes their failure

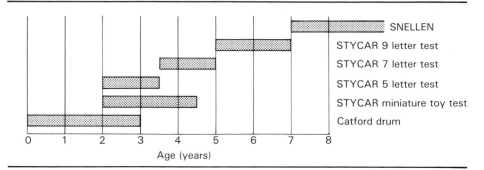

Most of the vision tests currently employed in child health clinics are those developed by Dr Mary Sheridan and are called STYCAR. STYCAR stands for Standard Tests for Young Children and Retardates. The first of these series is the graded ball test in which the child is required to follow a succession of white polystyrene balls ranging in size from $3\frac{1}{2}$ inches to $\frac{1}{8}$ inch, at a distance of 3 m against a black background. An alternative is to use the balls mounted on rods presented from behind a screen. A 6-month-old child should follow the balls down to the smallest one. The test is limited in its ability to detect minor or moderate defects.

The Catford Drum is a useful screening tool for this age group. The apparatus consists of a hand held screen with a central aperture behind which is a drum with varying targets of known Snellen type value. An electric motor operates the chosen target across the aperture with a slow transverse and quick return. The instrument is used at 60 cm in normal daylight conditions. Targets of decreasing size are presented until nystagmus is no longer elicited. It is possible to test eyes individually by putting a patch over one eye.

The toy matching test can also be used to test visual acuity. This involves the matching of miniature toys at a distance of 3 m. The test is useful particularly with handicapped children though an occasional obsession with one toy, such as the aeroplane, distracts the child from the other toys.

Under the age when letter cards can be used, the contribution of the graded ball test, the miniature toy test and the 'hundreds and thousands' test for the detection of visual defects is limited. Hall et al (1982) assessed the sensitivity and specificity of these tests with the following results.

| Test | Sensitivity for detection of (%) | | Specificity |
	Moderate defects	Severe defects	
Fixed balls	5	68	100
Rolling balls	12	70	100
Miniature toys	58	95	91
Matching letters	98	100	64

Development of visual acuity

Age	Average visual development	Late
2 months	3/60	2/80
6 months	6/18	6/36
1½ years	6/12	6/24
2 years	6/9	6/18
3 years	6/6	6/12
5 years	6/6	6/9
7 years	6/6	6/6

From the age of 3, the STYCAR single letter cards are in routine use by school nurses in most nursery schools. They involve the matching of single letters at a distance of 3 m. The letters used are those which are symmetrical and most easily identified by this age group. The child progresses through a series of tests which involve using more and more letters. Clearly the larger the number of letters, the less likely it is that the child will select the correct one at random. However, the visual acuity for single letters is better than that for a line of letters, especially in amblyopic patients. From the age of 3, most children will allow each eye to be tested separately by using a simple occluder. The Sheridan Gardner test corresponds more accurately with the Snellen letters as it is designed for use at 6 m. From the age of 7, the standard Snellen chart can be used.

Visual acuity of school entrants using STYCAR (from Ismail & Lall, 1980). The STYCAR single letter test can be misleading

	Distant vision			Near vision		
	Better eye	Other eye		Better eye	Other eye	
Normal	6/6–6/9	6/6–6/9	96.6%	N5–N6	N5–6	99.2%
Unilateral (moderate)	6/6–6/9	6/12–6/18	1.9%	N5–6	N8	0.3%
Unilateral (severe)	6/6–6/9	6/24–6/60	0.4%	N5–6	>N8	0.2%
Bilateral (moderate)	6/12–6/18	6/12–6/60	0.8%	N8	>N8	0.1%
Bilateral (severe)	6/24–6/60	6/24–6/60	0.2%	>N8	>N8	0.2%

Visual acuity at ages 7,11,16 using Snellen charts (from National Child Development study)

		7	11	16
Normal/minor defect		92%	88%	83.8%
Unilateral	(medium)	3.25%	3.6%	3.8%
	(severe)	1.42%	2.1%	2.4%
Bilateral	(medium)	2.5%	3.1%	4.3%
	(severe)	0.86%	3.2%	5.6%

The STYCAR near vision test is available for children from 4 years of age onwards and is used by letter matching with a seven or nine letter card at 25 cm.

In children who are too young to cooperate with letter tests, it is probably wise to confine oneself to a history, inspection of the eyes, a properly performed cover test and recognition of abnormal visual behaviour.

Abnormalities of refraction

In hypermetropia the eyeball is slightly shorter than normal so that parallel rays of light are brought to focus behind the retina. Hypermetropia is the normal state in the infant and diminishes with growth. Minor degrees of hypermetropia may be overcome by the normal powers of accommodation. If the hypermetropia is too great, difficulty will be experienced on normal vision screening when distant vision is tested. In severe hypermetropia, near vision is usually quite good, though the child may need to bring his eye very close to the object he is looking at. Hypermetropia may produce frontal headache or a convergent squint. It may be associated with astigmatism. It is treated with glasses using convex lenses to aid convergence of the light source.

In myopia the eye is marginally too long so that parallel rays of light are brought to focus in front of the retina. The myopic child has difficulty with distant vision. Myopia usually develops between the ages of 5 and 15 years due to excessive growth of the eye. There is often a family history. The condition is treated with glasses, and the defect is corrected by means of a concave lens. Rarely, congenital myopia occurs and may be associated with retinal detachment.

Hypermetropia and myopia

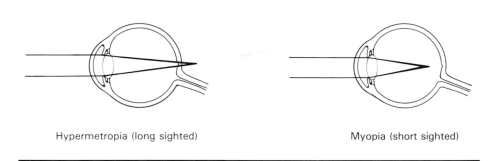

Hypermetropia (long sighted)   Myopia (short sighted)

Astigmatism arises when the curvature of the cornea and lens is different in the horizontal and vertical planes. Minor degrees of astigmatism have no significant effect but greater degrees of astigmatism produce difficulties in focusing horizontally and vertically simultaneously. Such a defect will produce difficulties in reading and a dislike of prolonged close work. Some children screw up their eyes in an attempt to improve acuity.

Amblyopia (lazy eye) is a defect in acuity that is not corrected by glasses. It arises from suppression of a poor image received by that eye. Amblyopia occurs early, the most sensitive period for its development being within the first 6 months of life, and it probably does not develop after the age of 5 years. Amblyopia with straight eyes occurs when there is an inequality of refraction between the two eyes, with a clear image in one and a blurred image in the other. It also occurs when stimulus is not received from one eye, as in ptosis, corneal opacity, cataract or vitreous opacity. The response to late surgical treatment in this group is poor.

Assessment of a refractive error

Having measured the defect in visual acuity, it is necessary to measure the degree of refractive error causing that diminution in acuity in order to apply appropriate correction. In young children this is generally done by retinoscopy following the use of drops to dilate the pupil and paralyse accommodation. With the eye in this condition, the underlying properties of the lens may be determined. If there is no error of refraction, parallel light entering the eye will emerge as parallel light. If the eye is hypermetropic the rays are divergent, if the eye is myopic the rays are convergent, and if the eyes are astigmatic the rays emerge in a band. Trial lenses are then applied in front of the eye until the rays emerge parallel, indicating that the refractive error has been corrected. This method is generally used for children under the age of 6, older children may be assessed using a trial frame and a chart.

Acceptance of glasses

Children frequently do not wear the glasses that have been prescribed for them. However on occasions these may be unnecessary. In the adolescents followed up as part of the National Child Development Study, 27% of the children prescribed glasses had normal unaided distant vision or only a minor defect. These constituted 42% of those who were not wearing glasses. If we exclude this group however, there remain children for whom the wearing of spectacles for near or distant work is important. In these cases close cooperation between doctors, parents, teachers and the children themselves is required. Attempts at educating all children about the value of spectacles will probably be more successful than putting pressure on individuals. For children with marked errors of refraction in one eye the failure to wear glasses to correct that error may give rise to amblyopia in that eye.

SQUINT

A squint occurs when the visual axis of one eye is not directed at the same point of fixation as the other. This interferes with the fusion of the two images of the object perceived and with the development of stereoscopic vision. Stereoscopic vision develops in the first 6 months of life and is a cortical function dependent upon appropriate sensory input. In the young child presentation of two differing images causes suppression of that which is less clear and the development of amblyopia. Later correction of the error will not improve visual function in that eye. The majority of squints in childhood are concomitant due to errors of refraction and of these over 85% are convergent.

Causes of squint

Squints fall into four aetiological groups.

Neurological disorders. In this type of squint the deviation is caused by underaction of one or more of the extra-occular muscles. This results from a congenital or acquired cranial nerve palsy, and is particularly common in children with mental handicap or cerebral palsy.

Eye disease. Any severe eye disease may give rise to squint. These may be divergent in type in contrast to the more common convergent squint. A divergent squint in a child under the age of one year is often associated with severe visual problems. Severe disease such as corneal scar, cataracts, optic atrophy or retinal disease can give rise to squint.

Refractive error. Refractive error, by preventing the normal development of binocular vision may precede the development of amblyopia and/or squint. Hypermetropia and unequal refraction in the two eyes (anisometropia), are particularly important in this respect. It is thought that in this condition, over-accommodation results in the convergent squint developing.

Failure to develop normal binocular vision. A family history is very common and the majority of children with squint probably fall into this category. The squint is usually convergent and is not entirely related to errors of refraction.

Descriptive terms for types of squint

Alternating squint	Either eye can take up fixation
Accommodative squint	One which is influenced by whether or not accommodation is taking place or by wearing of glasses
Concomitant squint	Deviation is constant, non-paretic, afferent, sensory
Incomitant	Deviation depends on angle of gaze, paretic squint, motor afferent, sensory

Clinical detection and assessment of squint

Facial appearance. Squint may be obvious on general inspection; however broad epicanthic folds can give the appearance of a convergent squint, and other facial asymmetries may have a similar effect. In the uncooperative young child, this may be the only clinical information that one can get in the clinic. Photographs may be helpful and the description of parents is most important in deciding the need for further assessment.

Corneal reflections. These should be identical in position in both eyes. This is a reliable test for detecting small degrees of squint. A small source of light held about 12 inches from the eye or a small object that will encourage the child to accommodate, are both suitable.

Ocular movements. Ocular movements should be tested in both horizontal and vertical axes using a small fixation object. Limitation of movement in one direction suggests a paralytic squint.

The cover test. The cover test, although easy to understand, is frequently difficult to perform. A young child may object to the intermittent occlusion of either eye, and the associated head movement of the child to avoid this, makes small eye movements very difficult to detect. In the test, each eye is encouraged to take up fixation separately whilst the other is covered. If a squint is present, the eye will move to take up fixation when it is uncovered, and retreat to its deviated position when occluded. Fixation should be tested for a near object at ap-

Testing for squints. When examining a child for a manifest squint watch the uncovered eye. When examining for a latent squint watch the covered eye

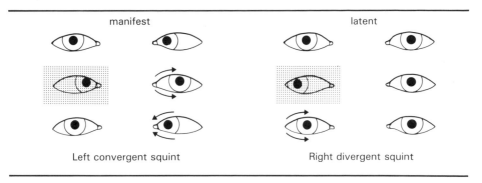

manifest   latent

Left convergent squint   Right divergent squint

proximately 33 cm, and a distant object at 6 m or optical infinity. The occluded eye must be completely covered and any abnormal head posture corrected.

Head tilt. Compensatory head tilts occur in squints in order to attempt to maintain binocular fixation. Head tilts are also seen in the presence of field defect, ptosis and torticollis.

Refraction is most important in the child with a squint. Over half the children with amblyopia have no detectable squint.

Examination of the optic fundi is manditory to detect retinal or optic nerve pathology.

Management of squint

Any squint after the age of 6 months should be referred to an ophthalmologist. Before that age, vertical or oblique squints or a constant horizontal squint should be referred. The first priority is the treatment of amblyopia, second, the treatment of the squint itself. Four approaches to management are possible.

— **Occlusion.** Occlusion of the good eye encourages the use of the squinting eye and the development of fixation. Some children may not tolerate this. Atropine drops daily to paralyse accommodation in the good eye may be used as an alternative.

— **Prescription of glasses.** Correction of the refractive error by glasses may be all that is required in many cases of squint.

— **The orthoptist** is predominantly involved with amblyopia therapy and the assessment of the state of binocular vision. Orthoptic exercises are of doubtful value in convergent squints. They also require cooperation from children which is only possible in the older preschool child.

— **Surgery** corrects the appearance and there is evidence that early surgery allows some degree of binocular function to develop. Surgery is aimed at lengthening, shortening or transplantation of the extra-ocular muscles.

Causes of blindness in childhood (after Schappert-Kimmijser et al, 1975)

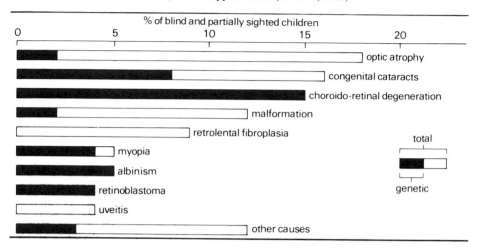

VISUAL HANDICAP

So far we have been concerned with visual disorders which, although important in their recognition and treatment, do not leave a residue of handicap significant enough to affect education and everyday life. This section covers the problems of blindness and partial sight. In 1977 in the UK, there were 2196 children registered as blind, and 2635 registered as partially sighted. Of the causes of blindness reported in a sample of 100 blind and partially sighted children in 1975 in the UK, 45% were genetic. Blindness is frequently associated with other handicaps. Fifty per cent of visually handicapped children have no additional handicap, but 37% are mentally handicapped, and others have hearing losses, cerebral palsy or epilepsy. Up to a third have serious social problems.

Clinical features

Enquire about photophobia and look for nystagmus and visual field defects. Photophobia is experienced with congenital glaucoma and albinism, and with achromatopsia, in which there is an absence of retinal cones and thus reduced visual acuity and total colour blindness. Keratitis and iritis also give rise to photophobia. Nystagmus may occur when central vision is poor, for example in albinism, congenital cataracts, optic nerve and macular abnormalities. It is usually pendular. There may be tunnel vision, a loss of central vision or other field defects. Children with hemiplegias may have a homonymous hemianopia.

Registration of people as blind is done by the Director of Social Services on the advice of the consultant ophthalmologist.

Development

Deprivation of vision affects many aspects of learning, behaviour and development. Bonding is facilitated by eye contact between the mother and the child. The development of fine motor skills starts with hand regard. The size of the environment that the child can see is reduced to that immediately around him.

Sound is a poor substitute for vision in terms of understanding distance. Objects are named by attaching a verbal label to a particular object that is seen. The labels have no meaning or significance if the child cannot understand the nature of the object to which they are attached. Gross motor development is delayed because the child does not have vision to guide him. Obstacles are unexpected and frightening.

Social development, feeding, dressing, and play are also impeded by lack of vision. The child needs to develop a sense of touch and hearing to compensate for the deficit in vision. He needs to be spoken to constantly so that things around him can be explained, which the sighted child discovers for himself. Examples are doors opening and closing, footsteps, the chink of bottles being picked up, the sounds of curtains being drawn. He needs to be shown these objects, and encouraged to explore and feel them. Toys need to be robust, bangable and chewable and such that the child can perceive his effect upon them. For instance, mechanical toys or a dolls house would be unsuitable. Water, rattles, a collection of objects differing in size, shape, texture, etc, are useful in developing fine motor discrimination. Talking, explaining, encouraging the child to handle and feel objects and helping the child to use any residual vision are the keys to learning. Nearly all blind children do have some residual vision and the child must make the best use of this, just as a deaf child must use his residual hearing. The child with visual handicap must be physically strong to deal with the unperceived obstacles and falls which he may have. His personality must also be able to deal with the problems of coping with an environment which he cannot always understand or perceive. He needs the confidence to move about in this environment, to deal with others and to ask for help. We have only to imagine ourselves deprived of our vision, trying to go through our daily lives or our journey to work. Our awareness of these needs of the visually handicapped, and the effects on gross motor, fine motor, language and social development enables appropriate advice to be given to parents on care and education.

Assessment
Assessment of the visually handicapped child must include paediatric, ophthalmic, psychological and social assessments. Ophthalmic assessment involves the clinical assessment of vision and the underlying pathology. General

Management of blind or partially sighted child

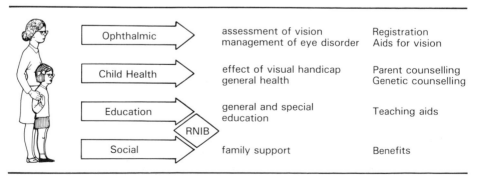

paediatric assessment is required, for visual handicap is often associated with other handicaps or may be part of a wider clinical syndrome. It is important to ensure that the hearing is normal. Although visually handicapped children do not as a rule have a high incidence of deafness, because hearing is so important to the education of the visually handicapped child, it is essential that adequate information on hearing is available. Psychological assessment is needed to determine the level of ability of the child and any particular problems in learning. Social work support is important to enable the family to come to terms with the handicap and to deal constructively with the problems that it presents.

Management

Medical management involves the clinical follow-up of the child's visual and other associated conditions. Specific management may be required with regard to surgical problems such as cataracts or corneal opacities. Glasses must be prescribed as needed. As many of the conditions giving rise to impaired vision are inherited, genetic counselling will be indicated in many cases.

Education needs to provide the child with the confidence to act in his environment and to make decisions. He may need to be taught living skills which other children just pick up. He needs opportunities for real experience of the world around him.

Numerous classroom aids are now available. The simplest of these are large type books for partially sighted readers. School resource centres should be able to reproduce standard texts in larger form. Special desks of an easel type to hold the written work are most valuable in allowing the child to get nearer to the text. Good illumination is essential. Low vision aids, for example magnifiers, may also enable the child to use more standard classroom material. Tape recorders can be used as a substitute for reading, and typewriters as a substitute for writing. Blind people may make excellent audio-typists and typing is a skill which can be taught early. Other low vision aids of great value are closed circuit television to magnify type up to the size of a TV monitor. Talking calculators are also available. The curriculum in schools provides a broad range of subjects not only English and mathematics, but languages, home economics and in some schools, sciences. Physical fitness is important, and sports, such as rowing and swimming, are applicable. Mobility training is an important part of education and the child needs to learn the route to school just as he would need to learn the route to work. Visual handicap can limit the child's understanding of the layout of the town and he may need to learn routes as sequences. He may not realise, for example, that one corridor is parallel to another.

Types of school

Most countries provide day or weekly boarding care for young and secondary school age children. The staff ratio needs to be high, almost 2:1. They and other schools operate as resource centres for parents and for professionals. Advice is also available from resource centres for those visually handicapped children within ordinary education. The Royal National Institute for the Blind provides many of the advisory services.

Some children with visual handicap go on to university and obtain degrees, particularly in art subjects. Some may become physiotherapists, others piano tuners, and others audio-typists. Some may work using closed circuit television magnifiers and others may use braille writing and shorthand machines. However, many children with visual handicap have added handicaps and the chances for future employment for them is poor.

DEAFNESS

Much effort is rightly directed to the early detection and management of hearing losses. For the severely deaf child, early detection and auditory training are essential for producing the best results. Mild and moderate hearing losses are equally important and far more common. Their importance in respect of delayed language development, often combined with other problems such as poor educational performance and behaviour problems, is not always appreciated.

Epidemiology and classification

Hearing losses are classically divided into sensori-neural hearing losses due to nerve deafness, and conductive hearing losses due to middle ear dysfunction. The first group is small but contains the children with very severe hearing losses likely to require special education. Children in the second group are common and may comprise 5–10% of the total population. About 1.8 per thousand children are sufficiently deaf to require a hearing aid, and 1 per thousand will require special education. Children with sensori-neural hearing losses may also have an added conductive element to their deafness. Conductive hearing losses may fluctuate from day to day. Diagnosis and treatment rest upon an understanding of the natural history of the underlying condition. The finding of a conductive hearing loss on a single occasion, without obvious long term pathology on history and examination, requires follow-up, but no treatment at that stage. Many are transitory and associated with upper respiratory tract infections.

Causes of deafness

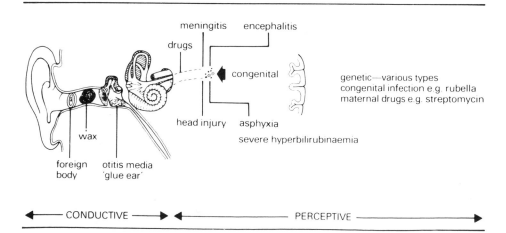

Auditory screening

Any formal screening procedure requires good, comfortable physical conditions, and a low level of background noise. Although specially sound treated rooms are desirable, they are seldom available. The child should be in a comfortable, alert and receptive mood, and clearly mealtimes and sleeptimes must be avoided. Although the screening tests are apparently simple to execute, they are full of pitfalls, and special training is necessary before staff should be considered competent in their execution.

The acoustic cradle. The detection of hearing losses early on in the maternity unit is obviously an attractive proposition. The acoustic cradle measures the motor response of the babies to auditory stimuli. The baby lies on a mattress which is sensitive to movements. The head rests in a moulded headrest which detects head turning and postural reactions. A band over the abdomen detects respiratory movement. Ear probes carry the stimulus into the child. The cradle detects changes in motor patterns during the stimulus period and compares them with those in the periods before and after stimulation. On the basis of up to 20 stimulation tests, the responses are analysed and an overall pass or fail determined. Further assessment by auditory evoked response must be available for those who fail this screening test.

Newborn infants at risk of deafness. The 6% of newborns at a high risk of being deaf includes 60% of those subsequently found to be severely deaf

Family history of deafness
Low birth weight
Significant birth asphyxia or severe jaundice
Congenital rubella, cytomegalovirus infection or neonatal meningitis
Malformation of the face or external ears

Distraction test. For this test the child sits on the parent's knee. The distractor sits in front of the child, and the person making the test sounds behind the child. The child's attention is attracted by the toy used as a distraction object, and then when the child is alert and has his attention focused on the object, the object is removed. In the interval when the child's level of attention is aroused, a test sound is made at minimal intensity about 3 feet from the ear and at a level with it. The child's response to this sound is recorded. The distractor is able to observe the child's reaction to the sound and also determine whether the reaction was auditory or visual. The test sounds usually used are minimal voice (ooh) to detect low frequency, and S as in yes to detect high frequency. Alternatively, a high frequency rattle such as the Manchester rattle, and cup and spoon which does not test any specific frequency, can be used.

Although simple in concept, skill is required in carrying out the tests properly. Attention to detail is most important. The child may react to the shadow of the person approaching, or hear the person's shoes, or react to creaking floorboards. The child may respond to the tester's perfume or aftershave, or visual clues. Skill is also required in presenting the sounds at the required low level. It is as well to check from time to time using a sound level meter. Children who do have hearing loss are more alert to other forms of stimulation, and unless tests are carried out with obsessional attention to detail, some of these children will apparently

Screening tests for hearing

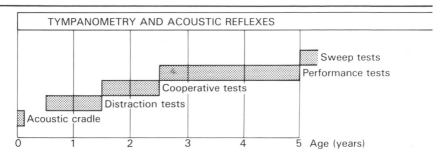

pass their hearing test using 'the eyes in the back of the head'.

Performance tests come in a variety of shapes and sizes. In the simplest type the child is conditioned to perform some motor act in response to the sound stimulus. For instance, the child is conditioned to drop a brick into a box at the command 'go'. 'Go' tests low frequency. Once the child is conditioned, the tester can reduce the test sound down to threshold level, behind the visual field of the child. The 'S' sound can be used to test high frequency, and pure tones can also be used from various sources. The game is first played with the mother and the child learns from the mother's example. Speech is therefore not required for this test. Clues to the child must be avoided. These may be in the form of a fixed interval between subsequent sounds, or a change of expression of the examiner, or the actual observation of the examiner's lip movements.

The mouth must therefore be completely covered if the sound is made from in front of the child. Speech discrimination tests involve the child identifying pictures by names. The pictures used are chosen so that the sounds may be easily confused, for example 'ship', 'brick', 'chick' and 'fish'. The words are mono-syllabic so that the rhythm of the word does not give a clue. The words must be within the vocabulary of the child to be tested, and it is first necessary to know that the child knows the names of the pictures. The tester should be 6 feet from the child and his lips must be covered, again to ensure the child does not lip read. These tests are very sensitive in detecting hearing losses. The Reed test supplied by the Royal National Institute for the Deaf is designed for use in school entrants and is remarkably useful in detecting hearing losses in this age group.

Toy discrimination tests work on the same basis as the speech discrimination tests, though using objects. They are therefore applicable for use with younger children if required down to a mental age of 2. The objects used in the toy test are cup, duck, plate, plane, shoe, spoon, house, cow, horse, fork, lamb, man,

Children at risk of developing deafness

Children who have had meningitis or encephalitis
Children with cleft palate
Children with a history of recurrent otitis media
Children with significantly delayed or unclear speech
Children with cerebral palsy
Children whose parents suspect deafness

key and tree. As with the previous test, it is first necessary to determine which of the objects the child knows and can identify by name. Children with normal hearing should be able to distinguish between all the test items at a listening level of 40 dB. Again the mouth must be covered to prevent lip reading. The examiner must also be careful not to look at the particular toy that he is requesting. This is a very useful test and one which children enjoy doing.

The sweep test is widely used for auditory screening of 5 year olds in school. The sweep test registers children's ability to hear test sounds at a 20 dB level over the range covered by the normal audiogram. This test has been subject to several criticisms. Many non-auditory factors are involved, such as intellect, constitution and motivation. It is a fairly difficult task for many children who may see the exercise as fairly meaningless. Much skill and patience is required to carry it out.

Tympanometry is a convenient and rapid method of detecting middle ear disease. It requires little cooperation from the child and can be performed at any age. It is also able to identify children with fluctuating conductive hearing losses who may be missed on a simple sweep test. In the normal condition, a sound introduced into the external auditory meatus is mainly transmitted through the middle ear. Where there is middle ear disease, less sound is transmitted and more is reflected. The ability of the tympanic membrane to conduct sound depends upon the pressure difference across it. It is maximal when the pressure is the same on each side. Therefore if the pressure is raised or lowered in the external auditory meatus, the amount of sound conducted will vary with the pressure with a peak when the pressure is equal at both sides. The peak would be normally around atmospheric pressure, though it will occur at a negative pressure in the case of middle ear disease when there is obstruction to the Eustachian tube. In this condition the peak will also be lower as the amount of sound conducted is decreased. If there is a perforation in the tympanic membrane, pressure will always be equal on both sides and hence will not be affected by attempts to alter pressure in the external meatus.

Tympanometry can therefore give a good indication of the function in the middle ear. It can also indicate integrity of the sensori-neural pathway by recording the acoustic reflex. However, acoustic reflexes may be physiologically absent in some subjects. In the stapedial reflex the stapedius muscles contract in

Tympanometry. Examples of normal and abnormal tympanograms are shown on page 276. The rest is sensitive but non specific.

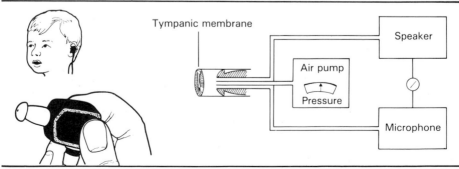

Tympanic membrane

Speaker

Air pump

Pressure

Microphone

both ears in response to a unilateral intense sound stimulus. Contraction of the stapedius muscle tenses the tympanic membrane and therefore alters the conductive properties of the middle ear. This can be detected using the same measuring equipment as is used for the tympanogram. In sensori-neural hearing losses, the acoustic reflex threshold indicates the level at which the phenomenon called 'recruitment' occurs. Above this level, amplification causes pain, and results in diminished and not improved hearing. The acoustic reflex may be unobtainable in conductive deafness.

Perhaps the simplest and most reliable screening test is to ask the parents. A parent's conviction that her child is deaf must never be lightly disregarded. Parental assessment may be improved by the use of a clues list.

Hints for parents produced by Dr Barry McCormick, Nottingham Hearing Services Centre

---

CAN YOUR BABY HEAR YOU?

Here is a checklist of some of the signs you can look for in your baby's first year:-

	Tick if Response Present
Shortly after birth	
Your baby should be startled by a sudden loud noise and he should blink or open his eyes widely to such sounds.	☐
By 1 Month	
He should show the additional response of becoming still if you make a sudden prolonged sound.	☐
By 3 Months	
He should quieten or smile to the sound of your voice even when he cannot see you. He may also turn his head or eyes towards you if you come up from behind and speak to him from the side.	☐
By 6 Months	
He should turn immediately to your voice across the room or to very quiet noises made on each side.	☐
By 9 Months	
He should listen attentively to familiar everyday sounds and search for very quiet sounds made out of sight. He should also show pleasure in babbling loudly and tunefully.	☐
By 12 Months	
He should show some response to his own name and to other familiar words. He may also respond to 'no' and 'bye bye'.	☐

IF YOU SUSPECT THAT YOUR BABY IS NOT HEARING NORMALLY EITHER BECAUSE YOU CANNOT PLACE A DEFINITE TICK AGAINST THE ITEMS ABOVE OR FOR SOME OTHER REASON THEN CONTACT YOUR HEALTH VISITOR FOR ADVICE. SHE WILL PERFORM A SIMPLE HEARING SCREENING TEST ON YOUR BABY BETWEEN SEVEN AND NINE MONTHS OF AGE AND WILL BE ABLE TO HELP AND ADVISE YOU AT ANY TIME IF YOU ARE CONCERNED ABOUT YOUR BABY AND HIS DEVELOPMENT.

Early diagnosis using equipment such as the acoustic cradle, the clues list and attention to suggestive clinical abnormalities such as malformation of the ear has made it possible for some children to have hearing aids fitted in the first weeks of life. This has enabled appropriate stimulation, the development of the auditory pathway and impressive language development to occur.

Audiometry

Audiometry is the standard method of accurately recording hearing. Reliable audiograms are difficult to obtain before the age of 5 years. Sound are fed to each ear using headphones and the child is asked to indicate when the sound is heard. Audiograms may record air conduction which is abnormal in both conductive and sensori-neural hearing losses, and bone conduction which is normal in conductive losses. 'Masking' may be needed to prevent sounds being conducted to the opposite ear.

Measurement of deafness

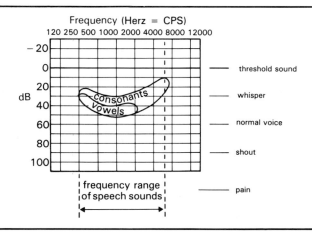

Difficulties in diagnosis

Most commonly the diagnosis of deafness is missed because the child's hearing is not tested at all or is tested inadequately. On other occasions the diagnosis of physical handicap deters us from looking for the additional handicap of deafness as may occur commonly in Down's syndrome. Indeed some children have been labelled as mentally handicapped where none existed and the correct diagnosis was severe deafness! Children from a background of emotional deprivation may appear unresponsive to test sounds but in fact have normal hearing. Where there is a severe developmental language disorder resulting in auditory imperception, differential diagnosis for deafness may again be very difficult.

Development in the deaf child

Loss of hearing affects development in two principal ways. Firstly, it denies the child a wide range of experience that comes through sound in the environment. Secondly, it prevents the acquisition of language and the use of language as a form of communication. Language is required to give shape to ideas, for internal reasoning and for the expression of ideas.

Sound is a useful distance sense that provides security for the young child. Although he may not be able to see his mother, he may be able to hear her out of his line of vision in the next room. For this reason deaf children like to keep their mothers within sight. They lack clues to understanding their environment, such as hearing dinner being prepared, the newspaper arriving through the door, or their parents' step on the stairs. Loss of hearing may prevent the child from mixing fully into family activities. That aspect of family life which is conducted at a verbal level will be completely missed. Because they tend to be shut off by their hearing difficulty, deaf children can become solitary and cling to toys rather than people. In their play, either alone or with other children, they again miss the important verbal element. In everyday life, verbal encouragement by the parents or words of approval or disapproval which help them mould behaviour and encourage learning are missing.

For all these reasons the experience of a deaf child may be severely limited. Awareness of this and the ways in which it occurs enables us to structure help in an appropriate way.

Management of the deaf child

Assessment of the deaf child is based on a multi-disciplinary approach involving a wide range of professions in the audiology clinic.

Assessment of the child and his family is not limited to the hearing loss but must also involve all aspects of growth, development, behaviour and family dynamics. The type of intervention recommended depends very much on this general assessment. We must know if the hearing loss is an isolated clinical finding, or whether it forms part of a syndrome with other clinical features. It is most important to know that the vision is normal, in view of the importance of vision in the education of the deaf. It is also required to know the general level of development so that work with the child is at his appropriate level of understanding and at a rate which takes note of his general intelligence. Many tests of IQ are heavily weighted towards verbal items. It is important that deaf children are assessed by educational psychologists familiar with their problems. Certain tests such as the Snijders-Oomen have been standardised on deaf children. Development, ability to communicate and understand, using spoken language and the child's use of and understanding of gesture all need to be assessed.

Services for deaf children

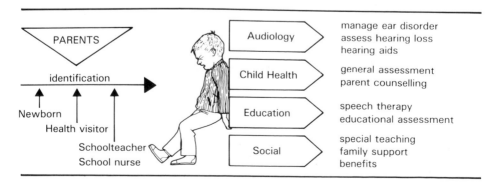

Early oral training in the home is vital. For this one needs to know the level of understanding of the family and ensure that the nature and consequences of their child's hearing loss is properly appreciated and to support them during their times of anxiety and despair as they care for their deaf child. Parent counselling and support is the first and most important aspect of management, without it success and everything else is likely to be limited.

Early auditory training starts at home during the regular visits of the peripatetic teacher of the deaf and during visits to the audiology unit. The child must experience a speaking environment so that he becomes aware that the residual sounds that he hears have meaning. Resort to gesture instead of speech does not encourage the child to develop the useful hearing that he has. Parents should be encouraged to talk to the child face to face and arrange themselves so that the child is not distracted by other movements. Good clear speech helps, but it is not necessary to shout or produce exaggeratedly slow speech. Lively facial expressions and the visual demonstration or reinforcement of a word used are important. Parents need to know that comprehension must precede expression. The child should be praised and encouraged for the initial fragments of speech or sound that he produces.

The deaf child, even with amplification, does not hear sounds in the same way that a hearing person does. He must learn to associate the fragments of distorted speech that he picks up, with the object. He must also attempt to produce with his own voice, speech sounds which he cannot fully monitor himself.

Oral versus manual methods of teaching. Management of the deaf child has for long been divided into the oral and the manual schools of thought. In the oral method, which is widely advocated, gesture is greatly discouraged for the use of gesture for communication will deter the development of speech. It is argued that only through the development of normal or as near normal spoken language as possible, will the child be able to communicate properly with normally hearing people. According to the manual method a system of signing such as the Paget-Gorman signing system, which is a complete language, has many advantages. They argue that in the young deaf child, the narrow channel for communication due to his poor language development, places a restriction upon his ability to communicate and receive information. A signing system provides a rapid and effective method of communication which can be used for all sorts of teaching purposes and to develop reading and writing skills. Its critics argue that those who are taught on a manual system can only communicate with those who know the system and thus they are limited in their day to day activities to those with a similar handicap. However, a combination of the oral and manual systems has no adverse effect on speech and does have advantages in terms of reading and general academic achievement.

There are various forms of signing including the Paget-Gorman sign system, cued speech where the signs augment information from the spoken word and finger spelling. Signing may be particularly valuable with the deaf child who has additional handicaps, particularly mental handicap.

Lip reading is of course an important adjunct to oral training.

Hearing aids. It is important to emphasise that hearing aids will not restore normal hearing and that in sensori-neural hearing losses above a certain level of

Sensori-neural hearing loss

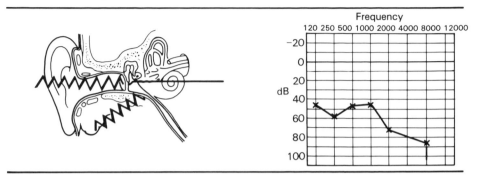

amplification the intelligibility of sounds will in fact decrease. It is also important to appreciate that excessive amplification can actually further damage the child's hearing. Aids may be either post-aural or body worn, the latter giving better amplification. They may have either an ear mould or a bone conduction facility. Each hearing aid consists of a microphone, an amplifier and a small speaker. The ear moulds must fit correctly or 'howling' will occur, which is caused by sounds leaking from the speaker back into the microphone. The provision of two aids enables better localisation of sound. As children are growing, their ear moulds need to be changed fairly frequently. The new moulds need to be delivered before the children have outgrown them! The aids must be serviced regularly. Children need to be encouraged to accept their aids and to wear them. A service to adjust and maintain the aids is essential.

Radio aids are expensive but very flexible in their use. They have the advantage of a range of up to 300 m between the child's amplifier and speaker, and the teacher's or parent's microphone. They permit communication with the child under a wide range of conditions which would not be possible with the conventional aid, for example language stimulation during play.

In the partially hearing unit the teacher can communicate with the pupil by a microphone and amplifier connected to a coil of wire around the classroom. The coil energises the hearing aids with a minimum of disturbing reverberant sound or noise from other children.

In sensori-neural hearing loss, children benefit from amplification. However excess amplification leads to distorsion and loss of benefit

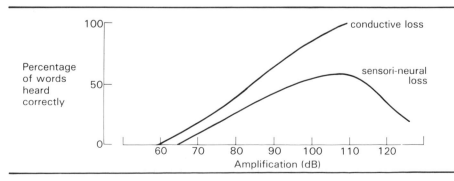

Types of hearing aid

Body worn

OL56 — 20–4000 Hz. Sturdy
OL57 — induction loop facility. For use in classroom.
Only hears teacher's voice via microphone, not his own
OL58 — more powerful version of OL56 (tone control)
OL58c — more powerful than OL58 (tone control)
OL63 — bone conduction (tone control)
(NB Tone control can raise or lower low frequency sound)

Post-aural aids

BE12 — similar to OL56
BE11 — has tone control facility
BE13 — more powerful aid

Commercial aids and radio aids

These are more expensive (the radio aids very expensive), but are available if there is not a suitable NHS alternative

---

Educational provision. A decision on the type of schooling required, is made jointly by the audiology team in conjunction with the family, and the members of staff of the local schools for the deaf. The type of school chosen depends upon the availability, the travelling distance for the child, the desirability or otherwise of residential schooling for a particular child, and the presence of other social, developmental or behavioural handicaps. Most important, school placement should not be a once and for all exercise as the child's needs may change or his progress may require transfer to another type of school. Children with very severe hearing loss require special schools. Children with lesser degrees of hearing loss may manage in partially hearing units attached to a normal school. Here, for some part of the school day, certain lessons, meals, etc, the child will mix with normally speaking and normally hearing children. Many children with mild or moderate hearing losses can be managed within the ordinary school setting, with the peripatetic teacher of the deaf providing an advisory service for the child's class teacher.

Disability associated with various degrees of deafness

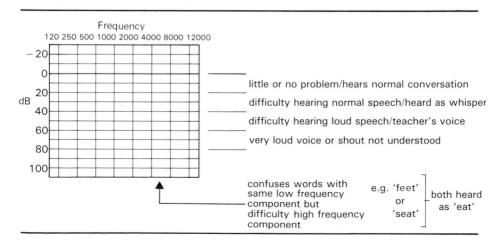

The following notes may be of value to teachers of children who have hearing losses in their class:

— the child should sit in a front seat with the better ear directed towards the teacher if there is deafness in one ear only, or in a favourable position if seats are not arranged in rows;

— the child should be able to watch the face of the teacher whilst he is talking to the class. Also the teacher should try to face the hard of hearing child particularly when important instructions are being given;

— the child with the hearing loss should be allowed to turn around to see the faces of other children participating in class discussions;

— it is not necessary for the teacher to shout or use exaggerated lip movements;

— the teacher must be aware of the increased concentration required of the deaf child to understand speech;

— the child must be encouraged to participate in all activities involving language and be a full member of the class;

— the teacher must be aware of the hazards that face the deaf child from teasing and other forms of reactions from children in the classroom;

— the teacher should try to avoid talking with his back to the class;

— if the child does have a hearing aid it is necessary to check every day that the aid is working;

— in some situations such as games, a child with unilateral deafness may miss some instructions. Likewise there are hazards for the child crossing the road and he must look for oncoming traffic;

— where there is a high frequency hearing loss, children often fail to hear the quieter consonants. Omission of certain letters in spelling and mispronunciation of words can be expected, for example the words choose and shoes may be confused;

— all special attention given to a child with a hearing loss should be handled and given as unobtrusively as possible so as not to call attention to the defect.

In spite of the prominence and long tradition of special education of the severely deaf and the normal intelligence in many children, their final reading ability is poor compared to normal children. They may start above average, but the growth of reading ability with time does not keep par with other children. In spite of much research, more effective teaching methods have not yet been developed.

Medical and surgical management of conductive hearing losses

Glue ear (chronic secretory otitis media)

This is an extremely common condition which is found far more often in deprived children living under poor conditions. As the hearing losses fluctuate, the condition may be missed by once only screening. However it has important implications in terms of impaired educational achievement, and a high incidence of emotional disorders, possibly as high as 30%. The initial cause is Eustachian tube dysfunction which causes accumulation of fluid in the middle ear. The dysfunction may be associated with enlarged adenoids, cleft palate, chronic sinusitis or allergic rhinitis. The long term consequences of serous otitis media are ossicular

Otitis media. In acute otitis media the drum is pink, in chronic otitis media the vessels are more obvious and the drum is dull

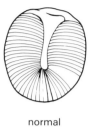
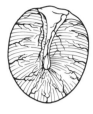
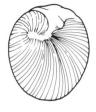

normal   injection of vessels   retracted

fixation through fibrosis, severe conductive hearing loss, tympanosclerosis, re-traction pocket formation, tympanic membrane perforation, cholesteatoma, os-sicular necrosis and mastoid process destruction. The tympanic membrane is dull and immobile, with dilatation of the peripheral vessels.

Conductive hearing losses are amenable to medical and surgical treatment. They may be superimposed upon a sensori-neural hearing loss. It is particularly important in unilateral hearing losses also to detect any middle ear disease de-veloping in the contralateral ear. Children with persistent conductive hearing losses should be initially treated with an antihistamine/beta adrenergic stimulant mixture such as actifed, benylin decongestant or dimotapp for a period of six weeks. Hearing will return to normal in many with this management. However they will require continued observation and follow-up.

Surgical management may involve improvement of middle ear drainage by ad-enoidectomy, removal of middle ear secretions by myringotomy and the insertion of a grommet into the tympanic membrane to aid aeration. Grommets are of un-certain benefit. Up to 21% of patients may still have unsatisfactory hearing fol-lowing insertion. As secretory otitis media frequently recurs, grommets may re-quire to be inserted on several occasions. The grommet is eventually extruded and areas of tympanosclerosis result. As co-trimoxazole with an antihistamine de-congestant mixture has produced very encouraging results, surgical management should perhaps only be considered after a 6 week trial of co-trimoxazole and de-

Tympanograms. In middle ear disease the curve flattens and the peak moves to the left

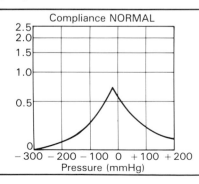
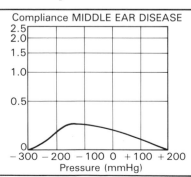

Conductive hearing loss

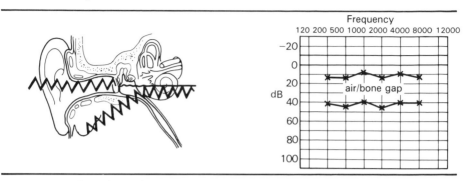

congestants. Acetylcysteine to loosen thick secretions may also be of value. Temporary hearing aids are useful.

SPEECH AND LANGUAGE PROBLEMS

Speech is probably the most highly developed of all human skills. Large parts of the brain are involved with speech, sound production, understanding speech and coding ideas into language. Language is required as a vehicle for thought and to convey ideas. Inner language enables us to think through, rather than act out problems and outer language enables expression of feelings. The next table shows just how common severe speech disorders are, as found in the 7 year olds studied in the National Child Development study. It also shows the high incidence of associated educational difficulties. At age 5 at school entry approximately 5% of children are recorded as unintelligible.

Epidemiology of speech disorders in 7 year olds (from the National Child Development Study). In children with marked speech defects, 38% had emotional problems, and boys were twice as common as girls. They were more likely to be preterm, younger children of large families and from social classes IV and V

Intelligibility	Difficult to understand (%)	Many or all words unintelligible (%)
Teachers' reports	10.7	2.4
Doctors' reports	13.5	1.4
Associated problems	Incidence (x expected)	
Non-readers	×12	
Poor number work	×9	
Poor design copying	×8	
Behaviour problems	×4	
Clumsiness	×3	
Impaired visual acuity	×3	

Children with delays in development of spoken language, will also be delayed in acquiring the written form, as children can only read or write with an understanding of those words that they have already acquired in the spoken form. A cycle has been described of children with delayed language leading to delayed reading and writing, which cuts the child off from gaining satisfaction in his schooling and leads to truancy in the early secondary school.

Because of the importance of language as a yardstick of general intellectual development and as a predictor of future educational performance, doctors involved in child health need a good knowledge of normal and abnormal language development, and to be able to assess language development and to describe areas of difficulty. Unfortunately there is no rapid test of speech and language development. The command from the parents 'speak for the doctor' is almost certain to ensure that no spoken language is heard. We must be aware of any differences in levels of ability between comprehension of language and expression of language. There are some children, for example those with spina bifida, who may have a vast 'cocktail party conversation' but little comprehension of the meaning of the words which they use. Parents' descriptions of their children's language ability can be misleading in that the mother's conclusions may be distorted by the child gaining many situational clues of the meaning of the mother's words, often supplemented by gestures from the mother. We need to be able to assess the development of pre-language skills such as attention control and understanding of symbols. Obviously language development must be assessed in the child in his own language.

Skills required for communication

Hearing — to listen to others
      — to monitor one's own voice
Auditory discrimination — to recognise (centrally), the differences between sounds
Phonology — the ability to reproduce these sounds
Semantics — the ability to ascribe meaning to patterns of sound that are remembered
      (vocabulary)
Grammar — the ability to use words within a framework of knowledge that modifies the
      ending of the word according to use e.g. tense (morphology) and constructs
      sentences according to particular rules e.g. affecting word order
Encoding — translating objects, actions, etc into the words that symbolise them
Decoding — the ability to relate the spoken word to the object or action for which it is a
      symbol

It is quite remarkable how the young child learns to distinguish a wide range of sounds in his environment, to imitate them, to attach meaning to them and to put them together into recognised grammatical constructions. We have only to recognise the difficulties that adults have in learning languages with a different vocabulary and grammatical structure. All the above skills are dependent upon intact sensory and motor systems, upon the integration of these systems, and upon complex coordination of motor activity in speech sound production. The child also must have listening skills and an understanding of gestures and symbols from cues such as toys and pictures. This whole collection of skills needs to be supported by appropriate intellectual development, the will to communicate and an environment in which the necessary opportunities for language acquisition are available.

Normal language development

Some of the major milestones in language development are shown in the accompanying diagram. The diagram represents a fairly gross over-simplification of a fairly complex development of skills.

The newborn is not only able to hear but also has some ability to discriminate sound. The baby's cry is not a single uniform ability. Mothers learn very quickly to

Stages in speech development

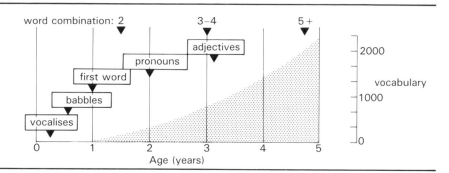

distinguish the cries of their baby from the cries of other babies in the hospital and to know which cries mean anger and frustration. The baby also rapidly develops a whole range of vocalisations, coos, glugs, grunts, laughs, in response to the appropriate situations.

In the first year the baby learns to discriminate sounds and in his babble practises them. The number of sounds that the child produces rapidly increases but some sounds such as the 'th' sound may not be produced until the child is 5 or older. Vowel sounds develop first, then the back consonants such as 'g' followed by the lip and tongue consonants. In the first year of life comprehension of words must develop before there can be meaningful expressive language. At first the child can only understand the words when there are heavy clues as to the context in which the word is used. At first this only amounts to reflex labelling of the object when the object is in sight and other clues are available.

Later the child acquires the proper meaning of the word in that the word is internalised as a symbol for the object. He may then use the word as a means of acquiring the object, for example drink, biscuit. At first words have very narrow meanings, for example dog may only mean the dog present in the household, though the meaning will gradually widen to include all other species of dogs, toy dogs, models of dogs, pictures of dogs. The first meaningful words appear on average at the age of 1 year though with a very wide range of normal.

Between 18 months and 2 years most children will be saying simple two word combinations. These are usually of the noun-pivot type in which a small series of pivot words such as bye-bye, can be linked to a wider number of nouns, such as daddy bye-bye, milk bye-bye. Sentences gradually increase in length and other parts of speech, adjectives, adverbs, pronouns, are introduced. The child will want to listen to increasingly complex speech such as nursery rhymes and stories, and develops quite an amazing memory and frequently verbatim knowledge of fairly long stories. Language is increasingly used in play in which children animate their toys and converse with them. However most of the speaking of young children in play is a monologue rather than an attempt to communicate. Language is increasingly used in the pre-school child to ask questions, initially of the 'what' variety but by 3 years extending to the 'where' and 'who' variety and at 4 the 'why' variety.

Language

4½ yrs (Range 2½–5 years)
Repeats story/knows colours red, blue, green, yellow
Explains picture using sentences, e.g. Ladybird
Talkabout book

3 yrs (Range 2–3½)
Gives full name/simple conversation
Listens to stories

2 yrs (Range 15/12–2½)
Simple word combinations
Asks for drink, food, 'toilet'

18/12 (Range 15/12–2)
Five + words (not mama etc.)
Points to parts of body — shows hands/shoes

12/12 (Range 9/12–18/12)
Two-three words with meaning
Gives a toy (request and gesture) simple command, e.g.
"give it to me, wave bye-bye"

9/12 (Range 6/12–12/12)
Two syllable babble – ma ma, da da, ba ba, ab ba/
copies sounds
Understands 'no'/where is mummy/daddy

6/12 (Range 5/12–10/12)
Unintelligible babble
Responds to different emotional tones in mother's
voice

3/12 (Range 2/12–4/12)
Laughs/squeals of pleasure
Looks around meaningfully when spoken to

6/52
Stills to mother's voice
Vocalises (coos and glugs)

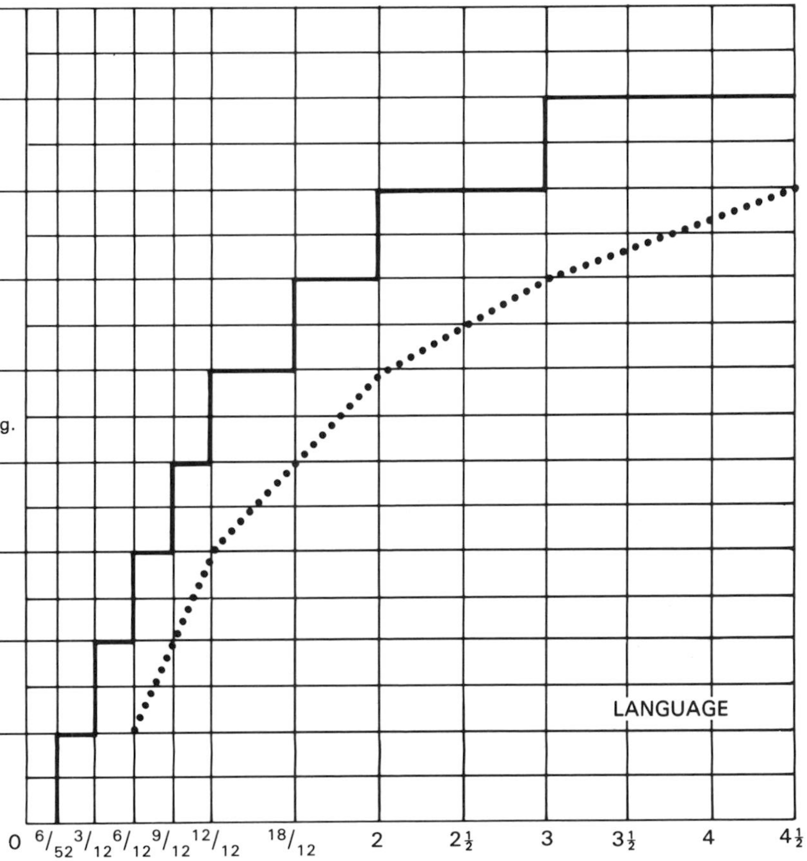

LANGUAGE

0   6/52   3/12   6/12   9/12   12/12   18/12   2   2½   3   3½   4   4½

The boxes are filled in for each item completed opposite the chronological age shown on the horizontal axis. 10% of children below their 'developmental step' require further investigation. Those below the dotted line are severely delayed.

In the preschool child sentence length gradually increases. Word length and the range and intelligibility of speech sound also increase. Language development is intimately related to general intellectual development and to the use of language in the home. In families using a so-called restricted code, speech is often limited to single word utterances related to immediate needs. In such settings the opportunity for language learning is severely limited.

Types of abnormal language development

Speech disorders fall into several categories. The most common is delay in language development with the speech produced resembling that of a younger child. Comprehension and expression must be assessed separately using procedures such as the Reynell Developmental Language Scale, for comprehension and expression may be affected to different degrees. In a second group, language development in terms of vocabulary, understanding and grammatical structure are normal but there is a problem with the intelligibility of speech and speech sound production. In a third group language development is deviant and abnormalities of structure and word combination occur which are not typically found in the speech of younger children.

Differential diagnosis of language delay

The principal conditions which need to be considered in a child with speech problems are mental retardation, deafness, environmental and emotional deprivation, elective mutism and infantile autism. Language delay is a common presentation of mental handicap. Mentally handicapped children have a high incidence of hearing loss and are also more susceptible to social deprivation. The speech therapist may see clues to a hearing loss from the pattern of speech production. It is essential that all children who are referred with delayed speech have careful audiometry performed. An analysis of the home environment and the degree of language stimulation received is most important. Such children particularly benefit from individual language programmes designed to increase the appropriate language input in the clinic, nursery or home. Children with elective mutism only fail to speak in certain situations such as in school. However when seen in other situations it is clear that speech development is normal. Even rarer than elective mutism is autism. It is in the diagnosis of rare conditions that we might not have met before that we are most likely to make errors. In autism in addition to the delays in speech and language development, there is a failure to develop interpersonal relationships. This means a failure to cuddle or comfort, lack of eye to eye contact, lack of attachment, or separation anxiety. The children seem to lack interest in people and do not tend to discriminate between them. Other forms of communication such as gesture and facial expression also seem to be lacking. Behaviour is often ritualistic and compulsive, and the child strongly resists any change in routine or alterations in his environment. The onset of such behaviour should be before $2\frac{1}{2}$ years of age.

Assessment of language ability

Language ability is not as easy to measure as height, weight, vision or hearing. Observation of the child in the clinical setting will provide useful information as

Clinical assessment of language. The following lists the sort of observations that can be made in a clinical setting of a child's language development. It enables a description to be made of the child's speech and areas of difficulty to be highlighted

To test comprehension ask the child to:	— identify objects on request — 'find me the ball, cup, spoon' — link objects and ideas — 'put the spoon in the cup','put the doll on the chair'. 'put the dog next to the man' — follow simple commands — 'where's mummy', 'give the ball to mummy', 'close the door', 'show me your nose' — react to more complicated concepts — 'show me the biggest balloon','show me what we drink from', 'what we draw with'
To test expression ask the child to:	— names simple objects or pictures — forms word combination — uses nouns, verbs, objectives, adverbs, etc

a basis for assessment. The 'tools' for doing this are miniature toys which can be used to test expression, comprehension, articulation, symbolic understanding, and the child's ability to understand commands related to the miniature toys or pictures.

Standardised clinical tests require time, patience and cooperation from the child.

The Reynell Developmental Language Scale is very commonly used and covers children from the ages of 6 months to 6 years. There is an alternative version of this test for use with handicapped children. The test gives scores for both verbal comprehension and expression. These results are recorded in 3 ways. These are a raw score, an equivalent age representing the level of language development, and a standard score representing the number of standard deviations from the mean for that child's chronological age.

The Edinburgh Articulation Test consists of 41 coloured pictures. It is concerned with recording the child's ability to produce consonant sounds. Pictures are presented one at a time and the response of the child is noted. The score is derived from the number of consonants correctly pronounced and is converted into a standard score. An articulatory age can be determined.

The English picture vocabulary test is designed to assess comprehension in terms of recognition of pictures. Four pictures are presented and the child is required to point to the correct one in response to a similar word. The vocabulary tested becomes more and more difficult. The number of words correctly identified is again compared with normative data and expressed as a vocabulary age and percentile equivalent. This test begins at a 3 year level.

Disorders of articulation — dysarthria
Disorders of articulation may be due to structural abnormalities of the lips, tongue or palate, or neuromuscular abnormalities. For these reasons articulation problems are common in handicapped children. A special mention should be

made of palato-pharyngeal incompetence in which the palate is inadequately formed to close off the nasopharynx completely during speech. This may be associated with a sub-mucous cleft of the palate where there is a deficiency of the bone of the hard palate or in the muscle of the soft palate. In this condition there is nasal escape of air. This causes difficulty with all vowel sounds and all the consonants except 'n', 'm' and 'ng'.If the child is asked to utter an 'e' sound, nasal escape of air is demonstrated by holding a mirror or wisp of cotton wool beneath the nose. The mirror will cloud or the cotton wool will move. Many of these patients have a history of nasal escape of milk. Adenoidectomy is contraindicated as this increases the degree of palatal disproportion and the degree of incompetence. Palatal X-rays (palatogram) are most useful to assess the degree of movement of the soft palate and closure of the naso-pharynx.

Causes of disorders of articulation

Structural defects

Tongue   — congenital hypoplasia (small immobile tongue)
           — macroglossia in Hurler's syndrome, Down's syndrome, Beckwith's syndrome
Palate   — cleft palate: often associated with a conductive hearing loss
           — palatal disproportion and submucous cleft
Nasal obstruction   — difficulty with 'n', 'm', 'ng': no air entry when asked to sniff
                 — adenoidal enlargement
                 — displacement of nasal septum
                 — chronic rhinitis
                 — partial choanal atresia (rare)
Malocclusion of the jaws   — micrognathia: a small lower jaw with protrusion of the tongue between the teeth in speech. . Occurs in association with cleft palate in Pierre-Robin syndrome
                          — prognathism: protrusion of the lower jaw
                          Malocclusion causes difficulty with the 's' and 's' blend sounds

Muscular defects

Myotonic dystrophy
Facio-scapulo-humeral dystrophy
Myasthenia gravis

Neurological defects

Cerebral palsy   — 50% have defects in articulation
                 — spasticity of tongue, lips and palate gives rise to slow laborious speech
                 — feeding problems, drooling
                 — involuntary movement
                 — incoordination of movements
                 — associated mental retardation or hearing loss
Nuclear   — failure of development of the nuclei of the cranial nerves
agenesis

Stuttering

Stuttering, stammering or speech dysrhythmia is a very common finding in preschool children at the stage when there is a rapid expansion of vocabulary and increase in sentence length. Persistent stuttering occurs in about 4% of children. The development of the stutter goes through several well defined stages. Initially there is simply repetition of initial speech sounds, and these increase in frequency with the prolongation of sounds, hesitation and blocking, in which speech completely stops. Associated with blocking there may be grimacing movements of the face. As the stammer develops, hesitation and blocking become more severe and the problem becomes one of absence of speech rather than the initial repetition. Particular words which are apt to set off the stammer are specifically avoided. The stammer becomes an increasing handicap in terms of oral work in the classroom and social relationships outside the classroom. It obstructs any form of employment in which communication with the public is essential. Stammering can be a source of great unhappiness and worry. Other children can be particularly unkind.

Below the age of 8 direct treatment is not required and parents should be recommended to avoid correcting the child. Drawing the child's attention to the stutter is likely to exacerbate it rather than improve it. Older children may benefit from intensive courses using the technique of the syllable timed speech in which a regular unaltering rhythm is imposed. Cutting back auditory feedback of the child's own voice also helps stuttering.

Developmental language disorders

This covers a wide spectrum of delay in language development in children who are either normal or who have only minor problems in other areas, and where the delay cannot be accounted for by mental handicap or environmental causes. There is often a family history, and boys are more commonly affected. There may be associated delay in lateralisation or minor neurological signs. In its mildest form there is delay in acquisition of speech sounds though language itself is normal. If the child is more severely affected, expressive language is delayed though comprehension is normal. The more severely handicapped have retardation in both expression and comprehension, and at the most severe end of the spectrum auditory imperception as well. There is failure to discriminate between sounds in the presence of normal hearing. Indeed these children initially are often thought to be deaf. They are very rare indeed. Most show improvement with age, but many will need to be educated using a signing system such as the Paget Gorman system, in the place of spoken language.

In developmental articulatory dyspraxia, voluntary movements only of the lips, tongue and palate are impaired. There is often a history of feeding difficulties and the children have trouble with such pleasant tasks as blowing bubbles or licking ice lollies.

Language programmes

Children with delays in language development, whether due to mental handicap or lack of environmental stimulation, may be helped most dramatically by specific language programmes. These are aimed at building up the child's language ability on a systematic basis and also the development of other skills such as attention control required for speech. Such a daily programme carried out by a parent or a nursery nurse in the child's everyday setting is a far more effective method than the 'traditional' once weekly speech therapy session. Such programmes may form part of a generalised enrichment programme. Examples are 'the first words' language programme produced by Dr Bill Gilham for use with severely mentally handicapped children, the developmental language programme of Cooper,

Moodley and Reynell and those used by Dorinda Bath among the day nursery children.

REFERENCES AND FURTHER READING

Vision
Gardiner P A 1982 The Development of Vision. MTP, Lancaster
Hall S M, Pugh A G, Hall D M B 1982 Vision screening in the under fives. British Medical Journal 285: 1096–1098
Ingram P M 1977 Refraction as a basis for screening children for squint and amblyopia. British Journal of Ophthalmology 61: 8–15
Ismail H, Lall P 1981 Visual acuity of school entrants. Child: Care, Health and Development 7: 127–134
Taylor D 1978 The assessment of visual function in young children: an overview. Clinical Paediatrics 226–231

Language
Bath D 1982 Developing the speech therapy service in day nurseries: a progress report. British Journal of Disorders of Communication 16: 159–173
Butler N R, Peckham C, Sheridan M 1973 Speech defects in children age 7: a national study. British Medical Journal 1: 153–257
Cooper J, Moodley M, Reynell J 1978 Helping Language Development. Edward Arnold, London
Gillham W 1978 First Words Language Programme. George Allen and Unwin, London
Jeffree D, McCorkey R 1976 Let me Speak. Souvenir Press, London
Reynell J 1980 Language Development and Assessment. MTP Press, Lancaster
Rutter M, Martin A, 1972 The Child with Delayed Speech. Clinics in Developmental Medicine No. 43. Heinemann Medical, London

Hearing
Brooks D N 1977 Auditory screening. Time for Reappraisal. Public Health 91: 282–28
Ferrer H P 1974 Use of impedance audiometry in school children. Public Health 88: 153–163
McCormick B C 1977 The toy discrimination test: an aid for screening the hearing of children above a mental age of two years. Public Health 91: 67–69
Taylor I G 1974 Deaf children. British Journal of Hospital Medicine 12: 440–451

16
Health and Learning

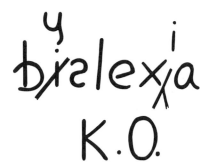

Educational medicine is concerned with the different ways that health and education interact. In its crudest sense it involves the general fitness of children to receive education and in its more specific sense it is concerned with the ways in which particular health problems or disabilities produce learning difficulty.

The doctor attending child health clinics will be able to identify children who will have learning problems before school age. These need to be discussed with educationalists and with the child's parents. The doctor attending school is in a position to give expert advice on medical matters which might affect the child's education or behaviour in school. For the chronically ill child, the health service can be an important source of continuity, as the child progresses from nursery to primary and then into secondary school. Expert advice is also required at school leaving, with respect to the limitations a child's disability might place on future employment. It is essential if the school careers service is to point the child towards suitable and rewarding occupations or appropriate further education.

The concept of routine medicals of a repetitive and unselective nature has now largely been abandoned other than for school entrants, although routine screening for disorders of vision and hearing remains important. The school nurse is the most appropriate agent for total population screening where it is required.

Expected disabilities per 1000 children entering infant school (Newcastle Upon Tyne, 1952)

Mental dullness	50
Severe speech defect	50
Growth failure	50
Squint	50
Behaviour disorder	40
Enuresis	90
Chronic otorrhoea	24
Chronic respiratory disease	6
Recurrent fits	6
Miscellaneous (including blindness, deafness, cerebral palsy)	2

Development

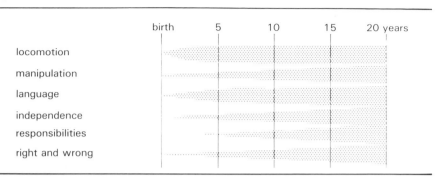

THE INFLUENCE OF EDUCATION

Children spend 10 years of their lives at school and it would be surprising indeed if the quality and content of this education did not have some, if not a major, effect on their final behaviour, academic achievement and functioning as an adult. There appears, however, to be a greater inequality in educational achievement than would be expected from examining children at school entry, and some would argue that this is due to the very strong influence of family and social background on outcome. Put crudely, good education does not compensate for social disadvantage. However, schools do have an effect for better or for worse. Rutter et al (1979), in their book '15 000 Hours', looked at the intake of 12 London comprehensive schools in 1970, and compared assessments at age 10 in primary school, with those at age 14 and the examination results at age 16. They showed that children did much better in some schools than in others, and that these differences could not be explained by differences in intake. For example, the intake of one school contained 31% of children with behaviour difficulties, which was reduced to 10% by the age of 14, whereas in another school the intake contained 34% of children with behaviour difficulties but this had risen to 48% by the age of 14. The kind of school which produced the best results largely followed the traditional model of firm and consistent discipline, high academic standards, homework, school uniform and a wide range of extra curricular activities in which children could engage and take responsibility. Other characteristics such as modern build-

Learning

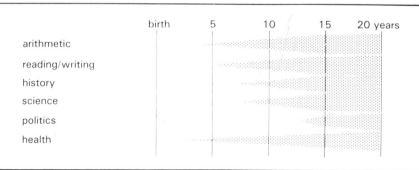

ings and facilities were not demonstrated to be important factors.

The pastoral side of education in both primary and secondary schools can do much to compensate for deficiencies at home or to supplement the positive influences of family life. Indeed the hallmark of many successful schools is that they not only influence their children, but also that they influence parents and the community around them as well. In return, parents and community can make a great contribution to the life of the school. The strength of such feeling becomes evident when the school is deprived of resources, or is threatened with closure.

The broader aims of both paediatrics and education are identical.

THE WARNOCK COMMITTEE AND THE 1981 EDUCATION ACT

In the UK, the Warnock Committee report (Special Educational Needs, 1978) reviewed the current position for children with learning difficulties and made new recommendations concerning their management. Many of these recommendations are incorporated in the 1981 Education Act. Their concept of special educational needs covered a much wider group than the 2% of children who attend special schools; it includes about 1 in 5 of the school population at one time or other in their education. This is in accordance with figures from the Isle of Wight Study (Rutter et al, 1970) which looked in detail at 2199 children aged between 9 and 11. The children were classified into four main groups; (1) physical handicap — being those children with a chronic disorder lasting for greater than one year; (2) intellectual retardation — being those with an IQ of below 70; (3) educational backwardness — being those with a reading age of more than 28 months below their chronological age; and (4) psychiatric disorder. Grouped together, they constituted 16% of the total population of 9 to 11 year olds.

Using this broader concept the committee recommended that provision should be made according to the educational needs of the child, rather than the category of handicap. This took a positive look at the child's strengths rather than his deficits. Previous policy has required children to be fitted into categories such as ESN (M), ESN (S), Maladjusted, Physically Handicapped, Blind, Partially Sighted, Deaf, Partially hearing or Delicate.

The Warnock Committee also recommended that children should be educated in ordinary schools as far as is reasonably practical. This move towards a broader

Services for the pre-school child

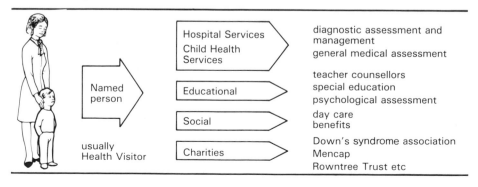

integration of handicapped children gave the children a wider choice of curriculum, a broader opportunity for normal social contacts and avoided the isolation that has been experienced by many handicapped children in the past. Bringing more handicapped children into ordinary schools means more support for the staff and increased resources.

The Committee supported the established need for multidisciplinary assessment so that all possible professional advice is obtained and coordinated in the interests of the child. They introduced the idea of a 'named' person, who might be the health visitor for children not yet in school, and the head teacher for children in school. The 'named' person acts as a lay adviser to the parents who are often bewildered by the wide range of professionals who become involved with their child.

The Committee also proposed a substantial increase in nursery provision, thus recognising the importance of early education for disadvantaged or handicapped children. They recommended the setting up of resource centres where information and expertise could be concentrated.

The 1981 Education Act embodies many of the recommendations made in the Warnock Committee Report, including integration within ordinary schools wherever possible, multidisciplinary assessment and a broader concept of special educational need.

Much of the assessment of children's individual needs can be obtained within the school. However, under section 5 of the 1981 Act, where provision, additional or otherwise different to the facilities and resources generally available in ordinary school is needed, a statutory assessment must be made. The provision of such a statement of special educational need is not confined to those over 5; it is applicable to a child of any age. A statement on children under two may only be prepared with the parents' consent. If such parents specifically ask for a statement, the education authority has to comply.

The statement consists of three parts. Part A represents the views of the parents, Part B represents the assessment made by the local educational authority, containing as a minimum, the views of the teaching staff, the educational psychologist and the school medical officer, and Part C states the special provision that needs to be provided. The parents are formally told that such an assessment is being made and are given the name of the person within the education authority

Services for the school child

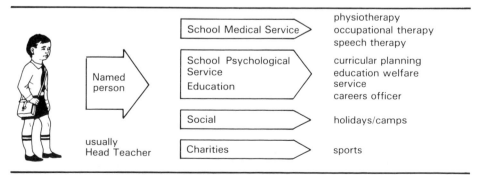

with whom to communicate. It is hoped that by involving parents throughout, disagreement is less likely to occur. However, appeals committees deal with any disputes. Assessment is not a single event but is a continuous process. The position is reviewed annually with a full reassessment at 13½–14½ years to determine further educational and vocational requirements. District handicap, mental handicap and child guidance teams may also act as the organisation or framework within which such assessments take place, though decisions on the provisions required are always made by the education authority.

Assessment

It is recommended that a professional assessment should consist of three parts. The first part is a description of the child, the second part the broad aims of provision, and the third part the facilities and resources that are required. Each professional is requested to base his own recommendations within his individual professional framework. In the past, doctors have been responsible for ascertainment of children's special educational needs. The habit of performing functions better suited to an educational psychologist must be resisted. The description of the child should involve his strengths and weaknesses. Areas that need to be covered are:

— physical state and functioning (physical health, developmental level, mobility, hearing, vision, emotion or behavioural disorders)
— adaptive skills and functioning
— cognitive functioning
— speech and communication
— educational attainment
— approaches to learning
— self image and interests
— social skills and interaction
— behaviour.

It will not be within the knowledge of an individual doctor to comment upon all these particular areas, though collectively they all need to be covered. Factors in the child's environment which lessen or contribute towards his needs in the home, family or school, must also to be stated.

Rates on formal ascertainment of handicapped pupils at ages 7 and 11 from National Child Development Study

Rate per 1000 Age 7 (1965)	Category	Rate per 1000 Age 11 (1969)
0.3	Blind and partially sighted	0.6
1.1	Deaf and partially hearing	1.3
5.3	Educationally subnormal	17.4
2.4	Severely subnormal	3.3
0.4	Epileptic	0.5
0.6	Maladjusted	3.1
1.8	Physically handicapped	1.8
1.9	Speech defect	0.3
1.0	Delicate	1.4
Rate 13.3/1000		Rate 27.8/1000

Handicapped children by category and placement (England and Wales, 1979) The 1981 act has changed all this:

	In special schools and on waiting list	In special classes in ordinary school
Blind	1 052	8
Partially sighted	2 224	154
Deaf	3 529	292
Partially hearing	2 235	3 474
Speech defect	1 295	799
Autistic	826	89
Moderate learning difficulty	66 025	8 330
Severe learning difficulty	31 328	212
Physically handicapped	14 040	473
Delicate	5 470	321
Epileptic	1 005	80
Maladjusted	17 274	1 548

Educational aims can be described within the following framework. Firstly the general curriculum needs to be defined. For example, if the ordinary curriculum is to be used, does the child require special access due to sensory or motor disabilities, or should the curriculum be modified for slow learners, or specifically adjusted to meet the needs of children with severe learning difficulties. Special features, for example teaching for the blind or deaf through specialised methods must be stated, and any specific requirement for an individual child defined. Adjustment of the emotional climate and social regimen may be just as important for other children. The need for specific strategies with regard to behaviour control in class, or areas for special training, like independence or continence should be outlined.

The facilities and resources that are to be made available are given in the third section. Equipment such as walking aids, wheelchairs, auditory and visual aids, is specified. Many children in special education require additional resources from nursing, social work, speech therapy, occupational therapy, physiotherapy, psychotherapy, audiology or orthoptics. This provision must be included within the statement of educational needs. The physical environment is important in the education of handicapped children, and physical conditions such as access and facility for non-ambulant pupils must be given, together with needs if necessary for appropriate lighting, alterations of the acoustic environment or health care accommodation. Transport to school is required by many handicapped children and others require particular forms of organisation and attendance such as weekly boarding, termly boarding or ordinary daily attendance.

Distribution by age of pupils in special schools (England and Wales, 1979)

Age group (years)	Percentage of all handicapped pupils in special schools
2–4	2.8
5–7	12.1
8–11	32.0
12–16	51.2
17+	1.9

POOR SCHOOL PROGRESS

The following scheme is offered as a framework for the medical assessment of children referred because of poor progress in class.

Limited intellect

If teachers and educational psychologists consider that the child's intellect is poor, ask the following questions.

Is there a specific syndrome associated with mental retardation, for example tuberose sclerosis? Positive identification of a named syndrome helps in establishing a prognosis, alerts one to looking for associated handicaps, provides an explanation for parents and teachers, and may indicate the need for genetic counselling.

Are there any events in the past medical history which may be the cause of mental retardation. For example is there a history of severe birth asphyxia, congenital infection, neonatal convulsions, head injury or encephalitis?

Are the parents likely to be within the ESN (M) range themselves? Many children in the ESN (M) group are functioning at this level because genetically they resemble their parents, rather than because of specific pathological conditions that they have inherited or that they have acquired.

It is not always the case that a presumptive diagnosis of mental handicap made by teachers or educational psychologists is correct. Parents may have other views and the answers to many of the questions given below relating to perceptual difficulty, the effects of chronic illness or the effects of treatment, may serve to alter the educational view of the child's learning difficulties.

Perceptual difficulties

It is essential to establish whether or not the child has perceptual problems.

Vision. What is the near and distant visual acuity? Are the visual fields normal? Assessment of visual fields is not routinely required, though it is most important in children with neurological defects such as cerebral palsy where, for instance, a hemiplegia may be associated with a homonymous hemianopia. The hemianopia if unrecognised, will certainly inhibit the development of reading and writing skills. In any statement to teachers it must be remembered that their training does not include the ability to understand medical shorthand, so that telling a teacher that a child's visual acuity is 6/36 may not be helpful. The teacher in a special school for visually handicapped children may understand this, but teachers working within ordinary schools will not. The teachers really want to know what size of print the child can be expected to read on a blackboard and in a book, and this can form a working base from which to begin to sort out the child's particular special needs.

Hearing. Hearing losses of as little as 20 dB have been demonstrated to impair school work and produce behaviour problems. Children should never be labelled uncooperative in hearing tests, as this avoids making a diagnosis of either deafness, a behaviour problem or a degree of mental handicap which renders the child unable to perform a particular hearing test that he should be expected to complete for his age. For the same reason the label 'uncooperative' cannot be accepted as an endpoint in vision testing either. Teachers need practical advice on appropriate seating for the child, an indication of the degree of hearing loss, the type of hearing loss, for example high frequency loss and its effects, and the difficulties that the hearing loss produces for the child.

Can the child comprehend what is said? It may be considered easy to identify children who are non-English speakers. However some children may have considerable delay in their own language. Failure to test the child in his own language may result in us assuming that the child is able to speak fluent Punjabi, Urdu or Italian, whereas in fact all we are really identifying is our own ignorance of that language. The parents may also speak little English which imposes added difficulties in assessment of a child. However this challenge is one which needs to be taken up earlier rather than late in the child's school career. Investments in terms of time, patience and an interpreter are essential.

Children who speak English as a second language quite commonly enter school with some knowledge of English but one which is not equal to their own native language. Within primary schools extra help is usually provided from specialist 'English as a second language' teachers and secondary school children are often able to attend a separate language unit with other non-English speaking children until their skills are sufficient for them to be integrated within an ordinary classroom. A superficial examination of such children does not reveal the depth of their difficulty and that their comprehension is inadequate for educational purposes.

Bilingual children are fortunate, for to speak two languages is an advantage. It is important to recognise and nurture this advantage rather than ignore it.

Dialect problems were once considered to be important in the difficulties of West Indian children in school, however its relevance was probably overstated. Other factors such as low expectation, low self-esteem, deficiencies in experience in the pre-school years and the view that many schools provide an inappropriate cultural setting for West Indian children may be far more important. Children from one part of the country moving to another where there is a strong regional accent, may also experience temporary difficulties in comprehension of that accent.

The combination of difficulties such as minor hearing loss in a non-English speaking child, may produce a major handicap. It is important to recognise the existence

Developmental scores of non-immigrant and West Indian 3 year olds in a deprived inner London area and their subsequent reading attainment at 9 years of age (from Pollak, 1972, 1980)

	Adaptive	Language	Personal/ social	Motor
West Indian children	3.48	3.85	6.97	12.91
Non-immigrant children	10.32	12.04	8.92	13.27
	p<0.001	p<0.001	p<0.001	NS

Follow-up of the same children at age 9 revealed the following results in terms of non-reading:
West Indian children   31.8%
Non-immigrant children   1.3%

of more than one factor.

Specific language difficulties are the least common of this group. They are also those most likely to be missed. Incorrect diagnoses of autism, deafness or subnormality may be made when a more appropriate diagnosis may be an expressive or receptive language problem, or auditory inattention.

Other perceptual difficulties include disorders of visual perception, for example figure-ground, disorders of body image, dyspraxias, the 'clumsy child' and children with some specific reading and writing difficulties (dyslexia). Up to 5–15% of children fall into the clumsy group. These various perceptual difficulties which are becoming of greater interest within education are discussed in detail later.

Chronic illness

The mechanism by which this occurs can be considered under a number of headings.

Genuine absence from school. This may be because the child is ill at home or requires frequent hospital appointments. There is an obvious conflict between the demands of treatment and education though clearly they are inter-dependent. School doctors are frequently asked by education authorities to adjudicate on school attendance records, stating whether non-attendance is or is not acceptable on the medical grounds stated. These are difficult issues; it is important that the doctor is not seen by the child or the family as an inquisitor whose job it is to establish guilt or innocence. The doctor's task is to see how a particular child's medical management might be modified so that his educational needs can be met as well.

A pretext to keep the child at home. In this situation the children do have a chronic illness but the degree of disability it causes or apparently causes, is out of proportion to that which would be expected. This may be due to excessive anxiety by the parents, combined with an attitude of over-protection towards any actual or potential adverse factor or symptom, for example bad weather or a minimal cold. The child's anxiety may act to exaggerate the effect of organic illness. There may be a degree of collusion between parents and children in such a situation.

Other children may be kept at home when perfectly well, under the pretext of illness, though with the real intention of helping mother look after a younger child or elderly relative. A sympathetic and helpful attitude towards these difficulties is more successful than a critical or punitive one.

'Present but ill'. In some situations the treatment is inadequate, for instance children with asthma may be either inadequately or inappropriately treated. Children with asthma may be too busy wheezing, children with eczema too busy scratching, children with petit mal too busy having absence attacks to follow the lessons properly. In others adequate treatment has been prescribed but compliance by the parents is poor. This may be because the parents do not understand the treatment or the technique for administration. Alternatively they may not be sufficiently organised to ensure they have a continuous supply of medicine, although they might realise the need. Occasionally parents may deny the existence of a specific diagnosis in their child and therefore withhold treatment. Sometimes the child rebels against the treatment, or may manipulate or sabotage the effects of treatment. This is particularly common amongst adolescents with chronic conditions such as diabetes. Finally, the treatment may be having its desired effect, there is a good compliance, but there remains some residual disability, for example in motor, sensory, or respiratory function, which has an influence on education. Under these circumstances additional educational rather than medical resources are required.

Treatment is interfering with the ability to learn. This is common with the use of antihistamines which are still frequently used for hay fever. Unfortunately hay fever often coincides with the times of important examinations. Similarly, anticonvulsants may make the child drowsy or ataxic. The possible effects of any drug that the child is taking must be considered in appreciating the possible role that they may have in producing or contributing towards existing learning difficulties.

The child's reaction to his illness. Some children in response to chronic illness adopt a 'sick role', so that the concept of disablement is generalised into many other areas of activity where it does not apply. Parents and teachers may to some extent collude with this by regarding the child as 'delicate', and having low expectations of him. They shield him from pressures such as education. Handicapped children need more education and not less, if they are to be able to compete for jobs on leaving school.

The reactions of other children. Children may be protective to a handicapped classmate and indeed on occasions over-protective, doing too much for him. However, we are more commonly drawn to the unhappy situation when the child with a handicap or disability has become a source of amusement, or a source of fear or has been rejected by his classmates. Peer group pressure may dictate that it is unsightly to wear glasses or a hearing aid or to take medication in school. Children may be amused by the abnormal gait or speech problems of a child with cerebral palsy or a stammer. Children may be frightened by the appearance of a skin complaint or the child convulsing. All these issues need to be handled sensitively within the classroom situation. They first of all need to be noticed; many children suffer in silence. Indeed most will not tell the teacher, which is another effect of peer group pressure. It is good for all children to learn how to be sensitive to the feelings of others. However, one should not under-estimate the skills required to handle this sort of situation. Too often, perhaps inevitably, the solution is to remove the victim to more secure surroundings rather than deal with the victimisers. The child can be taught that it is not necessary to tolerate abuse and that it is possible to combat this and to maintain self-esteem. It is often this lack of self-esteem and lack of emotional robustness that makes the child such an easy victim. To some extent such problems can be prevented by positive effort at the earliest age to encourage self-esteem, to provide support and an open channel for communication about the child's hurt feelings.

Unnecessary restrictions. Teachers in their general training receive little or no instruction in childhood illness. Without proper knowledge they may not wish to take the responsibility for what they may regard as 'risks'. Thus a child may be excluded from certain lessons such as chemistry, metalwork, and PE, and may be sent to a medical room or home for negligible reasons. The loss in education may be very significant and it is the doctor's role with parental permission to explain fully to the teacher the nature and consequences of the child's problems, to discuss any limitations that should be imposed (and there should usually be none), and that following discussion the doctor accepts responsibility for the decision that has been made. Teachers may not see their role as looking after children who are other than fully fit. Inevitably the implementation of the 1981 Education Act will increasingly expose them to children with chronic illness and handicaps.

Social and environmental factors.

Children who are tired, from whatever reason, are likely to perform poorly at school. Lack of sleep may be caused by a combination of noise and overcrowding. More commonly, lack of family discipline results in the child not having a suitable bedtime. It is accepted that children vary widely in the amount of sleep that they require in order not to feel tired the following morning. A survey of television programmes that children claimed to watch provides a good indication of bedtime. Many children who cannot tell the time do have a built in clock which tells them precisely when particular programmes are going to be on. Older children are tired because they are out late at night.

Not all children want and eat breakfast. However some children who do want breakfast do not get one, and they are hungry at school. In the 'no breakfast syndrome', the child is often tired and seems pale and unwell. Occasionally they are seen because they have fainted or have abdominal pain. These children usually perk up after their mid-morning milk break or school dinner.

Some children are tired because they have to do too much work at home. This is now very uncommon, but occasionally children do live a Cinderella life at home, doing much housework or work within a family business. Occasionally the parents force their child to do school type work at home, beyond the limits where any useful return can be expected.

The most common problem in this category, is due to lack of early childhood stimulation, coupled with little support for the child and teachers, limited contact

Adverse social circumstances related to education as revealed in the National Child Development Study

	Percentage at age 11 years (1969)	Percentage at age 16 years (1974)	Percentage of those at 11 with some adversity at 16 years
None	71	73	
One parent/large family	20	19	69
Poor housing	15	10	46
Low income	13	12	52
All three	4.5	2.9	1.6

Children in the disadvantaged group were:
— *twice* as likely to be absent from school for 1–3 months in the year
— *five times* more likely to be absent for more than 3 months
— *seven times* more likely to be unable to do basic arithmetical calculations
— *ten times* more likely to be unable to read well enough for everyday needs
— *six times* more likely to attend a special school especially for moderate learning difficulties
— *three times* more likely to display behaviour unacceptable at school

Effects of early intervention with deprived mothers and children upon later educational achievement at 14 years of age (Perry pre-school programme, 1980)

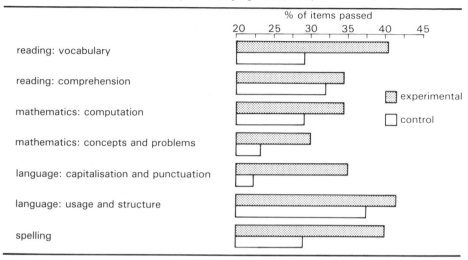

between parents and school, and no encouragement to do well. Neither the parents nor the child expect to succeed, and they don't.

Emotional problems

Some children are able to dissociate themselves in school from disruption and turmoil at home. More commonly, family disharmony may be translated in school into either depression and withdrawal, anxiety or aggression. Violence in the home, drunkenness, prostitution, the comings and goings of parents' boyfriends or girlfriends, and the reception into and out of care, provide an unstable background from which it is difficult for many children to make educational progress.

School refusal.

This is fairly frequently seen by those working within school health. School refusal is not a single entity. The cause may be anxiety about separating from the parent, it may be caused by anxiety related to the journey to school, by the transport, or dogs on the way, or it may be related to anxiety directly associated with school. At school children may be frightened of being bullied, of other children, of particular lessons or just the general scale of the buildings. Among primary school children, school lavatories are often identified as a source of fear, as the children may regard them (and often rightly so) as smelly and unclean. Children may be frightened by lack of privacy and some children may actively avoid using the lavatory for the whole school day, or soil or wet themselves when they are unable to accomplish this. Also, lack of privacy with regard to changing for PE may provoke great fear.

The more school that children miss, the further they are behind with their work, and this realisation produces secondary factors, which tend to potentiate school refusal. The management of school refusal is covered in the chapter on Child Psychiatry.

Depression
This is commonly seen at the upper end of the secondary school. It is often described as 'boredom' and can consist of a general withdrawal and inactivity. The child is often very easily upset and cries for reasons he cannot explain. Although usually a transient phase in adolescent development, it comes at an unfortunate time when examinations are taking place.

Poor attention control
Whether or not this is a psychiatric entity, it is certainly a problem within an educational setting. Children with a limited attention span, poor concentration and who fidget, are going to do badly whatever the subject matter taught. They also tend to be punished for their lack of concentration, which, if it is a basic problem, is not a very constructive approach. Aetiological factors include lack of stimulation in the child's early childhood, mental handicap, and neurological disorders.

Conduct disorders
Children who are truanting from school or who whilst at school present behaviour disorders, are commonly seen by those working within the school health service. The outcome for these children is poor in terms of educational achievement, and criminal activity in adult life often results. The keys to success are a warm, caring attitude from the school and an improvement in self image. They require firm and consistent discipline, counselling, and particularly a stimulating education. It is common knowledge that children tend to be described as having a conduct disorder in one school class and not in another and this probably relates to the quality of teaching received. Lastly, continuity of child — adult relationships is important in managing this group of children.

Psychotic disorders.
These are extremely uncommon. Occasionally these odd children are not correctly identified. In one instance, a senior secondary school girl's written work was labelled a 'lively and imaginative essay', whereas in fact, the writing showed elements of thought disorder and delusions, and she stabbed the teacher the following week.

CULTURAL DIFFERENCES

Cultural differences in outlook, behaviour, and social norms, not to mention problems of differences in clothing, language and climate, often cause difficulties in adjustment to the school environment. Children may adapt by staying within their own racial group at school, or schools which have a large number of children belonging to racial minority groups may go out of their way to absorb some of the culture into the school institution. Conflicts may develop between standards and patterns of behaviour expected at home and experience at school of the freedom which many of their peer group may have. In order to attempt to handle many of these problems the school doctor needs to acquire a lot of information about the cultural background of the families with which he is dealing. Much useful information can be obtained from two books 'Children of Immigrants to Britain, their Health and Social Problems' by Edwin D H Lobo and 'Asian Patients in Hospital and at Home' by Alix Henley.

BRIGHT CHILDREN

It is not exceptional to see very intelligent children referred because of poor progress in school. In some cases their poor progress may result from boredom and an insufficiently challenging educational programme. Others may have emotional problems and feel socially isolated from their peer group at school, and others may have such a great fear of failure that this overcomes their ability to concentrate.

In order to contribute towards the management of children with such a broad range of difficulties resulting in failure to learn, the school doctor obviously has to work closely with the others involved, particularly parents, teachers, psychologists, general practitioners and hospital paediatricians.

CLUMSY CHILDREN

Various estimates have given an incidence of clumsiness from 5 to 15% amongst the school population. Boys are more often affected than girls. These children show difficulty in motor coordination which is out of proportion to their general ability. They often have secondary emotional problems and learning difficulties. The difficulties in motor coordination may involve fine motor or gross motor skills. The label has become a popular one and may hide children with specific pathologies such as mild cerebral palsy, cerebellar ataxia or lower motor neurone disorders. A careful neurological examination is therefore required in order to ensure that such conditions are not missed. Management could very crudely, and perhaps unfairly, be described as finding out what the child cannot do, and then making him practise it over and over again. However, prior to this the child's difficulties are analysed and a therapeutic programme is developed in a graded series of steps starting with what the child can accomplish. Success in the early part of the programme does much to restore the child's confidence.

Aetiology

Much of what is said about aetiology of clumsiness is speculative. The children may well form the lower part of the normal distribution of manual dexterity. Genetic factors may be involved. However it is difficult to separate these from environmental factors, in that parents with high degrees of fine and gross motor skill tend to provide these activities for their children in early life, and provide a good model for copying. Some children go through a transient state of clumsiness during periods of rapid growth such as adolescence, when they are unable to adapt to the effects of changing body size. Organic factors such as birth asphyxia, insufficient to cause any gross neurological impairment, may in some cases contribute towards later clumsiness.

Presentation

Clumsiness may present with difficulties or delays in developing self help skills such as dressing. The child has difficulty with buttons, shoes, assembling a zip and some children may virtually strangle themselves trying to put on or take off a pullover. The child may be very untidy or poor at feeding himself, either missing the target area of the mouth or being unable to capture the food on the plate or transfer it to the mouth without spilling. In terms of play the child may have trouble with such materials as jigsaws, building blocks and drawing. Climbing through a hoop may be an impossible task as the child tries to put both feet through at the same time. Some children may present because of frequent falls. From the educational point of view, they may be seen by the school doctor because of learning difficulties, poor handwriting or extremely poor performance at PE. Such skills are important in terms of their position within the peer group and the child may find himself isolated. Likewise emotional reaction in the parents and the subsequent tension in the clumsy child may give rise to earlier referral. Punishment is often the response to damage, instead of sympathy, understanding and practice.

Examination

Fine motor skills The clumsy child may have difficulty in brick building, repetitive fast tapping, pronation and supination exercises or finger-thumb opposition sequences. The movements are irregular and not precise. Drawing may be difficult and such exercises as tracing or colouring within lines again demonstrate the child's particular difficulty. Threading beads which involves accurate eye-hand coordination is a useful test. Although standardised and timed tests for clumsiness have been developed, a simple approach is usually adequate for most situations.

Gross motor. The child usually has problems with such exercises as standing on one leg, hopping, kicking a ball, skipping, or heel-toe walking. The clap-catch test, in which the child is required to throw a ball in the air, clap the hands and then catch the ball, may be quite impossible. Walking on the lateral aspects of the feet is another useful test. Associated involuntary movements of the upper limbs are often seen in clumsy children.

Examples of simple tests for school entrants to identify the clumsy child. Watch for associated movements.

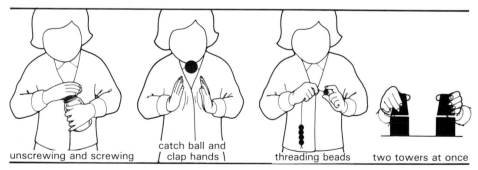

unscrewing and screwing | catch ball and clap hands | threading beads | two towers at once

Mouth coordination. The difficulties with motor coordination may also affect the muscles involved in speech. The child may have difficulty with exercises such as blowing, whistling, tongue protrusion, licking, clenching the teeth or rapid in and out movements and side to side movements of the tongue.

Laterality and handedness. Although clumsy children are frequently slow to develop laterality, the suggested association of handedness with neurological or perceptive deficits cannot be supported. Those left handers who do have difficulties are usually those with some dysfunction of the preferred side and hence transfer to the non-preferred side. Likewise, a number of right handers have difficulty with functioning on the left and have hence transferred to the right. As the right handed group is much larger than the left handed group, unless the function of the non-preferred hand is examined, incorrect conclusions can be drawn about the significance of left-handedness. Further examination of the subject of laterality has also established the unimportance of cross-laterality as a reason for poor gross or fine motor functioning.

Management

Management involves the practice of appropriate tasks in order to improve those areas where the child is having difficulties. These tasks start within their own level of ability so that confidence can be boosted and success ensured. Specific measures aimed at relieving tension or anxiety both within the child and the family may be needed. Remedial education may be required to enable the child to overcome his specific difficulties. A detailed assessment by physiotherapists or in some cases by a particularly interested educational psychologist or PE teacher, will determine the present level of functioning and outline in some detail the areas of difficulty. Without this, the blind stab at improving motor functioning may in fact involve the child in attempting tasks which are quite impossible for him at present.

Training in general awareness of body image, e.g. drawing around the whole body, identifying parts, or singing games in which imitation of posture or gesture is important. Other activities introduce awareness of rhythm such as in dancing, and swimming, though confidence in the water is a prerequisite for the latter. Eye-hand coordination may be practised with activities such as drawing, tracing and work with scissors. Practical training of self-help skills related to eating or dressing is required. By a series of exercises related to developing skills in these areas (eye-hand, manipulative, body image and independence), improvement in functioning can be expected.

GENERAL READING DIFFICULTIES

It is estimated that in the UK approximately two million, that is 6% of the adult population are illiterate. Twenty-five per cent of children leaving infant schools have reading difficulty and 10% of those leaving primary for secondary school still have difficulty. In many the problem is part of a general retardation in learning achievement. In others, however, there is a specific reading delay, with learning in other areas at a much higher level. Reading difficulties are likely to give rise to a loss of confidence, a sense of failure and result in secondary emotional problems. There is a strong association between reading difficulties and later delinquent behaviour. A third of the children with conduct disorders are described as having reading problems. Early identification of children with language delay at a pre-school age and the provision of appropriate help might have a beneficial effect upon later reading difficulties.

Skills required for reading

The following skills are required for the reading process:

— the ability to understand and use spoken language. Delays in speech and language development are the most commonly found associated difficulties in children with reading problems

— the ability to recognise visual symbols. Difficulties with visual perception are found less commonly than those of delayed language development. However the task of sorting out similar letters such as p's, b's, d's and q's, differentiating the m from the w and correctly orientating letters such as s may provide difficulties not only in reading but also in writing. Children with visuo-spatial difficulties may also have sequencing difficulties. They may be unable to remember a telephone number or the order of the months of the year. They may have important spelling problems, having difficulty with order of letters, or even complete reversals

— they must have normal sound perception and discrimination

— they must be able to relate written symbols to oral sounds

— they require a well established lateral preference. This does not mean that left handedness or cross laterality causes problems in reading or writing but confusion over laterality does

— normal emotional development. Defects in concentration, and impulsive behaviour are found more commonly in children with reading problems

— normal memory

Reading, writing and spelling problems are often related but not rigidly so. Some children can read words which they are unable to spell, and some children can spell words which they are unable to read.

Reading difficulties are also associated with low IQ, low social class and ascending birth order. They are increased in schools with a high rate of teacher and pupil turnover.

Assessment

Some 'reading' tests score the ability to read individual words. They are not really tests of reading as the words are used out of context. Speed in reading is obtained by scanning the text rather than by recognition and interpretation of individual letters. The Neale reading test involves errors accumulated whilst reading a particular passage.

Management

Remedial systems have been devised which depend upon an analysis of basic difficulties, for example visuo-spatial discrimination, and the introduction of programmes designed to improve these skills. However, studies of the effect of such programmes have shown that although they improve the underlying skill they do not improve reading itself. The results of remedial teaching programmes are generally most disappointing. Having made this statement, however, the needs of poor readers cannot be ignored. In general the child needs individualised teaching and the teacher must gain his confidence and interest. Any programme must be preceded by an accurate assessment of the child's ability and should be planned in very small steps where progress can be monitored and early success can be

The pictogram system — one way to teach children to read developed by Lyn Wendon

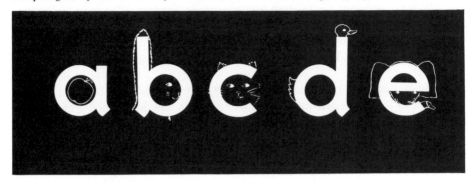

ensured. Success needs to be systematically rewarded and accurate feedback of achievements maintained throughout.

SPECIFIC READING RETARDATION

Specific reading retardation (sometimes called dyslexia or word blindness) is a common problem, with estimates of its incidence varying from 2 to 5% of school children. The condition is quite distinct, although there are overlaps with speech and language problems and with clumsiness, as mentioned in the previous section. In specific reading retardation, difficulties are seen despite conventional education, adequate intelligence and socio-cultural opportunity. Boys are far more likely to be affected by a ratio of 3 or 4 to 1. There is frequently a family history of reading problems.

The children in addition to difficulties with reading, often have trouble with writing and sometimes arithmetic. Although some features, such as reversal of letters may be regarded as immaturity, others such as mirror writing or bizarre spelling are highly deviant. Left/right confusion, (which is distinct from crossed

The results of good and poor readers, and a dyslexic sub-group from the poor readers using the Aston Index (from Newton & Thomson)

	'Poor readers and spellers' (Experimental group)	'Good readers and spellers' (control group)	Dyslexic group
Chronological age	9 y 1 m	9 y 0 m	9.3
Reading age (Schonell)	7 y 2 m	10 y 8 m	5.7
Spelling age (Schonell)	6 y 9 m	10 y 1 m	5.2
Draw-a-man	8 y 8 m	8 y 11 m	8.9
Vocabulary	9 y 3 m	10 y 6 m	10.4
Copying designs	6.22	6.78	6.02
Laterality	4.97	8.05	3.67
Memory pictorial	5.84	7.83	5.49
Visual sequential memory (symbolic)	6.55	8.14	5.92
Auditory sequential memory	5.83	7.46	4.36
Sound blending	7.02	8.02	6.42
Sound discrimination	9.19	9.97	9.53
Free writing	2.59	6.67	1.75
Total score for performance items	43.51	57.05	39.57

laterality) is common and the children show difficulty in sequencing from left to right which is necessary for reading and writing in English. The sequencing difficulties may affect order as well as direction, producing difficulty in memorising tables or other sequences such as days of the week. Handwriting is often very poor and becomes very untidy due to alterations and indecision. Misuse of grammar is also seen.

Secondary problems may arise if the child's intrinsic reading difficulties are not appreciated. Pressure, criticism or even punishment may be applied when an obviously intelligent child is failing to progress as he might be expected to do. This response may come from parents or teachers. The child's reaction to this results in the setting up of emotional barriers, which may themselves be formidable obstacles to progress.

Aetiology

A large amount of educational and psychological research has been carried out in order to identify 'a cause' for specific reading difficulties. The result has been the recognition of a series of associations but no single factor has been isolated that can be harnessed into a successful remedial system. There may be coding/decoding difficulties, but this perhaps represents a description of the problem rather than a formulation of cause. Neurological causes have been proposed particularly with relation to abnormalities in left or right cerebral hemisphere location of function. There are perceptual difficulties resulting in problems with correctly orientating letters such as p,b,d,b,q. The ability to retrieve visual or auditory information from the short and the long term memory may be lacking. Thus connecting auditory perception to written symbols is a problem. Integration of senses, vision, hearing (speech/sound), fine touch, and spatial awareness, is clearly important in the reading/writing process and some have argued that the defect in specific reading problems lies at this higher level.

Management

Based on these findings, various strategies have been developed to deal with dyslexia. Some are exercises designed to overcome difficulties with visual and auditory perception or short term memory. All approaches depend upon an analysis of the child's individual ability and difficulties. They build on the child's strengths and begin with tasks that he can be expected to achieve. This is important as many children have lost confidence by the time they receive help. They need to find again the pleasures that reading and writing can give.

Not all teachers accept the category of specific reading difficulties. However, parents can request assessment through the Director of Education or directly from the Educational Psychologist. When a diagnosis of specific reading or writing difficulty is made, the educational psychologist can then apply to examination boards for a special allowance to be made in respect of reading and written work produced in public examinations.

SPECIAL UNITS

Although the hope is to integrate children with learning difficulties within ordinary schools, a variety of special units either separately or attached to ordinary schools is needed. Remedial classes exist in many schools in which smaller groups can be withdrawn for special help in reading, writing or spelling.

CAREERS ADVICE

Careers advice is certainly not the province of any one discipline. Within ordinary secondary schools it is the practice to see selected fourth year pupils with medical problems to discuss the influence that their problem might have on their future career, and with parental permission, to provide the necessary information to the careers service (on form Y9). A more complicated system (Form Y10) is involved for handicapped school leavers with a broad consultation between teachers, doctors, parents and careers officers. The prospect for employment for many normal and handicapped school leavers is limited at the present time and although it is desirable that they should avoid occupations which might aggravate their medical condition or where their disorder may affect the quality of work produced, it is also important not to over-estimate the effects of the health problem. Irrelevant medical information such as a past history of epilepsy or febrile convulsions which could influence the employment of the child should be put into a proper perspective. More detailed information on career is obtained in the chapters covering various types of handicap and the chapter on chronic illness.

REFERENCES AND FURTHER READING

Bowley A H, Gardner L 1980 The Handicapped Child. Educational and Psychological guidance for the Organically Handicapped. Churchill Livingstone, Edinburgh

Davie R, Butler N, Goldstein H 1972 From Birth to Seven. A report of the National Child Development Study. The National Children's Bureau. Longman, Harlow

Department of Education and Science. Statistics of Education. HMSO, London

Gordon N, McKinley J 1980 Helping Clumsy Children. Churchill Livingstone, Edinburgh

Miller F J W, Court S D M, Knox E G, Brandon S 1974 The school years in Newcastle upon Tyne 1955–62. Oxford University Press, Oxford

Newton M, Thomson M Learning Development Aids: Materials for Children with Learning Difficulties. LDA Wisbech

Pollak M 1972 Today's Three-year-olds in London. Heinemann, London

Pollak M 1979 Nine Year Olds. MTP Press, Lancaster

Rampton A 1982 West Indian Children in our Schools. Interim report of the Committee of Enquiry into the Education of Children from Ethnic Minority Groups. HMSO, London

Rutter M et al 1979 Fifteen Thousand Hours. Open Books, Shepton Mallet

Rutter M, Yule W 1976 Reading difficulties. In: Rutter M, Hersov L eds Child Psychiatry. Modern Approaches. Blackwell Scientific Publications, Oxford

Rutter M, Tizard J, Whitmore L 1970 Health, Education and Behaviour, Longman, Harlow

Schweindart L J, Weihart D P 1980 Young children grow up. The effects of the Perry Pre-school Programme on Youth through age 15.Monographs of the High/Scopes Educational Research Foundation, No. 7

Seglow J, Pringle K M, Wedge P 1972 Growing up Adopted NFER

Spence J C, Walton W S, Miller F J W, Court SDM 1954 A Thousand Families in Newcastle Upon Tyne. Oxford University Press, Oxford

Tansley P, Panckhurst J 1981 Children with Specific Learning Difficulties. NFER. Nelson, Walton on Thames

Warnock M 1978 Special educational needs. Report of the Committee of Enquiry into the education of handicapped children and young people. HMSO, London

Wedge P, Prosser H, 1973 Born to Fail? National Children's Bureau. Arrow Books, London

Wedge P, Essen J 1982 Children in Adversity. National Children's Bureau. Pan Books, London

17
Mental Handicap

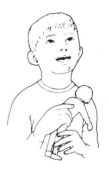

The discovery, assessment and management of mental handicap requires a high degree of cooperation between health, education and social services if the mentally handicapped child and his family are to be given the best care that current resources can provide.

The 1959 Mental Health Act defines severe mental subnormality as 'the state of arrested or incomplete development of mind which includes subnormality of intelligence, and of such a degree and nature that the patient is incapable of living an independent life, or of guarding himself against serious exploitation, or will be unable to do so (when he reaches an age where these abilities are normally achieved)'. In the same Act subnormality was defined 'as a state of arrested or incomplete development of mind (not amounting to severe subnormality) which is of such a nature or degree that it requires or is susceptible to medical treatment or other special care or training of the individual'. This classification corresponds broadly to the educational division in to ESN (M) with IQs from 50 to 75 and

Population distribution of intelligence and classification of mental handicap

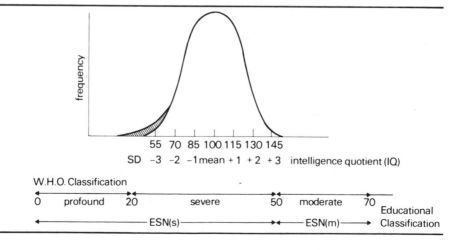

Prevalence and social class distribution of mental handicap (after Birch et al, 1970)

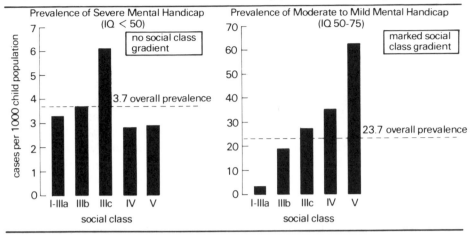

ESN (S) with IQs below 50. The current terminology is moderate and severe learning difficulties. Clearly there is a very wide variation in ability and attainment within the groups. Many other factors such as visual handicap, hearing loss, physical handicap, behaviour problems, speech problems, epilepsy and the quality of care, stimulation and opportunity both within and outside the home, also have a large influence on the final outcome.

Of the mentally handicapped, 75% have IQ in the range 50–70, 20% in range 20–50, and 5% less than 20. Studies of the prevalence of mental handicap give figures for severe mental handicap of around 3.7 per thousand with no relationship to social class. Estimates of the prevalence of moderate to mild mental handicap range from 20 to 30 per thousand of population. In this instance there is a steep social class gradient with the prevalence in social class V being three times the mean level. Neuropathological causes are far more likely to be found amongst the severely mentally handicapped than the mildly mentally handicapped. In the ESN (M) group, psychosocial factors such as degree of opportunity, stimulation and child rearing practices, together with the tendency to resemble their parents, many of whom are also in the bottom end of the normal distribution curve for intelligence, are important. In social classes I and II, an IQ score of less than 80 is rarely found without a pathological cause being identified.

Diagnosis by percentage of 450 children with severe learning problems (born 1968–77) (from Oxfordshire mental handicap register)

Down's syndrome, other chromosomal abnormalities	26.5	Cultural, familial	1.0
Non-chromosomal abnormalities of CNS	9.0	Heredofamilial, degenerative	1.5
Cerebral palsy	6.5	Epilepsy	1.0
Birth injury	2.0	Recognised symptoms of unknown aetiology	1.5
Infection, post-infection, immunological cause	2.0	Other conditions	3.0
Nutritional, metabolic	2.0	Subnormality (not elsewhere classified)	4.0
Psychiatric syndromes	4.0	No known cause	34.5
Cerebral anoxia	1.5		

CLINICAL FEATURES

Diagnosis consists of firstly the realisation of developmental delay, secondly a functional assessment indicating the severity of handicap and thirdly, investigations to determine the aetiology.

Development is a dynamic process. Assessment on one single occasion can be misleading. Thus a child who appears to be at one time somewhat behind his peer group, may be making very rapid progress and on a subsequent occasion be found to be within normal limits. For this reason a series of assessments is most valuable. The shy, quiet, fearful or introverted child may demonstrate very little of his actual ability in the formalised testing situation, particularly if the child is unfamiliar with both his surroundings and the person seeing him. It is most important to get to know the child, often in a less formal situation, before any assessment can be made.

Doctors working in isolation just as any other profession, may make errors in the diagnosis of mental handicap. It is therefore essential that multidisciplinary assessment at a Children's Assessment Centre or by a District Handicap Team, should be made. The content of such an assessment will be described later. With many children, observation in a play situation may be more valuable than formal assessment. The contribution that the parents have to make to assessment must never be forgotten. The parents have far more information on the development and ability of their child and will know what he can do at his best in his most relaxed setting at home. Likewise the stresses on the parents of the assessment and the care of a handicapped child must be recognised. These factors also have a powerful influence on the child's progress.

In addition to all the difficulties already mentioned in diagnosis, the label of mental handicap may be falsely applied in a variety of circumstances. Errors have occurred in the past where a hearing loss or an expressive language problem have not been identified and the child simply labelled as 'severe mental handicap'. The child with severe physical handicap may be extremely difficult to test and very careful assessment over a long period of time may be required. The effects of chronic illness, admissions to hospital, neurological disorders such as petit mal,

Comparison of aetiological factors (in subjects with moderate and severe learning problems aged 15–19 years
(from Wessex Region and Wiltshire, 1963)

Aetiological factor	Moderate(%)	Severe(%)
Infective (rubella, meningitis, encephalitis, etc)	3.6	5.8
Toxic (jaundice, rhesus incompatability, etc)	4.9	3.0
Injury (definite or suspected birth injury)	13.0	10.4
Metabolic (muscular dystrophy, lipoidosis, hypothyroidism)	0.7	0.8
New growth	0.2	0
Congenital malformations (mongolism, hydrocephaly, etc)	34.7	8.1
Neurological (epilepsy, motor disturbance)	11.5	10.0
Non-neurological (cultural, familial, psychotic, severe personality disorder, other non-neurological factors)	25.9	49.2
No information	4.9	12.9
Total	100.0	100.0
	(N = 608)	(N = 539)

gross emotional deprivation, nutrition, and lack of early experience or stimulation must all be considered. In the case of deprivation, improvement in the environment will result in improvement in the level of development of the child, and the effects of early intervention programmes with such children have been most rewarding. Maternal depression or family discord may be cause or effect in the family with a mentally handicapped child.

The diagnosis of a specific syndrome should not necessarily be equated with mental handicap. Predictions seem to be self-fulfilling. In conditions such as Down's syndrome, Turner's syndrome, Kleinfelter's syndrome and tuberose sclerosis there is wide variation in the level of intelligence attained. Individuals with some of these conditions may have intelligence within the normal range. Many of the early studies were made on patients in mental subnormality hospitals and the conclusion incorrectly drawn that mental handicap and the condition identified were always associated.

History

The medical records of the mentally handicapped frequently go into several volumes spread over many years. They tend to get scantier as time goes by. Recently a patient died in a long-stay hospital for mentally handicapped patients with no note written in the last 30 years! It is therefore useful to have a summary of the history of past events with a list of current problems from which to work.

Antenatal and birth history. The previous obstetric history including miscarriages, stillbirths and any difficulties with conceiving, the ages of the parents at the time of birth, and any consanguinity should be recorded. Was the baby born after an unplanned pregnancy in a single mother, or a much wanted child conceived after many years of investigation? Major events in the pregnancy, pre-eclampsia, infection, bleeding, premature labour, drugs given in pregnancy, and evidence on fetal growth and movement are noted, followed by details of the labour and any evidence of fetal distress during delivery. Baby's birth weight, condition at birth and need for resuscitation complete the birth history.

Neonatal history. Here we need to summarise major problems encountered in the neonatal period, for example respiratory distress, jaundice, neonatal convulsions, poor feeding, etc. The time spent in the special care baby unit should be known and the feelings of the parents about the child and any problems encountered at this time recorded.

Past medical history. Major medical problems and interventions to date should be recorded.

Developmental history. Retrospective developmental histories are not always accurate. It is useful to supplement the parents' account of the child's development to date with serial clinical records.

Family history. It is important to know about the general health of other members of the family, both physical and mental, as this may determine their ability to look after their child. Also the presence of disorders or handicaps in other members of the family must be ascertained, for many have a genetic component.

Social history. We need to know about the general background and upbringing of the parents as this may enable us to understand the parents' reaction to the handicap and the resources or difficulties that they may have in dealing with it. Housing is important in terms of difficulties of access for a handicapped person, transport to and from the house and the suitability of its general layout. We need to know the sources of help that the family are using in terms of the extended family, voluntary groups and official agencies involved with health, education, social services and social security.

Current problems. These may be divided up into those that primarily affect the child, those that affect the parent and those that affect the family as a whole.

Current management. Therapy must be recorded and this includes speech therapy, physiotherapy, occupational therapy, as well as medication that the child is receiving. It is also important to know the educational programme that the child is following, plus any special programmes that may have been organised with the day nursery or home programmes or from the Schools Psychological Service. Current management strategies in terms of support, counselling, and relief of parents must also be recorded.

THE EXAMINATION

The doctor's examination should concentrate on general health, growth, level of function, aetiology and nature of handicap and recognition of any syndrome.

General health. Everyday health problems can be overlooked in the mentally handicapped child. Loss of sensation or inability to communicate could be the reason. Important areas to be considered are nutrition, because of feeding difficulties and the possibility of deficiencies such as iron deficiency anaemia occurring, dental problems, constipation, particularly impacted faeces and overflow, and skin problems, pressure areas and infection.

Growth. Distortion of growth is often seen in handicapped children either as an intrinsic part of the cause, for example short stature in some chromosomal disorders, or as a consequence of paresis or immobility. A small immobile child is clearly easier to manage than a large child similarly handicapped. Obesity should be avoided especially in children with motor handicap. The onset of puberty may be advanced in conditions where there is an inflammatory disturbance of the brain, for example due to neonatal infection, or signs of puberty may be delayed or absent. These are clearly important in the total management of the child. With growth, wheelchairs, walking aids, furniture and footwear need to be reviewed.

Functional assessment. This is somewhat different from developmental assessment, which records progress and the age equivalents of the child's current level of functioning, or a neurological examination which looks for the underlying pattern of sensory and motor disturbance. A functional assessment looks at the child's positive abilities, rating them for specific tasks that the child needs to perform.

Physique. The child's general physique and build should be noted. Upper limbs and lower limbs, tone, strength, voluntary movements and contractures should be noted. Within this the level of mobility of the child and the ability to manipulate objects such as spoons, cups, pencils, buttons, etc required for everyday living should be recorded.

Hearing and vision. Assessment of hearing and vision using appropriate tests often requires both skill and patience (see Chapter 16).

Speech and communication. This includes all verbal and non-verbal communication. An estimate should be made of the child's comprehension, expression and articulation, together with any secondary problems arising from difficulties in communication. The use of gesture or the adoption of signing systems or symbols should also be known.

Toileting. Whether the child is incontinent or continent, and whether the child can manage toileting independently, are major factors in the day to day management of the child. The child who always requires assistance from an adult or who is incontinent, requiring frequent changes of clothing, is very difficult for a parent to manage.

Behaviour. The presence of any behaviour problems, for example temper tantrums, aggressiveness, self-destructive behaviour, sleep disturbance, needs to be determined.

Intelligence. Measurements that are made by Educational Psychologists using standardised tests are described in the chapter on educational medicine. Functional assessments may be misleading in that the child may not have the motor ability to demonstrate his reasoning powers. Prolonged contact and familiarity with the child and his methods of communication are a far more rewarding way of assessing intelligence than a formal one-off examination.

Identification of syndromes

These may be made on the basis of examination, biochemical or genetic investigations, and by reference to standard text such as Smith's 'Recognisable Patterns of Human Malformation', which lists the clinical features of a large number of recognised syndromes. Identification of a syndrome may help in many ways. It helps in giving a prognosis. It alerts us to the presence of associated features which we may wish to investigate. It may also indicate the need for genetic counselling or the need for specific antenatal screening procedures.

SERVICES

In the UK three recent reports summarise current approaches to the needs of the mentally handicapped.

Better Services for the Mentally Handicapped, (Command 4683 HMSO 1971) recommended (a) a shift from hospital to community care, (b) a rapid expansion of local authority residential provision, (c) a concomitant reduction in numbers of mentally handicapped residents cared for within the hospital services and (d) the development of a decentralised hospital service which would link closely with community based services. The aim was to move away from the large residential hospitals isolated from the main community, which were built in Victorian times and were run on a large and impersonal basis with little continuity of care or relationship between staff and 'patients', to a more domestic setting. By the age of 15–19, 71% of severely subnormal people are continent and ambulant with no severe behaviour disorders. The predominantly medical and nursing model of care is inappropriate to their needs. The 'total institution' type of care is detrimental to the child's normal development. Within large institutions there was found to be a lack of clear objectives in the care offered and a uniformity of treatment which was not geared to individual needs. In the institution, children were bathed and toileted in a group and there was a uniform bedtime and getting up time every day of the week. Staff ate separately from the children and personal clothing and possessions were restricted.

The antithesis of this institutional type of care is setting up substitute family homes within the community. These would be the same as any other house, where individuals can live in a small group with their own interests and possessions. Dual responsibility for the mentally handicapped between health and the local authorities was recommended, with the health service providing care for those with physical handicaps who required special medical attention, and the local authority providing for the others. As well as encouraging the setting up of these new units, the report prompted changes in hospital residential care to a more personal and homely regime where individual needs and continuity of relationships were recognised.

A large majority of mentally handicapped children under the age of 16 are cared for at home. However once they leave school there is a large shift towards residential accommodation. This is caused by the increased demands placed on parents when school no longer provides whole day relief. As they grow bigger, their parents get older and so the physical demands of care increase. Other types of day care arrangements which act as a substitute or continuation of school will be discussed later.

The Jay report. Report of the Committee of Enquiry into mental handicap nursing and care, Command 7468, HMSO 1979, proposed total access by mentally handicapped people to all locally provided services, e.g. recreational facilities, public transport, home helps, etc. They recommended the right to enjoy normal patterns of life within the community, the right to be treated as individuals and the provision of appropriate help within the community to assist their individual development. They recommended the doubling of residential staff and that this staff should be trained to teach, that a common training for health and social services staff involved in residential care of the mentally handicapped be developed, and that positions of responsibility should only be given to those who are suitably qualified.

The Warnock Report. Special Educational Needs, the report of the Committee of Enquiry into the Education of Handicapped Children and Young People

HMSO 1978 and the current procedures in the UK for meeting children's special educational needs are discussed in the chapter on Educational Medicine.

Services for mentally handicapped pre school children

Services for the handicapped are always open to criticism. Parents may argue that they are insufficient or that therapists make too heavy demands upon them. They may complain of lack of specialist knowledge by many who advise them or that services are poorly coordinated. A district handicap service or a community mental handicap service will help to combat some of these criticisms.

A community mental handicap team or the district handicap team acts as a point of contact for parents, provides advice and help, and coordinates services to establish a close working relationship with all the various organisations and services relevant to both mentally handicapped children and adults. Not all children with mental handicap, particularly those with lesser degrees of delay, will be referred for full multidisciplinary assessment. Many will be seen in general paediatric clinics both in hospital and within the community. Wherever the assessment takes place, it is essential there should be continuity, easy access for parents and excellent communication between all those who are involved with the family. Good working relationships between medical teams involved with assessment, the social work teams and the education teams who will deal with the child's future and special educational needs, are the keystones to management.

Questions to be answered by assessment

To what extent is this child mentally handicapped?
What is the rate of progress?
Is there any evidence that this is a degenerative condition?
What associated handicaps are there?
   Vision?
   Hearing?
   Physical handicap?
   Epilepsy?
   Speech?
   Behaviour?
   Social environment?
What practical problems are the parents facing in caring for the child?
What are the stresses on the family and how may they be relieved?
What are the child's special educational needs?
Is there an identifiable cause for the child's handicap?
What investigations are necessary?
What is the opportunity for prevention of handicap in future siblings?

Bringing children to appointments is not always easy for parents and help and advice given within the home are very welcome by parents. The family health visitor with support from a resource health visitor with special knowledge or training in handicapping conditions, or direct help from the specialist health visitor provide a basis for this. The Warnock Committee saw the health visitor as the appropriate named person to provide the principal point of contact for the parents and the child. Home visits by doctors, such as general practitioners, or child health doctors, enable realistic assessment of family needs and support good continued relationships with them.

The teacher counsellors appointed by education authorities are specialised in the handicapped pre-school child and bring into the home practical advice on management and the appropriate activities for parents and children. They form a vital link between the home and the child's future school placement. Education departments may also provide small pre-school diagnostic and therapeutic groups. Toy libraries may be provided by health, education, social services or voluntary bodies and are particularly useful in meeting the needs of the pre-school mentally handicapped child.

Day care need not necessarily be in special nursery units. These do have the advantage that they can provide other services such as physiotherapy, occupational therapy or speech therapy where they are required. However, many mentally handicapped children will attend normal nursery school or play group where their needs can also be met. This avoids the isolation of the handicapped child and his parents, and provides them with a full range of opportunities that would be open to ordinary children. The dangers of early categorisation and the assumptions about future development that turn into self-fulfilling predictions are thus avoided.

Services for the mentally handicapped school child

School entry and assessment of the child's special educational needs is a very sensitive and stressful time for the parents. Just as at the time of diagnosis, the parents are faced with the realisation that their child is mentally handicapped, on school entry these feelings are reawakened. Entry to school may also be a time for a change in the professionals who are supporting the child and the family. Continuity of care over this period is essential. It should be the doctor or health visitor who has known the child from birth who discusses the child's special educational needs with the parents, rather than a stranger who arrives at the house and hurriedly fills in the relevant forms before disappearing. School placement not only involves an assessment of what would be the best education resource for the child but helps their parents to accept its conclusions too. It is therefore a process which cannot be concluded in one consultation in which a decision is 'handed' to the parents. The parents may have unrealistic fears about special schools and they need to visit the school in advance, accompanied by the doctor or health visitor or other worker who has known them for a long time. They need to know what curriculum the school offers and to be shown work that has been produced in the school and to see the standards achieved by children who are leaving the school. Many parents may not realise that children leaving ESN (M) schools will have acquired basic reading, writing and arithmetic skills. These will be sufficient for employment for many children. A few children attending ESN (S) schools at the upper end of the range will also acquire such skills. It is important to allay parents' fears and show them what is on offer in a particular school.

School placement is not a once and only affair and is subject to review. The parents must be aware of this. Particularly when a child is borderline in ability or, as is often the case, we are uncertain of the child's ability, the value of the day to day contact with the child and the progress made at school, may necessitate a change of educational programme.

In the past, assessment has been a separate exercise from management. The word ascertainment was used and the aim of the exercise was to provide a measurement of the IQ. of the child and then fit the child into the educational category which corresponded to this figure. Assessment is now regarded as the process whereby the child's special educational needs are determined and leads on to an appropriate educational programme. Doctors, psychologists, social workers and teachers are all involved in the assessment of the child.

Formal assessments are made by the educational psychologist but his role is primarily as an adviser of educational programmes rather than a measurer of intellect. Practical developments such as pre-school therapeutic and diagnostic groups are run by educational psychologists. The development of new material emphasises the direction of change.

With entry into school the head teacher is the key person (defined by the Warnock Committee as the named person) acting as a focal point for the parents. Many children will still attend normal schools, particularly at the infant stage. Others will attend a school for children with moderate or severe learning difficulties and those with profound mental handicap, which is often associated with physical handicap will attend special care units. Before 1971, children with severe learning difficulties were defined as ineducable. Now all children benefit from appropriate educational provision.

Progress at school and the type of curriculum provided depends not only upon the intellectual level but on the presence or absence of other handicaps. Thus the school may need to provide physiotherapy, occupational therapy, speech therapy, the teaching of a sign system for those with severe communication difficulties, or a behaviour modification programme for those whose behaviour problems prevent effective learning. Records of the child's progress are valuable in showing parents the new skills that the child is acquiring. Parents need to be constantly reassured that the children do learn, even if at a slower pace and with far more repetition

Curriculum for the child with severe learning problems

Mobility skills
Social skills: vital if the child is to be integrated rather than separated from society: understanding shopping, money, transport, use of public lavatories, crossing the road, meeting people
Self help skills: vital to reduce the load on parents: feeding, dressing, toileting, washing, cooking
Communication skills: essential to any form of education to relieve frustration
Occupational work skills: teaching of tasks, e.g. assembly work, working environment, working day
Leisure skills: productive use of leisure time has been forgotten in the past, sport, music, games, etc are just as important to the mentally handicapped as anyone else
Literacy and numeracy skills
Knowledge of the world about us
Personal relations/contraception/child care: many who have left ESN(M) schools in the past have had no knowledge of family planning or child care. Consequently their children have rapidly become patients through accidents, failure to thrive, etc or are received into care

than in an ordinary school. Small classes, a high number of staff to the number of children and their training in special education, ensure optimal progress.

Services for the mentally handicapped school leaver

School leaving represents another crisis period for the family with a mentally handicapped child. The period between 16 and 20 is the time of the peak rate for admission of severely mentally handicapped people into residential care. It is also the time of transition for many children from educational service provision to social service provision and from child orientated services to adult orientated services. Ideally this should take place in a number of small steps, rather than representing an abrupt change for the child. School leaving should be preceded by an assessment of the child's future needs, which should take place 1 year before school leaving to permit appropriate arrangements to be made. Many school leavers from ESN (M) schools will gain employment in manual occupations outside any special provision. The degree of provision available locally varies widely and many parents find themselves without the daytime relief and support which they had whilst the child was at school. Likewise the physical resources and staff resources available to the school may be more extensive than those in the adult training centre. The adult training centres are a social service and not an education department provision. A unified district mental handicap service would provide important continuity over the school leaving period.

Provisions for the school leaver with a mental handicap

Admission and assessment unit attached to an adult training centre
Bridging course into further education
Course at College of Further Education
Part-time and evening courses
Work orientation course
Work experience course
Non-vocational courses — teaching leisure skills, providing social contact
Sheltered employment (via disablement resettlement officer)
Enclave sheltered workshop in open industry
Employment rehabilitation schemes
Day units

Benefits

In the UK, attendance allowance may be claimed after the age of 2, if the child requires frequent attention or continual supervision beyond the ordinary needs of children. Mobility allowance is payable for children after the age of 5, if the child is unable to get around unaided for a period of at least 1 year. Families on a low income may also be entitled to assistance with hospital fares. The Family Fund, administered on behalf of the Government by the Joseph Rowntree Memorial Trust, will give financial assistance to families of severely handicapped children with such items as washing machines, holidays and telephones. (see Ch 14)

Management

Medical management. The continuity of care that the medical profession can provide is just as important as the more specific aspects of treatment. This need not necessarily be in the hospital paediatric department. The GP or community child health doctor is in an ideal position to provide continuity.

General medical problems probably occur more frequently in the mentally handicapped. Infections, nutritional problems, dental problems and skin problems are common. Maintaining a treatment programme may be more difficult in the mentally handicapped child. Also the presence of undetected general medical problems or inadequately treated ones may be a further impediment to the general developmental progress of the child.

Toilet training is a most important activity for the mentally handicapped. Successful toilet training increases the social acceptability of the child and decreases skin problems and the possibility of long term care. Before commencing toilet training it must be realised that the aim should be total independence for toileting and therefore the following steps should be recognised;
— to realise the need to pass urine or open bowels
— to get to the toilet
— to pull the pants down
— to sit on the toilet
— to perform
— to wipe bottom
— **to pull the pants up**
— to flush the lavatory
— to wash the hands.

A period of observation enables one to record the general level of ability in each of these areas. Knowledge about the times of spontaneous defaecation and micturition are important in setting up any training programme. Underlying problems like constipation, associated painful anorectal conditions such as fissures, or urinary tract infection need to be treated. It is also important to ensure the child is comfortable and feels secure when sitting on the toilet or pot. Successful toilet training needs to be a planned activity and needs to be fairly intensive. The principles are no different from those used to toilet train normal children. Indeed when the techniques developed for toilet training mentally handicapped adults were tried on normal children, they were dramatically successful.

The principles are simple. Added opportunity for practising micturition may easily be obtained by increasing the fluid load. Appropriate behaviour or approaches towards appropriate behaviour in each of the activities outlined above is rewarded. In a simple interval training routine the child is potted regularly, starting at half hourly intervals and rewarded for appropriate action. Elaborations of this scheme may involve the use of musical potties to play a tune as soon as the child urinates into them. Doll play, involving the use of wetting dolls and the child periodically checking the doll's pants, potting the doll and praising the doll are useful additions to teaching. These sorts of schemes can be great fun for the children.

The management of nocturnal enuresis is the same as for other children and this is described in detail elsewhere.

Communication. Delay in the development of language and communication skills is a central problem in the care of the mentally handicapped. Lack of understanding or expressive language provides barriers to further learning with immense frustration on the part of both parents and children in making their wishes or feelings known in everyday life. Many children will be helped using objects, photographs or pictures. Techniques such as the First Words Language Programme developed by Dr Bill Gilham in Nottingham, or developmental language programmes carried out by speech therapists, parents or nursery staff, greatly benefit the acquisition of language in these children. Such programmes require careful observation of the child to record current abilities. This means paying attention not only to comprehension, expression and articulation but also to other more basic skills of symbolic understanding and attention control. Based on these initial observations an individual language programme is constructed, to build gradually on the child's ability. Each step in the programme is structured so that the progress of the child can be easily monitored. Opportunities to acquire language skills must be available throughout the day and not concentrated into brief therapy spells on a weekly basis. The use of carefully chosen toys to encourage growth of attention and symbolic understanding is most useful. Toy libraries may be useful in this respect. Programmes such as 'Let me speak' and 'Let me play' provide a broader range of teaching programmes for parents to aid language acquisition.

Some children will not acquire spoken language and need to be taught some other communication system. Makaton contains a vocabulary of 350 signs developed from British Sign Language. Most of the signs relate visually to the idea that they depict. Picture boards have been in use for many years. In this the child can point to a picture of the required object, be it food, drink or toilet. On a more sophisticated level, symbols rather than objects may be used. A system of written symbols developed by Dr Charles Bliss has been used for this purpose.

Behaviour modification

The application of behaviour modification techniques in the mentally handicapped is extremely valuable in handling unwanted behaviour and in encouraging the development of desired skills. Behaviour modification is based on the theory that aberrant behaviour is due to faulty learning and that there is unintended reinforcement of these undesirable patterns of behaviour. The unwanted behaviour is maintained because the consequence of it is desirable to the child. Removing the positive reinforcements decreases the incidence of the unwanted behaviour. Likewise, giving positive reinforcements to desired behaviour increases the frequency of these behaviour patterns.

Any behaviour modification programme must start with careful assessment of a child. This depends upon making written observations of the child's behaviour.

Behaviour modification

Analyse behaviour
   Antecedents ——— unwanted behaviour ——— consequences
Define precise objectives
Define method
Decide reinforcers
Implement strategy, maintaining written records of the type described
Withdraw reinforcement when the required behaviour is established (learned)

The undesirable behaviour is recorded together with the antecedent events, and the consequences. Such records enable us to understand any triggers to the unwanted behaviour and the nature of the reinforcement which caused it to continue. Thus if the child's temper tantrum leads to mother coming into the room and giving him attention, then this activity is the reinforcer of the unwanted behaviour. Even the mother coming into the room in anger, but which results in him having more of her attention may be seen by the child as more desirable than being left alone. In the case of unwanted behaviour it is necessary to define carefully the behaviour that one wants to remove, or in the case of the development of new skills or behaviour, to define carefully what one wants to achieve and to analyse these into small steps. During therapy a written record can therefore be kept recording his behaviour, its antecedents and its consequences and the progress that the child makes towards the desired behaviour.

During a programme aimed at reducing unwanted behaviour, the behaviour increases in frequency before it is eliminated. The following analogy explains this. If, each time we walk through a door we are rewarded with a £5 note, this reinforcement would encourage us to walk through that door on more occasions. When the consequence of walking through that door are changed, for example receiving a cold shower, initially we may try even more frequently to go through the door in order to try and elicit the previous response. It is only after a period of increased activity that we would learn of the inevitable undesirable consequences of this action.

Routine records must be maintained and events recorded as they occur. It is only through the written record that progress can be charted and understood. When the required behaviour is established, the reinforcement can be withdrawn.

Procedures and Glossary of Terms

Positive reinforcers are really anything that is pleasant to the child. The choice will obviously depend upon the knowledge of the individual. *Negative reinforcement* is anything unpleasant to the child, such as parental anger or withdrawal as in the 'time out' situation. *Generalisation* occurs when behaviour learned in one situation is transferred to similar situations. *Shaping* is the process by which desirable behaviour is obtained by reinforcing successive approximations to that behaviour. The task is broken up into small steps, each leading towards the desired target. Thus if the required intention is for the child to sit on the pot successful stages might be, approaching the pot, sitting on the pot for short periods of time, sitting on the pot with pants down, sitting on the pot for longer periods of time. *Training* occurs by the connection of two or more different learned responses such as sitting on the pot and taking pants down. The reinforcement is given after the final response in the chain is gained. *Reinforcement schedules* define the relationship between giving the reward and the exhibition of the required behaviour. *Variable ratio schedules* in which there is not a precise relationship of the number of required responses to the reinforcement being given, have been shown to be most effective. Because the child cannot effectively anticipate when reinforcement will be given, he is likely to respond in anticipation of that. *Fixed ratio schedules* in which every response is rewarded or every two or three responses are rewarded, are not as effective as the variable ratio schedules.

Desired behaviour can only be reinforced if it is already present in some form. If it is not, then it may be initiated by the process of *modelling* in which the desired behaviour is demonstrated either by the therapist or a model, such as the use of the wetting doll when teaching bladder control. Much ordinary learning in childhood depends on the process of modelling. *Prompting* is the use of any strategy which helps to ensure the occurrence of the desired behaviour. It might be a direct instruction or it might be a gesture. In the process of *fading*, the prompt is gradually withdrawn until the required behaviour occurs spontaneously. Tokens may be used instead of the usual types of reinforcement such as sweets. These can be accumulated and exchanged for a wider range of more desirable objects.

Extinction of unwanted behaviour is obtained by withholding the reinforcements that support it. Alternatively a pleasant stimulus may be withdrawn as and when the behaviour occurs. In *satiation*, the child is encouraged to repeat the undesirable behaviour until it no longer occurs. Perhaps the resultant fatigue from its constant performance causes the undesirable behaviour to become painful to the child.

Examples of behaviour modification

Julie, hyperactivity. Julie was seen in the day nursery because of her restless, hyperactive behaviour. When observed she did not handle any particular toy for more than a few seconds. She was for ever up and down during meals and could not be held for any length of time by an adult in any situation that could facilitate learning. It was therefore decided that in order to get progress in any field of development, Julie's attention span should be increased and that her purposeless running about should be discouraged. Julie was rewarded for spending longer and longer periods of time sitting at a table, playing with toys. In this way her attention control increased and therapeutic language and other programmes could be commenced.

Barry, biting and aggressive behaviour. Barry was noticed to become increasingly aggressive in the nursery. There had been complaints of injuries from the parents of other children. The immediate intervention of an adult which he provoked was probably reinforcing this undesirable behaviour. It was decided therefore that future acts of aggression should be handled by a withdrawal from the room for 10 minutes after which he was allowed to return. He was also positively rewarded for any cooperative play or affection at play with other children. Using this means the episodes of aggression and biting gradually disappeared.

Ronald, constipation with overflow. Since having an anal fissure 1 year previously, Ronald had become progressively constipated and because of pain on defaecation tried to hold on to his stools. This always resulted in soiling. He was frightened of going to the toilet and screamed whenever this was attempted. A programme consisting of a graded series of steps was devised, whereby he first went to the toilet, then sat on the toilet for progressively longer periods of time. He was rewarded for each step in this programme. The programme was accompanied by the use of a stool softening agent to ensure defaecation would not be painful. Using this method the soiling ceased within the next 2–3 weeks.

Relief and support of parents

Because of the slower rate of development of mentally handicapped children, they remain dependent on their parents for round the clock care and supervision for a prolonged period of time. In addition, the amount of care required may be greater than that for a normal child of the same age. For example, problems of bowel or bladder control, associated physical handicap, moving or dressing a large immobile child, can impose enormous day to day stresses on families. Because of the greater level of care required, neighbours and friends who may also be frightened of the mentally handicapped child are less willing to offer their service for baby sitting or other activities. Day care, be it in a day nursery, play group, nursery school or special unit, in addition to the positive benefits for the child, provides relief for the parents and also an opportunity to do activities such as shopping or having their hair done which might be very difficult or impossible with the child. Organised babysitting services are also most useful. Holiday relief may be provided for parents in special home units, or in short-stay units devised for this purpose, or by hospital or fostering arrangements.

Prevention of mental handicap

Prenatal. Prenatal prevention would ensure that every mother was in an optimum state of health before conception. Obvious preventive measures such as rubella immunisation should have been carried out. Any potential teratogenic drugs can be stopped and genetic counselling provided in the case of familial disease. In some cases, for instance patients who have phenylketonuria, it will be necessary for them to resume their diet in the pregnancy in order to prevent severe mental handicap in their offspring.

Antenatal care. It is estimated that the application of currently available knowledge would greatly reduce the incidence of handicap. However, many still book late for antenatal care and the opportunity to correct abnormalities is lost. In the 1958 British Perinatal Mortality Study, the increase in mortality for those who had no antenatal care was five times, and in those who only attended on one to four occasions, four times that of mothers who attended regularly for antenatal care. The French have used incentive payments to ensure high uptake of antenatal care from the first trimester. Using this system 96% of patients are booked before 15 weeks. Attitudes towards health care in pregnancy and the value of early booking need to be taught long before pregnancy, as part of health education programmes in schools. During antenatal care, screening tests may detect disorders such as spina bifida and Down's syndrome with the opportunity for early termination if positive.

Perinatal care. Resources to monitor the progress of labour and to ensure 24 hour availability of resources for resuscitation of infants and special care baby units will reduce the incidence of handicap. However, the standard of such care needs to be high. Routine examination of the newborn provides early detection of abnormalities and a possibility for remediation. Routine biochemical screening such as those for phenylketonuria and hypothyroidism, permit the mental handicap associated with these conditions to be prevented.

Postnatal care. Good nutrition is essential for normal brain growth. The effects of early malnutrition cannot be prevented by improvement in diet later in age. Although the effects of early deprivation and disadvantage can be lessened by improvements in later life the importance of early learning cannot be underestimated. Early and appropriate treatment of general paediatric problems, such as acute dehydration states and meningitis, would lead to a diminution in the complication rate and a reduction of later mental handicap.

REFERENCES AND FURTHER READING

Birch H G, Richardson S A, Baird G, Illsey R 1970 Mental subnormality in the community. A clinical and epidemiological study
Brimblecombe F S W 1974 Exeter project for handicapped children. British Medical Journal 4: 706–709
DHSS Census of mentally handicapped hospital patients. Statistical and Research Report Series. No. 3. HMSO, London
DHSS 1971 Better Services for the Mentally Handicapped. Cmnd 4683. HMSO, London
DHSS 1979 Cmnd 7468. Report of the Committee of Enquiry into Mental Handicap Nursing and Care. (The Jay Report). HMSO, London
DHSS 1980 Mental Handicap: Progress, problems and Priorities HMSO, London
Elliot D, Jackson J M, Groves J P 1981 The Oxfordshire Mental handicap register. British Medical Journal 282: 289–292
Gilham B 1979 First Words Language Programme. George Allen and Unwin, London
Griffiths M 1973 The Young Retarded Child. Churchill Livingstone, Edinburgh
Jeffree D, McConkey R 1976 Let me Speak. Souvenir Press, London
Jeffree D M, McConkey R, Hewson S 1977 Let me Play. Souvenir Press, London
Kiernan C 1974 Behaviour modification. In: Clarke, Clarke (eds) Mental Deficiency — the Changing Outlook. Methuen, London
Kushlick A 1966 A community service for the mentally subnormal. Social Psychiatry 1: 73–82
Kushlick A, Cox 1968 Ascertained prevalence of mental subnormality in the Wessex region. Proceedings of the International Congress for the Scientific Study of Mental Deficiency. Montpellier
Mackay R I 1976 Mental Handicap in Child Health Practice. Butterworth, London
Mackay R I 1982 The causes of severe mental handicap. Developmental Medicine and Child Neurology 24: 386–388
National Development Group for the Mentally Handicapped 1977 Mentally handicapped children: a plan for action. DHSS, London
National Development Group for the Mentally Handicapped 1977 Helping mentally handicapped school leavers. DHSS, London
Smith W 1976 Recognisable patterns of human malformation. W B Saunders, Philadelphia
Wilson B 1980 Toilet training for the mentally handicapped child. Developmental Medicine and Child Neurology 22: 225–228

18
Behaviour

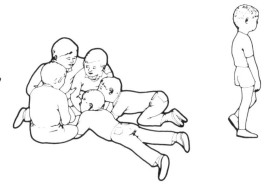

This chapter is concerned with those problems which are more likely to be referred to the child psychiatrist than the paediatrician. The majority of the common behaviour problems which are usually managed within primary care or general paediatrics are discussed elsewhere.

CHILD PSYCHIATRIC SERVICES

Child psychiatric services are more appropriately called child and family psychiatric services, for any form of intervention invariably involves the family. In the UK the services have developed in two ways: as a health provision largely within hospitals or as an educational provision in community based child guidance clinics. The sharp distinctions between these two types of establishment should no longer exist. Teamwork is a long established practice in child psychiatry and involves social workers, psychologists, teachers and nursing staff as well as child psychiatrists. The work is labour intensive.

Approaches to treatment
The concepts of mental illness as seen in adults are not easy to apply to children with behavioural problems. Some problems may be regarded as extremes of normal development, others due to unsatisfactory environment and others extremes of behaviour like naughtiness. A small group is due to organic brain disease and specific psychiatric syndromes. The children themselves rarely seek help, it is the concerns of either parents, teachers, social services or the courts which lead to referral. The same problem may arouse very different reactions and consequences in different families. Take non-attendance at school for example. In one family the situation may be accepted and no effort made whatever to make the child attend. In this situation the problem is likely to be dealt with by the courts. In another family the parents are able to ensure that the child does attend and to deal effectively themselves with any difficulties that arise. Thus no outside services are involved. In a third family, the parents may be unable to deal effectively

with the problem themselves, and in the unequal conflict that ensues, the child does not attend school and the parents may arrive at the family doctor with a variety of psychosomatic symptoms related either to themselves or to the child. In a fourth family, the parents may be sufficiently effective to ensure school attendance but educational achievement falls off and referral is made because of the concern of the teachers. More dramatic forms of presentation such as hysterical paralysis, loss of voice, hearing or vision, or attempts at self-injury may present to the emergency services, hospital paediatric services or directly to child psychiatric services.

In view of this variety of reactions and sources of referral, the initial problem may be defined from a single point of view only. However, for the appropriate management the assessment must be comprehensive involving the child, the family, intellectual ability, environment at home and at school and the presence of any physical handicap or disorder.

A variety of treatment methods is available which may be used either singly or in combination. This may include behaviour therapy, psychotherapy, casework help for the family, or family group therapy. Behaviour therapy is described in more detail in the chapter on Mental Handicap. Treatment may be by educational measures only if it is thought that by meeting the child's special educational needs more appropriately the behavioural problems will be eased. Sometimes the treatment may involve speech therapy, physiotherapy, occupational therapy, or general paediatric treatment where there is overlap with organic problems. Other measures such as reception into care, may also form part of the recommendation following assessment.

Psychotherapy is probably the main method of treatment used. This has been defined as 'a form of treatment in which the main therapeutic agent lies in the communication and in the relationship between the therapist and the patient' (Hersov & Rutter, 1977). This involves discussion within the family of the various conflicts that may be present at home or at school. Treatment involves application of the four following principles: firstly, a non-critical acceptance of the patient; secondly an empathetic understanding of the patient; thirdly, to help the child express those aspects of himself which his conscience and his ideal self has rejected; and fourthly, the use of communication between doctor and patient as a treatment tool.

Within the Child Guidance Clinic, psychotherapy is usually combined with case work from the social worker. This may involve tackling specific problems, trying to influence particular attitudes, providing resource or enabling the family to make better use of resources already available.

Family therapy is being increasingly employed within child psychiatry. This involves the therapist seeing the family as a group, to gain an understanding of family relationships and as a means of trying to resolve any family disharmony. This method of treatment is particularly applicable where the main problems lie in family communication or interaction.

Hospital admission is required where the abnormal behaviour is too extreme for the parents to cope with at home. It may also be necessary for diagnostic investigations or periods of continuous expert observation. In most health districts in-patient units are available for both adolescents and younger children, though some children may be cared for in general paediatric wards. In-patient and day patient units usually have an integrated school component. Causes for admission are excessive aggression, severe depression and anorexia nervosa. Day hospital facilities combine many of the advantages of in-patient treatment but with the child being able to maintain contact with his own family within the home.

EPIDEMIOLOGY AND NATURAL HISTORY

The Isle of Wight study, conducted in the 1960s, demonstrated a 6.8% incidence of psychiatric illness amongst 9–11 year olds in that population. Only one-tenth of these were actually receiving psychiatric treatment. Boys were represented more often than girls in conduct disorders but not for the remainder. They found a considerable overlap between psychiatric illness and other handicaps such as educational retardation and physical disease.

A wide range of social and family characteristics has been found to be associated with psychiatric illness in childhood. The existence of parental ill-health or psychiatric illness results in an increased incidence in the children. Lower social class is associated with an increase in antisocial disorders but not in other psychiatric illness. Broken marriages, discord and disharmony at home are also associated with an increase in childhood psychiatric disorders. More behaviour problems are found in schools where the staff turnover is high. Paternal criminality is also associated with a high incidence of psychiatric illness amongst the offspring.

O'Neil and Robbins in the United States, succeeded in following up and tracing 500 children 30 years after attendance at child guidance clinics between 1924 and 1929. Those who had been seen for neurotic disorders were fairly well adjusted and had the same incidence of psychiatric problems in adult life as a control group. Those who were seen because of antisocial problems had a poorer prognosis in adult life than the control group, with 28% being described as psychopathic and others having a wide range of other problems, such as divorce, unemployment and alcoholism.

Assessment of the overall effectiveness of child psychiatric services is a difficult task. Two-thirds of children improve significantly within 2 years whether or not treatment is provided. The response to psychotherapy was better in patients with high intelligence, those expressing a high level of anxiety, those with higher social achievements and those with greater self awareness, insight and sensitivity. It can be argued that this group may well be contained within the two-thirds who will improve spontaneously with or without treatment.

DEPRIVATION AND DISADVANTAGE

Many children are particularly vulnerable to environmental stresses because of the level of disadvantage that they and their parents have suffered. Those parents who through their own childhood, have not acquired appropriate skills in child care or experience of family life are less able to pass on these skills to their children. They often have so many unfulfilled needs of their own that they are unable to put the children's needs first. Many go straight from unsatisfactory childhoods with multiple problems such as family discord, educational problems and truancy, into parenthood which is seldom planned, and relationships which are intended to but do not succeed in replacing their previously unsatisfactory home life. The result is frequently a repetition of the type of problems that existed in the previous generation. In these households there is often low self esteem, low levels of personal expectation and a failure to recognise individual responsibility for control of themselves and their children's lives. Hence both support and guidance are lacking.

Ill health of parents, poverty, poor housing, overcrowding and poor management of the resources that are available, frequently result in a background of discord and disharmony at home. Nutrition and general care of the child may be poor. Individual parental interaction with the child and the aims of day to day life may be based upon 'keeping the child quiet' or minimising the child's interference in what the parents themselves wish to do. The result is frequently a very poor level of development, particularly language and social development, and the failure of the child to acquire rules of social behaviour and family life. In the pre-school years children may experience numerous changes of addresses and also changes of caretaker, if they are received into care at times of stress, or if a variety of relatives or change of cohabitee take place. The parents themselves may show a diminished adaptability to change and a low level of industry in solving problems such as ensuring the safety of a small child in a new home.

Some of the most gross effects of deprivation have been described in completely institutionalised children. Follow-up studies of such children brought up in institutions in the first 3 years of life where little continuous attachment could be formed with adult figures, shows that the children in adult life adjust poorly socially and have difficulty with emotional relationships. They are often apathetic, restless, unable to concentrate, emotionally detached, sometimes aggressive and often promiscuous in an attempt to find some compensatory loving relationship.

Children from these unhappy homes may present with a wide variety of problems ranging from delays of development to specific problems with behaviour. Thus some have enuresis or soiling whilst others show aggressive or difficult behaviour. At school there may be educational failure or truanting. They may be deliberately injured or abandoned at times of crises in the parents' life, such as eviction, hospital admission, a custodial prison sentence or psychiatric illness. It is often very difficult to engage the cooperation of parents in helping the child with his difficulties. Attendance records at hospitals and clinics may be poor. However, a broad based family approach recognising the needs of the parents as well as the children, is likely to be successful. It is also important to realise that many parents are unable to put into practice advice that is given on the management of their child. In our professional contacts with families, we should be aware of the devastating effect that criticism can have, with further loss of confidence and self-esteem.

Many children from disadvantaged backgrounds do not follow the course described above and do not have similar problems to their parents. Factors intrinsic to the child may compensate for a poor family and physical environment. Influences outside the home, particularly schools, may have a striking beneficial effect. Studies of early intervention programmes with parents and babies have shown a wide range of changes in families that receive help, compared to control groups. Children followed up to the age of 16 have shown better educational achievements, are less likely to have been in care, are less likely to go to prison than control individuals and are more likely to be employed when they leave school. The economic benefits of such intense early help are increasingly being shown. In addition, intervention at any stage of the child's life is likely to lead to an improvement, contrary to previous belief that only very early help could be effective in compensation (see Rutter, 1980).

CONDUCT DISORDERS

Conduct disorders are the commonest reason for contact between child psychiatry and families. Conduct disorders cover the entire range of ages, from the difficult baby to the negativistic toddler, the disobedient primary school child up to the secondary school child who is truanting and becoming involved in crime.

Whether a baby is difficult or not, depends upon his own temperament and upon the temperament of his parents. Parents may fail to appreciate the nature of the baby's needs. They may attribute to the baby feelings of rejection, persecution or hate. The effects of problems within the marriage may affect their relationship with the child. A tense, anxious, uncertain mother who reacts with hostility and anger towards problems such as feeding, vomiting or crying, conditions the baby to respond with difficult behaviour and thus a vicious circle develops. The ideal to provide good pleasant experiences leading to a sense of trust and contentment can be achieved by practical support for the mother.

In the toddler, negativism may be expressed in areas such as feeding, dressing, toileting, sleep and in numerous temper tantrums. The underlying attitudes of the parents towards the child needs to be explored. Are the parents' expectations of the child realistic?

Are the parents consistent in their handling of unwanted behaviour? Do parents through fear of the violence of the child's reaction, give in? Are the parents transferring hostility which should be directed elsewhere on to the child? Are the parents giving the child due credit and reinforcement of appropriate behaviour? Is there an underlying current of tension in the family which virtually provokes difficult behaviour in the child?

The issue of anger and punishment within the family needs to be discussed. Frequently parents punish a child as a vehicle for their own angry feelings, rather than an attempt to discourage particular behaviours. The fact that certain behaviour is unwanted is lost amid the barrage of the parents' temper. All that the child remembers is the parent being angry. The parental tantrum and demonstration of uncontrolled anger provides a poor model for the child. Among a child's greatest needs is the approval and affection of the parent. The presence of excessive anger tends to intensify angry disobedience by the child rather than compliance. Translating such a theoretical understanding of the causation and persistence of behaviour disorders in toddlers into an understanding by the parents, may frequently take many hours of discussion, many hours of work with the family, consideration of relationships outside the immediate one with the child and discussion of the parents' own upbringing and its shortcomings.

Once at school, behaviour previously confined to the home is transferred into another setting. In school the children are seen to have little self control in the face of provocation. They may obtain status with their peer group through an aggressive or defiant attitude. They frequently have educational difficulties. They have often come into school with a poor understanding of the nature of rules and the desirability of conforming to them. Some children become increasingly difficult to control as they grow stronger and become increasingly backward in terms of their educational achievement. In secondary school some start to truant and become involved in delinquent activity which leads them into trouble with the law.

In an educational context, the principles that seem to be of most importance are as follows: firstly, a warm caring attitude and continuity in child-adult relationships, the latter being more difficult to organise within a secondary than a primary school context; secondly, a stimulating educational programme and improvement of self-image through success in this programme; and finally, firm and consistent discipline combined with counselling.

TRUANCY AND DELINQUENCY

Truancy and delinquency are expressions of antisocial behaviour which extends outside school and where police and legal authorities may become involved. It is found more commonly in boys than girls, in those from large families and from those in social classes IV and V. There is frequently a family history of truancy and a negative attitude of the family towards education. Families may have a history of criminality and maternal depression. The families themselves may often be single parent families or families in which there is considerable discord. There is a noticeable lack of communal family leisure activities. In areas with a high adult crime rate, it has been suggested that the low level of social disapproval attached to delinquency is a direct factor in its causation.

Delinquency has been divided into the solitary delinquent where psychiatric factors are more likely to be present, and group delinquent behaviour. As well as stealing and aggressive activities, other problems such as glue sniffing or more serious drug abuse may be found.

Management of truancy and delinquency
Non-attendance at school which is not amenable to direct approaches by the

Factors associated with delinquency

Unhappy homes
Single parent families
Parental criminal records
Low intelligence
Poor self-image
Aggression

---

teacher is taken up by the Education Welfare Service. If there is not an appropriate response to verbal warnings then a court referral may be thought to be appropriate. This may be through the Magistrates Court, if the parents are thought to be mainly involved, or through the Juvenile Court under Section 1 of the 1969 Children and Young Persons Act. The object of the latter approach is to put the child under a Care Protection Order. Children involved not simply with truancy but delinquency, may also be referred to the Juvenile Court. Residential care may not be appropriate as it could expose the child to those who are further along the path of delinquent behaviour. Intermediate treatment schemes within the community or special fostering schemes may be more effective. Social work intervention with the family to enable them to understand and cope more effectively with the child's behaviour or to exercise proper authority or supervision over the child may also be effective. Social services observation and assessment centres can provide the complete assessment of a child in a residential setting, allow a period of relief for the parents and permit the formulation of recommendations for future action. However, there may be a wide gap between the ideal recommendations and the willingness of the parents to implement them or the availability of the required resources within the community, for example specialist fostering.

Educational guidance centres with a high teacher to pupil ratio within secondary schools cope with children who might otherwise be suspended from school because of behavioural difficulties. They operate in a rigid structural setting with emphasis on remedial work and the aim is full-time reintegration into the ordinary school.

For some children psychiatric treatment may be required, either on an individual or a family basis. In-patient treatment may also be indicated for some children.

Children and young persons found guilty or cautioned at all courts by type of offence, sex and age (England and Wales, 1981) (from Criminal Statistics)

Offence	Boys (thousands)			Girls (thousands)		
	10–14	14–17	17–21	10–14	14–17	17–21
Violence against the person	1.5	7.8	15.2	0.3	1.4	1.1
Sexual offences	0.4	1.6	1.8	—	—	—
Burglary	11.0	24.3	23.8	0.7	1.0	0.9
Robbery	0.2	0.8	1.4	—	0.1	0.1
Theft and handling stolen goods	31.6	53.7	55.0	11.9	15.5	11.0
Fraud and forgery	0.3	1.1	4.1	0.1	0.4	1.4
Criminal damage	2.0	2.7	3.9	0.1	0.3	0.2
Other	0.1	0.7	5.3	—	0.1	0.7
Motoring offences	0.1	2.3	6.5	—	—	0.1
Total	47.3	94.9	117.3	13.3	18.8	15.5

THE JUVENILE COURT

In the United Kingdom, the juvenile courts deal with offences committed by children (aged 10–13) and young persons (aged 14–17). The three magistrates in the juvenile courts are lay people but with direct practical experience of young people. The court clerk is a professional solicitor or barrister. The court is closed to the public. The identity of children appearing before the court cannot be disclosed publicly. Many children or young persons are not prosecuted and a decision is made after appropriate investigation by the juvenile bureau of the police not to proceed or for a caution to be issued by a senior police officer.

If the child is summonsed to the juvenile court, both he and his parents must attend. They may be legally represented. In addition to information about the child's alleged offence, the court also receives a school report and a social enquiry report containing specific recommendations. In addition to establishing guilt or innocence, the court must also satisfy itself that the child does understand that it was wrong to carry out the particular offence. Penalties available to the juvenile court are as follows:

Children: — Absolute discharge
         — Conditional discharge
         — Fine
         — Supervision order
         — Care order
         — Attendance centre order
Young persons : as above, plus Detention Centre order.

In England and Wales, about 2.5% of the age group 10–17 appear before the juvenile court. Boys outnumber girls by 6:1.

Young people either cautioned or found guilty of indictable offences. The graph on the left illustrates that males are more in trouble than females; the graph on the right shows the trend for males in different age groups over the last 15 years in England and Wales. (from Criminal Statistics)

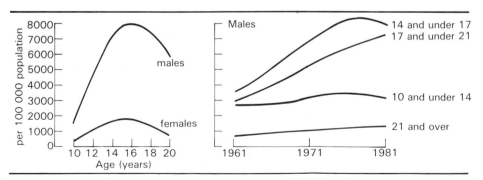

SCHOOL REFUSAL

This has already been mentioned in the chapter on the school child. Compared with other causes it represents a very small proportion of persistent non-attenders. Eighty to 90% of absence from school is due to illness, 1% due to school refusal and the remainder due to either truancy or active witholding of the child from school attendance by parents.

School refusal or school phobia may start with intermittent non-attendance and the manifestation of systemic symptoms when under pressure. The parents are unable to exert sufficient support or encouragement to attend school and the child shows a high level of anxiety or fear. Because of the variety of symptoms with which the child may present, he may in fact be sent home from school or spend much time away from the class in the medical room. School refusal in contrast to truancy is more common in small families and in social classes I, II and III. It is equally common in boys and girls and carries a better prognosis than truancy. Although many cases of school refusal, particularly if recognised at an early stage, may be managed by school doctors, more intractable situations need to be referred to a child psychiatrist.

School refusal contains a wide variety of individual elements. In some it may be anxiety about separation from the parent and there may be some degree of collusion that keeps the child out of school. In others anxiety may be related to the journey to school or to particular elements in school, individual lessons, individual teachers, relationship with other children, school lavatories, school dinners or changing for games.

The initial stage in management is to recognise that the problem is distinct from truancy and to be confident that somatic symptoms are not due to underlying disorders. These need to be confidently excluded and the parent and child reassured. Without the recognition of the psychosomatic nature of symptoms, the child may have a long series of fruitless investigations whilst remaining out of school. An early return to school is required with the help of the family or external sources such as the education welfare officer. Factors within the school environment, such as an inappropriate educational programme, may be dealt with and psychotherapy provides an outlet for the child expressing his fears. The pathology may also be within the parent, and appropriate help needs to be offered there too. In selected cases, treatment of the child with tranquillisers may be successful.

Insistence that the child must go to school under all circumstances, can prevent the establishment of a pattern of non-attendance that is accepted without resistance by parents. Missed lessons magnify the difficulties to be encountered by the child on return and discontinuity in relationships with classmates causes him to become an outsider within the peer group. In some centres it has been the practice to escort the children to school every day against whatever resistence is offered, fol-

Comparison of the backgrounds of children with school refusal and truancy (Hersov, 1960)

School refusal	Truancy
Small family	Large family
Social class I,II,III	Social class IV, V
Boys = girls	Boys > girls
Better prognosis	Poorer prognosis
Anxious, phobic	Antisocial
Fewer separations	More separations
Parental over-protection	Parental rejection

lowed by a party at the weekend. This form of 'implosion therapy' is highly effective. Others would plan the return to school in a series of small graded steps, often using such special aids as tutorial classes as intermediate stages.

For some children where this basic pattern of help fails, admission to hospital may be an effective alternative. This serves to break up family tensions and removes the child from the environment where the adults are unable to help. Separation of the parent and child may also enable the parents to make more objective judgements about their child's particular needs. Admission to hospital, although it may cause initial but often short-lived distress, provides a concrete demonstration that the child can survive and cope away from the parents and with others of his own age group. Whilst an in-patient, underlying problems may be dealt with, such as learning difficulties, psychiatric problems (neurosis, depression, personality difficulties) or social inadequacies.

ANOREXIA NERVOSA

Anorexia nervosa is an uncommon, though life threatening, condition associated with anorexia. There is a refusal to eat and associated endocrine changes giving rise to amenorrhoea. There may be a family history of mild obesity or aversion to food. The adolescents are usually emotionally immature and have an abnormal self-image. In spite of weight loss, some may not experience hunger. Food may be lost through vomiting or the use of laxatives, and periods of deprivation of food may be interspersed with times of bingeing.

The families are often found to be over-protective and to be rigid and unadaptable to new events. There is a poor ability to cope with conflicts. The family may present no model of self-sufficiency, the child is unable to become independent and grow away from a closely knit family unit.

Characteristics of families in which there is a child with anorexia nervosa

---

Enmeshment — insufficient individualisation
Over protectiveness
Rigidity
Inability to tolerate conflict

Management
The child nearly always requires admission to hospital, firstly because of the risk of death and secondly to put the child into an environment where proper control of food intake can be gained. The complex relationships at home may prevent such control being established. A contract is established in which restrictions are removed in response to an increase in weight. In combination with such a programme — which does not permit the manipulations which might occur at home — psychotherapy is required with the child and family in order to explore relationships and the child's attitudes towards growing up.

Following treatment, relapses can occur. Many patients continue to be underweight and have some persisting difficulties.

AUTISM

Autism is a rare condition affecting 4–5 per 10 000 children. The aetiology is unknown though a very large amount of research has been done in order to understand the nature of these children's difficulties and their cause. Both neurological and psycho-social factors have been suggested as possible explanations for the syndrome.

Children with autism are normal at birth but later develop the following four features described by Rutter, all of which need to be present for diagnosis.

- an autistic type failure to develop inter-personal relationships. By this he means a failure to cuddle or come for comfort, lack of eye to eye gaze, giving the appearance of aloofness or distance, relative failure to become attached to parents, little or no separation anxiety, sometimes little variation in facial expression, apparent lack of interest in people, a tendency when a toddler to treat all adults in much the same way, failure to make friends or join in group activities
- delay in speech and language development
- ritualistic and compulsive phenomena
- onset before 30 months.

In addition to these diagnostic criteria a number of other characteristics have been described in children with autism. They often seem to make a greater use of peripheral rather than central vision. This may advance to visual avoidance looking past or beyond objects or paying greater attention to things at the periphery of the visual field or introducing flicking fingers at the periphery of vision. The child may appear to be indifferent to noise and deafness may be difficult to exclude. In their speech echolalia is very common, as are problems with word order and nominal aphasia. In addition to difficulties with expressive language there are equal difficulties with comprehension. Some children may be hyperactive. Some may be obsessed by repetition of particular movements, e.g. twisting wrists, flapping arms, spinning, rocking, swinging, etc. Children commonly show difficulty in changing routines that are established. In their moods the children are often described as remote and aloof. They do not seem to demand affection and parents describe difficulties in getting through to them. Outbursts of crying and screaming also commonly occur. Many children may show a lack of fear of real dangers whilst at the same time developing fear of harmless things.

Differential diagnosis
Deafness, language disorders and mental handicap need to be distinguished from autism. Careful observation of the child will show that in none of the other conditions are all four diagnostic criteria met. Many children with autism do have concomitant mental handicap.

Management
Management to some extent may be described as empirical as we do not have an established understanding of the underlying disorder. Parents require practical advice on how to handle the child and support and help in understanding the

child's unusual behaviour. Much work is devoted to teaching communication and socially acceptable behaviour by means of a system of rewards. This would be a rational approach if an underlying deficit in language and communication were the cause of the syndrome.

Prognosis
Only about one-third of the children make a reasonable adjustment in terms of obtaining employment and leading an independent existence. However, even among these there may still be gross difficulties in relating to others. Good prognostic factors are the development of useful language before the age of 5 and an IQ of over 70.

LATE ONSET PSYCHOSIS

Many of these children have disorders which resemble schizophrenia in adults. They are extremely uncommon and the diagnosis is often not recognised. The children have auditory hallucinations, thought disorders and are socially isolated from their peer group.

HYSTERIA

Psychosomatic problems, abdominal pain, vomiting and headache, are commonly seen in paediatrics. True hysteria is a much rarer occurrence. It often starts with a genuine organic illness though the extent and duration of the symptoms continues for a long time after the initial cause has been removed. The range of presentation includes paraplegia, dysphonia, deafness and loss of vision. In part these children's symptoms could be explained by the conversion of anxiety into somatic symptoms.

In the management of these children an organic cause needs to be excluded through a minimum of examination and investigation. Some hysterical symptoms may be easily removed by demonstrating the normal function of the part. For example, if the child is 'paraplegic' demonstrating that he turns over in bed in his sleep. Others may be more resistant to treatment. Psychotherapy involving exploration of the underlying sources of anxiety is required.

PREVENTION OF PSYCHIATRIC DISTURBANCE IN CHILDREN

Health education and the positive promotion of mental health has much to offer in this field. Programmes intended to provide decision making skills, and helping individuals to understand and cope with stress and exploring the nature of family life and responsibility, may be valuable. Programmes aimed at preparation for parenthood may also be useful. The availability of resources for crisis intervention and provision of support for families under these circumstances, may prevent more chronic problems arising.

Certain groups of children, particularly those from disadvantaged backgrounds are more susceptible to psychiatric problems, particularly conduct disorders. Early intervention programmes with parents and children aim not only to provide enrichment of experience, but to modify child rearing practices towards a more favourable outcome. Other vulnerable groups may be identified, such as children with physical handicaps, chronic illness, children with educational difficulties and children whose parents have psychiatric illness. Maternal depression is common and may be associated with disturbance in the child. This occurs in mothers who may be socially very isolated. Such isolation may be seen in relation to modern high rise flats or in immigrant families. Community resources such as playgroups and nurseries have much to offer children and families under these circumstances.

A wide range of people can contribute towards prevention of psychiatric illness in childhood. These will range from professional groups, such as health visitors, social workers, teachers, counsellors and doctors, to local voluntary groups and youth clubs which give valuable resource and support to parents and children in their community.

REFERENCES AND FURTHER READING

Bentovim A 1976 Disobedience and violent behaviour in children: family pathology and family treatment. British Medical Journal 1: 947–949, 1004–1006
Fraiberg S 1980 Clinical Studies in infant Mental Health. Tavistock.
Rutter M 1975 Helping Troubled Children. Penguin, Harmondsworth
Rutter M 1973 Maternal Deprivation Reassessed. Penguin, Harmondsworth
Rutter M 1980 The long-term effects of early experience. Developmental Medicine and Child Neurology 22: 800–816
Rutter M, Hersov L 1977 Child Psychiatry. Blackwell Scientific Publications, Oxford

19
Protection
of Children

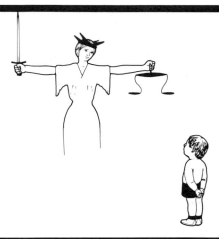

Towards the end of the 18th century, the public conscience was stirred by the plight of child chimney sweeps and an act was passed limiting the working day, which, even for a child of 5, could be 14–16 hours. The Factory Act 1833 went further and prohibited the employment of children under 9 years, and restricted the working day of 9–11 year olds to 9 hours. The Poor Law Amendment Act (1834) aimed to provide healthy living conditions, education and training for orphan children. In 1847, Liverpool appointed the first Medical Officer of Health, to be followed in 1848 by London. In 1888, the Local Government Act established elected County Councils and empowered them to appoint Medical Officers of Health.

However, prior to the the 19th century, in the UK the state took little interest in the education and health of children. It was philanthropic individuals like Robert Raikes, who, in 1780, started schools for children on Sundays, the only day on which factories were closed.

In 1880 elementary education was made compulsory and in 1891 it was provided free. In 1890 the London School Board appointed the first school doctor.

Ironically it was the Government's concern at the high rate of rejection of recruits for the South African War, 1899–1902, and the subsequent publication of three reports early in the 20th century, which were largely responsible for the setting up of the School Medical Service in 1907. The 1904 report in particular was a far sighted document, whose recommendations were very enlightened. There were fifty-three in all which covered among other subjects, anthropometric surveys, nurseries, smoke pollution, housing, medical inspections of workers in factories and coal mines, alcoholism, infant mortality, the employment of women, registration of still births, medical inspection of school children, feeding of elementary school children, juvenile smoking, vagrancy and defective children. This led to the passing, in 1907, of the Education (Administrative Provisions) Act which marked the beginning of medical inspection in schools, and in 1908 the first school clinic opened in Bradford.

Towards the end of the 19th century there was also increased awareness that some children needed protection from their parents. The NSPCC was first set up in the US, and its equivalent in the UK received a Royal Charter in 1895. The Prevention of Cruelty to Children Act in 1899 allowed the issue of warrants to enter a home and remove children if cruelty was suspected. Juvenile Courts were established in 1908.

In 1907 an Act was passed making notification of births to the Medical Officer of Health permissive, and thus enabling local authorities to offer advice and help to nursing mothers in rearing their babies. In 1915 this notification was made compulsory and local authorities were also given the power to undertake maternity and child welfare work. Also around the turn of the century, child health clinics evolved for the distribution of milk and for giving advice to mothers. The Maternal and Child Welfare Act in 1918 recognised the importance of safeguarding the health of mothers and children and empowered local authorities to establish free clinics.

In 1919 the Ministry of Health Act established the Ministry of Health, whose function would be 'to promote the health of the people', and it transferred to the Minister of Health all the powers and duties of the Board of Education for the medical inspection and treatment of children and young persons. Adults have always taken others' children to live with them but adoption only acquired a legal framework with the Adoption Act of 1926.

A major step in the legislation for the School Health Service was the Education Act of 1944, which, with various subsequent regulations, is still the legal background to some of the school health work of the Child Health Service. This Act gave local education authorities the duty to provide school meals and milk for pupils at schools maintained by them, to make medical and dental inspection and treatment available in all types of maintained schools, and to ascertain children needing special education. The NHS Act of 1946 enabled local education authorities to arrange with Regional Hospital Boards for free specialist and hospital treatment.

The Children Act of 1948 established Children's Departments staffed by social workers who were responsible for looking after children in Local Authority care. It placed an obligation on them to board out children in care where possible. In 1952 it became possible to bring care proceedings without first prosecuting the parents. The Nurseries and Child Minders Act regulated institutions or individuals caring for children under 5 years by requiring them to be registered with the local authority.

Immunisation procedures were governed by the NHS Act of 1946, and the Health Services and Public Health Act of 1968, which dealt with prophylaxis, care and aftercare. The former was repealed and replaced by the NHS Act of 1973. The NHS Re-organisation Act of 1973 brought together General Practitioners, Hospital Services, and Local Authority Health Services into a comprehensive National Health Service.

SCHOOL HEALTH SERVICES

The report of the working party on collaboration between the NHS and Local Government 1973 stated that the value of the school health service 'shall be fully recognised and sufficient resources devoted to it, and also that the medical and other staff shall continue to see themselves as part of the team responsible with the education service for trying to provide the best opportunity for each individual child'.

The Education Act of 1944 still forms the basis of some of the medical work in schools. Section 54 of the 1944 Act empowers the Education Authority to authorise a medical officer to see that children who are verminous, are examined and to ensure that appropriate action is taken. Section 59 and local bye-laws provide that a pupil shall not be 'employed in a manner prejudicial to his health or otherwise to make him unfit to obtain full benefit of the education provided for him'.

The 1973 NHS Act directs that medical and dental inspection must be available to all children in state schools and this may also be offered to other schools by arrangement. Education authorities have a duty to make accommodation available for this. The Education (Milk) Act 1971 makes provision for milk to be given on the advice of a school medical officer to certain children between the ages of 7 and 12 years.

Under the Disabled Persons (Employment) Act and the Employment Medical Advisory Service Act 1972, the school medical officer supplies information on forms Y9 and Y10 to the careers officer about handicapped school leavers, and those who may not be suitable for certain specific employment. If requested by the Employment Medical Advisor, the school medical officer has a duty to provide him with medical information relevant to a pupil's employment.

Special educational needs

The NHS (medical examinations-educationally subnormal children) Regulations 1974 laid down the qualifications needed by medical practitioners employed by health authorities to carry out, on behalf of the education authority, medical examination of a child who may need special schooling.

The 1944 Education Act made provision for ascertaining children who need special educational treatment. As a result of the report in 1978 of the Committee

Current legislation governing health in schools (England and Wales)

1944 Education Act	
Section 54	Examination of verminous children
Section 59	Employment of children
1971 Education (Milk) Act	Provision of milk to 7–12 year olds on advice of medical officer
1972 Disabled Persons (Employment) Act Employment Medical Advisory Service Act	Information supplied by Medical Officer to careers officer and Employment Medical Advisor
1973 NHS Re-organisation Act	Provision of medical and dental inspection in schools immunisation procedures
1974 NHS (medical examination — educationally subnormal children) Regulations	Qualifications required for medical officer examining children who may need special schooling for ESN chidlren
1978 Medical Fitness of Teachers DES circular 11/78	Examination of entrants to teacher training
1981 Education Act	Provision for children with special educational needs

of Enquiry into the Education of Handicapped Children and Young People (Warnock Report), the Education Act of 1981 was passed. This Act does away with the system of special educational treatment for children with certain categories of handicap, and introduces the concept of a child having special educational needs if he has a learning difficulty which calls for special educational provision to be made for him. It also establishes the principle that all children for whom the education authority decides to determine the special educational provision to be made, are to be educated in ordinary school, so far as it is practicable — provided that account has been taken of parental views, the school can meet the child's special needs, the efficient education of other children in the school is possible and the education authority's resources are being efficiently used.

Sections 4–10 of the 1981 Act cover identification and assessment and provide a new legal framework for the education of children requiring special educational provision. Section 10 specifically deals with the role of the health authorities under the Act. It places a duty on the authority to inform the parent and the appropriate education authority when they form the opinion that a child under the age of 5 years has or is likely to have special educational needs. The health authority must give the parent the opportunity to discuss their opinion before notifying the education authority. The provisions of section 10 apply from birth to 5 years. The parents must always be notified before the education authority, but if they do not agree with the health authority, or do not want to discuss it, then the education authority will nevertheless be informed.

Section 10 also requires that health authorities inform the parents of such babies and young children if they think that a voluntary organisation is likely to be able to help them.

The assessment process will involve medical participation in the multi-professional assessment of children with severe and complex problems, and in some cases there will be nursing and other paramedical involvement. The process will culminate in a 'statement' of the child's needs, which will be made by the educational authority. Part of this statement will set out the advice of the health professionals involved in the assessment.

CHILDREN IN CARE

There are a number of ways in which children may be received into the care of the local authority. Many are in *voluntary care* particularly for short periods (e.g. mother admitted to hospital or other temporary crisis at home). Here parental rights are given over to the local authority but can be claimed back by the parents at any time.

In an emergency a *Place of Safety Order* may be taken out. Any person can apply to a magistrate at any time of day or night for an order to detain a child for up to 28 days. It must be demonstrated that there is reasonable cause to suspect that

— his proper development is being prevented or neglected, or his health is being avoidably impaired or neglected or he is being ill-treated

— if another child in the household is subject to an order, similar conditions apply to this child
— he is exposed to moral danger
— he is beyond the control of his parents
— he is not attending school.

A *Supervision Order* is granted where the local authority is concerned about a child living at home. Here the social worker has a duty to advise and help the parents and child but there is no statutory right to enter the home or to remove him without the parents' consent. If there is further concern or lack of cooperation it should be fairly easy to return to court for a Care Order. The Supervision Order lapses after 3 years.

The local authority takes over the responsibility of the child compulsorily if a *Care Order* is obtained. The child may still be placed with the parents but the local authority can more easily remove him if thought necessary. The child who is the subject of a Care Order may also be placed in a children's home, residential nursery or with foster parents. The grounds for obtaining a Care Order are the same as for a Place of Safety Order with the addition that he is in need of care and control that he is unlikely to receive unless the order is made. This can also be used if a child is guilty of an offence. A Care Order remains in force until the child is 18 years unless it is discharged by the court on application from the local authority, child, or parents on the child's behalf.

An *Interim Care Order* can be applied for on the same grounds when evidence for a Care Order is not complete. This lasts for only 28 days but re-application can be made for an unlimited number of times.

A child may also be made a *ward of court*, in which case the court takes over legal responsibility for the child and must be consulted when major decisions are made concerning the child. The grounds are simply that the Order is in the best interests of the child. This remains in effect until the child is 18 years unless application is made to terminate it earlier.

Current legislation governing children in care (England and Wales)

1969 Children and Young Persons Act	
Section 1(3)	Care Order
Section 1(3)	Supervision Order
Section 2(10), 20 (2) 22,28(6)	Interim Care Order
Section 28	Place of Safety Order
1969 Family Law Reform Act	Wardship proceedings
1980 Child Care Act	Duty of local authority to provide voluntary
Section 1	supervision in the home
Section 2	Duty of the local authority to receive child into voluntary care
Section 3	Assumption of parental rights by local authority

Medical involvement

Doctors may be required to give evidence in court when an Order is applied for. All children received into care undergo a medical examination primarily to ascertain any immediate threat to the health of the child or those accepting the child (e.g. infectious illness). The children may well have had very poor medical super-

Children in care. Circumstances in which children came into care (Health and Social Service Statistics)

	Thousands	
	1976	1980
Admission to the care of local authorities	50.0	45.0
Section 1 of the Children Act 1948	37.7	30.6
Abandoned or lost	1.0	0.9
Death of parent, other parent unable to provide care	0.6	0.5
Incapacity of parent or guardian		
— confinement	1.9	1.4
— short-term illness	11.9	8.6
— long-term illness	0.8	0.6
Deserted by parent, other parent unable to provide care (including		
illegitimate, mother unable to provide care)	4.5	3.4
Parent dead (no guardian)	0.3	0.2
Parent or guardian in prison or remanded in custody	0.9	0.7
Family homeless (eviction or other cause)	1.2	0.6
Unsatisfactory home conditions	5.0	5.4
Other reasons	9.7	8.2
Care orders made under Sections of the Children and Young Persons		
Act 1969	11.5	5.1
Interim care orders or remands to care	-	8.7
Other court orders	0.8	0.6

vision prior to this because of a chaotic home background or neglecting parents, and this might be the first opportunity there has been to collect together any medical information previously obtained on the child and to diagnose and assess long term medical problems. It is also a good opportunity to measure height and weight for later comparison, to assess development, and to check for evidence of neglect or non-accidental injury.

Children in care by age group and manner of accommodation (Health and Social Service Statistics)

	Thousands	
	1976	1980
Total of all children in care	95.8	95.3
By age groups		
Under 5	11.7	10.1
5–15	64.9	62.1
16 and over	19.2	23.0
Manner of accommodation		
Boarded out	31.5	35.2
In lodgings or residential employment	1.7	1.8
In community homes provided, controlled or assisted by local		
authorities:		
with observation and assessment facilities	4.8	5.0
with education on the premises	6.4	5.2
residential nurseries providing accommodation for children under		
the age of 7	1.8	0.7
other homes	20.5	18.0
Voluntary homes	4.0	3.1
Accommodation for handicapped children	2.7	2.9
Hostels	0.7	0.5
Under charge of parent, guardian, relative or friend	17.0	17.3
Other accommodation	4.9	5.5

Figures may not add to totals because of rounding.

Children in foster care are required to have a medical examination every 6 months up to 2 years of age and then every year. Children's homes should have an appointed medical officer to supervise the medical care of the children and this will generally be a local general practitioner.

ADOPTION

Full parental rights are taken on by adopting parents and the child has all the rights of a natural child of those parents. The majority of adoptions involve one of the child's parents such as mother marrying or remarrying and the husband adopting the child.

The attitude to non-parental adoptions has changed over the years from an attempt to find children for childless couples to an attempt to find families for children in need. The 1975 Children's Act has acknowledged that the child's interests are paramount and puts a duty on the courts and adoption agencies to consider the child's welfare first, and to take account of the child's wishes if old enough to have sufficient understanding. There are fewer healthy newborn babies for adoption, but it is increasingly clear that older children and handicapped children in care benefit greatly from adoption. Adoption of older children now forms a greater proportion of all adoptions.

Table: Adoption in 1980 showing parental adoptions far exceed non-parental adoption of children over 5 years old (England and Wales)

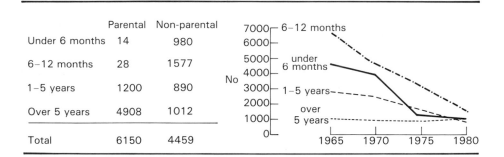

	Parental	Non-parental
Under 6 months	14	980
6–12 months	28	1577
1–5 years	1200	890
Over 5 years	4908	1012
Total	6150	4459

There is medical involvement at two levels. Adoption agencies have medical advisors. The Social Services departments are the largest agencies and here the advisor will usually be the Specialist in Community Medicine (Social Services). There may also be a specialist paediatric advisor, probably a consultant paediatrician. These specialists will act in a general advisory capacity, scrutinising reports, collecting further medical information if necessary, or discussing with the examining doctor findings of special significance. They will advise the social workers on the interpretation of the medical facts about the child and the prospective adoptive parents.

The second level of medical involvement is that of carrying out pre-adoption examinations. If a newborn child is to be placed for adoption, the first examination is normally during the neonatal period and will ascertain any congenital defects apparent at birth and give details of problems arising at birth or in the neonatal period. This is usually done by the paediatric or obstetric staff for hospital deliveries, or by the general practitioner. The baby will often be placed with the prospective adoptive parents directly from the maternity hospital. Adoption proceedings cannot start until the baby is 6 weeks old and the final adoption order will not be less than 3 months after this. The routine check at 6 weeks should be carried out as with all children. A further developmental assessment will often be done at about 3 months. The only statutory assessment is one required within a month of the court hearing to finalise the adoption which will be at about $4\frac{1}{2}$ months for a baby placed for adoption at birth. This statutory assessment may be the only one in an older child placed for adoption. The forms used for these examinations are often those provided by the Association of British Adoption and Fostering Agencies, apart from the statutory examination where a special form is provided. Other statutory requirements in England and Wales are the test for phenylketonuria done routinely on children at 6 days old, and a test for syphilis on mother *or* child when the child is 6 weeks old.

It is important to collect together information on both natural parents if possible, the pregnancy and delivery, neonatal problems, developmental progress, and any other problems that have arisen. The purpose of these examinations is *not* to see if the child is fit for adoption, but to have information available about any special needs that the child may have. These will then be discussed with the adopting parents so that they are fully aware of them. Alternative placing might be seen to be more appropriate in the light of these discussions or the parents may wish to delay adoption.

Adopting children with special needs
Many older children, and children with mental, physical, or emotional handicap are now being placed for adoption. The doctor examining these children has a special responsibility for assessing the children, discussing their problems with the adopting parents, and ensuring further medical care if necessary.

Problems in the natural parents
Children of an incestuous relationship are a group with a high risk of problems. Studies suggest that if the parents are first degree relatives there is a 14% risk of an autosomal recessive disorder, a 26% risk of severe mental retardation, and a 35% risk of mild retardation. Less than half the offspring were normal. It might be wise to test for the common recessive disorders.

Information about known inherited disorders in a parent must be sought so that advice on risks to the child can be offered to the adopting parents.

Psychotic, psychopathic, and alcoholic parents probably offer *no* increased risk of these disorders in the child, though if mother has been on drugs or drank heavily during the pregnancy there will be an increased risk of congenital abnormalities in the child.

Outlook for adopted children
Most adopted children do very well. There may be more psychological problems

Percentages of 'maladjusted' children according to whether they were born legitimate, and whether they were adopted or not (from Seglow et al, 1972)

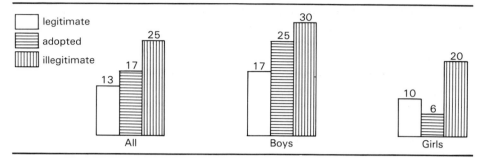

than average, but fewer than among illegitimate children staying with their biological mothers. In the National Child Development Study of babies born in 1958, 90% of those to be adopted had separated from their mothers by 3 months of age; at 7 years the adopted children were doing much better than those illegitimate children not adopted (Seglow, 1972). Children placed at an older age or those with special needs are more likely to have problems but most are successful.

FOSTERING

Fostering is covered by the Children Act 1958, Foster Care Act 1980, and Child Care Act 1980. Prior to long term fostering, children will normally undergo similar assessment to children being adopted.

CHILD ABUSE

This is an increasingly recognised problem. The incidence depends on the awareness of the problem and how it is defined. Physical injury is the most readily recognised, diagnosed and studied and the incidence has been estimated at 1 in 2000 children per year under 15 years or 5000 children per year of whom 65 are killed and 700 seriously injured.

The person injuring the child is usually a parent though it may be a cohabitee or child minder. The parents are often young and had unhappy childhoods themselves. The circumstances surrounding the incident have been summarised by Kempe as follows:
— something wrong with the marriage
— something wrong with the parent
— something wrong with the child (real or imagined)
— a crisis
— no lifelines — for geographical or social reasons.

In 1974 a recommendation was made for the setting up of Area Review Committees to bring together representatives of legal, education, housing and social service departments of local authorities, medical, nursing, dental, and administrative members of the health services, police, probation, and the NSPCC. These committees would establish local procedures and a manual should be available giving details. A register of children considered to be 'at risk' is generally kept locally and is available for consultation 24 hours a day. In some areas NSPCC Special Units take particular interest in non-accidental injuries and may be responsible for Registers and Case Conferences.

Diagnosis

Certain features in the history and examination should alert one to the possibility of non-accidental injury. With any injury a careful history should be sought.

In the history watch for:
— discrepancy with the injury seen
— changing story with time or different people
— delay in reporting
— unusual reaction to injury
— repeated injury.

The child should be examined all over if non-accidental injury is suspected, and injuries carefully charted (this may be needed for evidence in court later). Bruises are the most common type of injury and are not often caused accidentally in children under 1 year, particularly if not mobile. A quarter of all fractures under 2 years are probably not accidental and more of those under 1 year.

Injuries of particular note are:
— bruising on head and face and lumbar region (often finger marks)
— small circular bruises (finger marks)
— bruising around wrists and ankles (swinging)
— bruising inside and behind pinna (blow with hand)
— ring of bruises (bite mark)
— two black eyes
— torn frenulum (blow or force feeding)
— small circular burns (cigarette burns)
— burns or scalds to both feet or buttocks
— fractured ribs (shaking)
— epiphyses torn off (swinging)
— subdural haematoma (shaking)
— retinal haemorrhages (shaking)
— multiple injuries and injuries of different ages.

Sites where bruises are found by age group in normal children and children found to have non-accidental injuries (from Roberton et al, 1982)

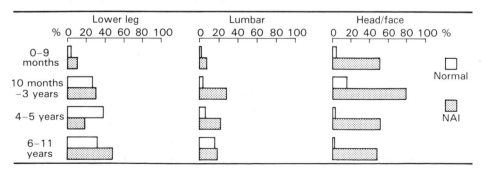

Pitfalls in diagnosis

Underdiagnosis is much commoner than overdiagnosis. However there are certain pitfalls to keep in mind. Mongolian spots may look very like bruises and are often over the buttocks. They are seen in coloured races but the racial origin may not be apparent. Bruises from a bleeding disorder and fractures from a bony disorder can also present in a similar way to non-accidental injury. Careful, sympathetic history taking and examination with these in mind should avoid mistakes being made, and if these disorders are suspected they need investigation in their own right.

Management

If a child is seen with definite or probable NAI he should be referred to hospital and will probably be admitted. This is usually accepted by the parents and relieves the immediate situation, but a Place of Safety Order may occasionally be required. Investigations such as a skeletal survey and coagulation studies are normally done in hospital. Other children in the home need to be examined and admitted to hospital if thought to be at risk. A case conference will normally be called soon after admission to collect information and plan further management, appoint a key worker, make recommendations to the police about prosecution and to decide about placing the child's name on the register of 'at risk' children.

In more minor cases of injury where there is significant doubt about the diagnosis, careful recording of the history, findings and discussion with the parents is essential. The register of children at risk should be consulted. The general practitioner, and health visitor or school nurse should be consulted and any other agencies involved. A referral to Social Services might be thought appropriate.

Prevention

Primary prevention involves identifying families at risk before any injury occurs. Certain characteristics are known to be associated with child abuse such as young parents, emotional disturbance in the parents, infant separated from mother at birth, recorded concern about mother's ability to cope with the child. Combinations of these factors are particularly important. There may be a 'cry for help' from the mother, such as frequent visits to the doctor for minor problems or complaints of excessive crying or difficult feeding. The mother may say that she thinks she will injure the child; this should always be taken seriously and steps taken to relieve the crisis by admitting the child to hospital if necessary. Once recognised as a family at risk, additional support from health visitor or social worker may prevent the crisis leading to actual injury.

Secondary prevention means identifying children who have been injured and taking steps to prevent further injury. Subsequent injury is likely to be more severe. Plans will normally be made at a case conference and may mean removing the child from home at least temporarily, but many children perhaps 35–45%, are able to be reunited with their parents.

Sexual abuse

It is becoming increasingly apparent that sexual abuse is not uncommon and affects perhaps as many as 1/6000 children/year or 1500 children a year. The children are often girls over 11 years old but much younger children can be involved. The majority of these are attempted or actual intercourse; the others being involvement in adult sexual activity or injury to the genitalia. There is often physical abuse as well. Presentation may be obvious with a complaint of sexual abuse by the child, parent or friend. However it may present as behaviour disturbance, psychosomatic symptoms, or associated symptoms such as cystitis or gonococcal infection.

Poisoning
This is another form of abuse more recently recognised and should be considered when symptoms and signs are hard to explain. Screening for drugs in the blood and urine should identify these cases.

Neglect
This is a form of abuse that has been recognised for some time by the health professions but has only more recently been accepted by the courts. It may manifest as failure to thrive, failure of normal development, or lack of normal emotional responses. Other causes will need to be excluded, but the diagnosis usually becomes apparent when the child progresses better in the far from ideal environment of hospital.

Management of any form of child abuse should follow the same pattern as that for physical abuse.

REFERENCES AND FURTHER READING

Child Sexual Abuse 1981 British Association for the study and prevention of child abuse and neglect
Education Act 1981 Circular 8/81. HMSO, London
Jones D 1982 Understanding Child Abuse. Hodder and Stoughton, London
Oliver J E 1983 Dead children from problem families in NE Whiltshire. British Medical Journal 286: 115–117
Oxtoby N 1981 Medical Practice in Adopting and Fostering. British Association for Adoption and Fostering, London
Rawston D 1981 Child Care Law. British Association for Adoption and Fostering, London
Robertson D M, Barbor P, Hull D 1982 Unusual injury? Recent injury in normal children and children with suspected non-accidental injury. British Medical Journal 285: 1399–1402
Seglow J, Pringle H M, Wedge P 1972 Growing up Adopted. NFR,
Wolhind S 1979 Medical Aspects of Adoption and Foster Care. Clinics in Developmental Medicine no. 74. Heinemann, London

Index